Shock: Biochemical, Pharmacological, and Clinical Aspects

ADVANCES IN EXPERIMENTAL MEDICINE AND BIOLOGY

Shock: Biochemical, Pharmacological, and Clinical Aspects

Proceedings of the International Symposium on Shock held at Como, Italy, October 10-11, 1969

Edited by

Aldo Bertelli
Institute of Pharmacology
University of Milan
Milan, Italy

and

Nathan Back
Department of Biochemical Pharmacology
School of Pharmacy
State University of New York
Buffalo, New York

℗ PLENUM PRESS · NEW YORK–LONDON · 1970

Library of Congress Catalog Card Number 77-122624

SBN 306-39009-4

© *1970 Plenum Press, New York*
A Division of Plenum Publishing Corporation
227 West 17th Street, New York, N.Y. 10011

United Kingdom edition published by Plenum Press, London
A Division of Plenum Publishing Company, Ltd.
Donington House, 30 Norfolk Street, London W.C.2, England

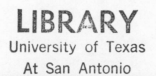

PREFACE

Few pathologic phenomena, as shock, can originate from so many causes and involve so many complex physiologic mechanisms: The complexity of the phenomenon, thus, has resulted in extensive study and raised many uncertainties. Different conditions, such as hemorrhage, trauma, burns, bacterial infection, and anaphylaxis, can cause a shock state which initiates a chain of biochemical events that tends to maintain the shock. Recent progress in biochemistry, physiology, and pharmacology has tended to clarify this chain of events, and elucidate the possible trigger mechanism. Besides the hormonal and catecholamine involvement, the possible intervention of various protease and lysosomal enzyme septems and kinin release introduces new elements into the characteristic mosaic of the shock state.

This International Symposium, organized at Lake Como by the Italian Society of Clinical Pharmacology and the International Society of Biochemical Pharmacology, is another in a series of symposia under the joint auspices of the School of Pharmacy, State University of New York at Buffalo, and the Institute of Pharmacology, University of Milan, Italy. The Symposium has gathered together eminent scientists from such varied disciplines as surgery and pharmacology, internal medicine and biochemistry, physiology and pathology, all focusing on the question of shock. The many researchers in these specialities had the possibility of meeting and discussing together in a multidisciplinary fashion the many theories and experiences associated with this problem.

The Symposium has provided an excellent setting for such discussion, and on the basis of the new information presented, new approaches have been proposed which may be of significant therapeutic benefit.

Grateful thanks are extended to all participants. It is hoped that our meeting together here will result in continued and new collaborative efforts in this clinically important problem.

Aldo Bertelli

LIST OF PARTICIPANTS

G. Antoni, Istituto di Patologia Medica, Università di Siena, Italy

Desiree Armstrong, Department of Pharmacology, Middlesex Hospital
    Medical School, London, England

N. Back, Department of Biochemical Pharmacology, School of
    Pharmacy, State University of New York at Buffalo, New York

Z. M. Bacq, Laboratory of Radiobiology, Léon Fredericq Institute
    and Laboratory of Physiopathology, University of Liège,
    Belgium

M. L. Beaumariage, Laboratory of Radiobiology, Léon Fredericq
    Institute and Laboratory of Physiopathology, University of
    Liège, Belgium

F. Benvenuti, Istituto di Patologia Medica, Università di Siena,
    Italy

Alvise Berengo, Istituto di Patologia Medica I, University of
    Milan Medical School, Italy

James L. Berk, Assistant Clinical Professor of Surgery, Case
    Western Reserve University School of Medicine, Cleveland, Ohio

H. Berry, Department of Pharmacology, Institute of Basic Medical
    Sciences, Royal College of Surgeons of England, London,
    England

A. Bertelli, Institute of Pharmacology of the University of Milan
    Medical School, Italy

G. C. Castiglioni, The Surgical Clinic of the Catholic University
    of the Sacred Heart, Rome, Italy

F. Cocola, Istituto di Patologia Medica, Università di Siena, Italy

J. G. Collier, Department of Pharmacology, Institute of Basic
    Medical Sciences, Royal College of Surgeons of England,
    London, England

Camillo Cortesini, Departments of Surgical Pathology and of
    Anesthesiology of the University of Florence, Italy

Clifford G. Crafton, Tulane University School of Medicine, New
    Orleans, Louisiana

P. L. Del Bianco, Department of Medicine, Division of Clinical
    Pharmacology, University of Florence, Italy

H. L. Dhar, Department of Pharmacology, Jawaharlal Institute of
    Postgraduate Medical Education and Research, Pondicherry,
    India

N. R. Di Luzio, University of Tennessee Medical Units, Memphis,
    Tennessee

L. Donati, Institute of Pharmacology of the University of Milan
    Medical School, Italy

M. Fanciullacci, Department of Medicine, Division of Clinical
    Pharmacology, University of Florence, Italy

L. Gallone, Istituto di Patologia Speciale Chirurgica, Ospedale
    Maggiore "Ca'Granda", Milan, Italy

G. Geissl, Department of Pathology, University of Munich, West
    Germany

A. Gerola, Istituto di Patologia Medica, Università di Siena, Italy

L. Gielow, Department of Pathology, University of Munich, West
    Germany

J. A. Gladner, National Institute of Arthritic and Metabolic
    Diseases, National Institute of Health, Bethesda, Maryland

E. Glaser, Department of Internal Medicine, Justus Liebig-
    University, Giessen, Germany

George J. Grega, Department of Physiology, Michigan State
    University, East Lansing, Michigan

Gert L. Haberland, Forschungszentrum, Bayer Wuppertal, Germany

Francis J. Haddy, Department of Physiology, Michigan State
    University, East Lansing, Michigan

Robert M. Hardaway, III, Medical Corps. United States Army General
    Hospital, Frankfurt, Germany

D. Hey, Department of Internal Medicine, Justus Liebig-University,
    Giessen, Germany

J. C. Houck, Biochemical Research Laboratory, Children's Hospital,
    Washington, D. C.

J. Karn, Department of Biochemical Pharmacology, School of
    Pharmacy, State University of New York at Buffalo, New York

Kurt Kramer, Physiologisches Institut der Universität Muenchen,
    Germany

H. G. Lasch, Department of Internal Medicine, Justus Liebig-
    University, Giessen, Germany

J. Lecomte, Laboratory of Radiobiology, Léon Fredericq, Institute
    and Laboratory of Physiopathology, University of Liège,
    Belgium

L. Lojacono, The Surgical Clinic of the Catholic University of the
    Sacred Heart, Rome, Italy

P. Neri, Istituto di Patologia Medica, Università di Siena, Italy

H. Neuhof, Department of Internal Medicine, Justus Liebig-
    University, Giessen, Germany

M. Neuman, Cochin Hospital, Paris, France

Gian Paolo Novelli, Departments of Surgical Pathology and
    Anesthesiology, University of Florence, Italy

Elio Pagni, Departments of Surgical Pathology and Anesthesiology,
    University of Florence, Italy

Carlo Palmerio, Department of Surgery, Harvard Medical School and
    Beth Israel Hospital, Boston, Massachusetts

M. Rocha e Silva, Department of Pharmacology, Faculty of Medicine,
    University of São Paulo, Ribeirão, Prêto, São Paulo, Brazil

A. Schauer, Department of Pathology, University of Munich, West
    Germany

Charles L. Schneider, Obstetrics and Gynecology, Wayne County
    General Hospital, Eloise, Michigan

James M. Schwinghamer, Department of Physiology, Michigan State
    University, East Lansing, Michigan

F. Sicuteri, Department of Medicine, Division of Clinical
    Pharmacology, University of Florence, Italy

John H. Siegel, Department of Surgery, Albert Einstein College of
    Medicine, New York

F. Spinola, The Surgical Clinic of the Catholic University of the
    Sacred Heart of Rome, Italy

R. Steger, Department of Biochemical Pharmacology, School of
    Pharmacy, State University of New York at Buffalo, New York

G. Stötter, Medical and Neurological Clinic I, City Hospitals,
    "Städt. Krankenanstalten," Augsburg, Germany

S. Thune, Medical and Neurological Clinic I, City Hospitals,
    "Städt. Krankenanstalten," Augsburg, Germany

P. van Caneghem, Laboratory of Radiobiology, Léon Fredericq
    Institute and Laboratory of Physiopathology, University of
    Liège, Belgium

J. R. Vane, Department of Pharmacology, Institute of Basic Medical
    Sciences, Royal College of Surgeons of England, London,
    England

H. Wilkens, Department of Biochemical Pharmacology, School of
    Pharmacy, State University of New York at Buffalo, New York

Bengt Wranne, Departments of Clinical Physiology, Anesthesiology,
    and Thoracic Surgery, University Hospital, Uppsala, Sweden

CONTENTS

SECTION 1: PATHOGENESIS OF SHOCK

SECTION 4: CLINICAL AND THERAPEUTIC ASPECTS OF SHOCK

SECTION 1

PATHOGENESIS OF SHOCK

EFFECTS OF HEMORRHAGIC AND CATECHOLAMINE SHOCK ON CANINE FORELIMB TRANSCAPILLARY FLUID FLUXES AND SEGMENTAL VASCULAR RESISTANCES[1]

George J. Grega, James M. Schwinghamer and Francis J. Haddy
Department of Physiology, Michigan State University

East Lansing, Michigan 48823

Although the literature on transvascular fluid movement in shock is conflicting, considerable evidence suggests that filtration of fluid from blood to tissue in hemorrhagic and catecholamine shock may be an important determinant in the development of irreversibility [Haddy, Overbeck, and Daugherty (1968); Bloch, Pierce, and Lillehei (1966); Chien (1967)]. This conclusion regarding filtration of intravascular fluid is based largely on measurements of blood volume with dilution techniques and/or hematocrit, and plasma protein determinations in dogs. However, in primates including man the available evidence, while sparse, suggests that hypovolemic shock is associated with hemodilution due to continuous fluid reabsorption [Chien (1967)]. If this apparent discrepancy between dog and man is true it would appear that the dog is a poor shock model. It is generally agreed that in the dog filtration of fluid does occur in the intestine. However, Porciuncula and Crowell (1963) and Smith, Crowell, Moran, and Smith (1967) reported that the volume of fluid lost via the intestinal route in dogs is relatively small, and that atropine administration prevents the hemorrhagic enteritis but has little effect on survival rate or time and on the hemodynamics of the shock state. This intestinal fluid loss appears to be a pecularity to dogs only for it does not occur in primates. Dilution measurements of blood volume may be misleading in states associated with profound vasoconstriction because of inadequate mixing of tracer substances. While the changes in hematocrit and plasma protein concentrations in dogs are compatable

[1] These studies were supported by grants from the Michigan Heart Association and the National Heart Institute (HE 12421-01).

with transvascular fluid loss, no light is shed on the mechanism
of their occurrence. For example, the dog has a large spleen and
contraction of this organ will itself increase hematocrit significantly. Finally other investigators employing dilution techniques in dogs have failed to observe progressive blood volume loss
[Chien (1967)]. Mellander and Lewis (1963) and Lundgren, Lundwall,
and Mellander (1964) reported that in cats (utilizing organ volume
as an index of transvascular fluid fluxes), hemorrhage is associated with fluid filtration in skeletal muscle. However, the question arises as to whether this is simply another species peculiar-
ity. With this is mind we began a systemic study of the direction
and possible mechanism of transcapillary fluid movement in the dog
utilizing a gravimetric technique. The forelimb was selected as
the test organ because it contains skin and skeletal muscle which
compromises over 60 percent of body weight. Hence, transvascular
fluid movement in these tissues, if representative of all skin
and skeletal muscle, must be of paramount importance in shock states
initially as a compensatory attempt to restore blood volume (reabsorption) and possibly later in the development of the irreversible
shock state (filtration). This paper summarizes our work on transvascular fluid movement and segmental vascular resistances in
hemorrhagic and catecholamine shock.

All animals utilized in these experiments were anesthetized
with sodium pentobarbital and allowed to breathe spontaneously
through a cuffed endotracheal tube. The right forelimb including
humerus was completely sectioned except for the brachial artery,
forelimb nerves, brachial and cephalic veins (Figure 1). Catheters were inserted into the aorta and in a small artery, small vein,
and large vein in both muscle and skin in order to calculate segmental pressure gradients. The brachial and cephalic veins were
cannulated with polyethylene tubing and the venous return was
directed to a reservoir, and subsequently returned to the animal.
Anatomical and pharmacological evidence suggest that in this
preparation, after ligating the median cubital vein, brachial
venous outflow is largely from muscle while cephalic venous outflow
is largely from skin [Abboud, (1968); Abboud, and Eckstein (1966);
Daugherty, Scott, Emerson, and Haddy (1968); Miller (1964)]. Therefore, muscle and skin blood flows were measured by timed collections
of the venous outflows. Total and segmental (large artery, small
vessel, large vein) vascular resistances in both skin and muscle
were calculated by dividing appropriate pressure gradients by
appropriate blood flows. In addition the forelimb was suspended
on a sensitive I-beam balance in order to follow changes in forelimb weight. All animals were well heparinized prior to bleeding
or catecholamine infusion.

The segmental resistance technique does not provide a direct
measure of the pre/postcapillary resistance ratio. The small
vessel segment contains both pre- and postcapillary components

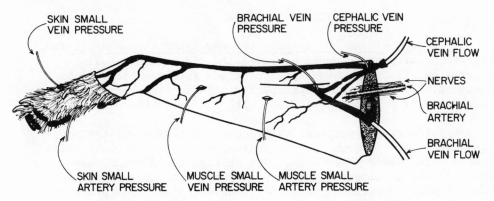

Figure 1. Canine forelimb preparation used in this study. The
          forelimb is shown partially skinned only to better
          visualize vessel and catheter positions. In actual
          practice, the skin remained intact.

but the proportion of resistance residing in the pre- and postcapillary vessels of this segment cannot be determined. However,
the large artery resistance is exclusively precapillary and the
large vein resistance is exclusively postcapillary; hence the large
vessel pre/postcapillary resistance ratio reflects the relative
degree of constriction of the two large vessel components of the
pre- and postcapillary segments. The prevenous (large artery plus
small vessel) resistance is a maximum for precapillary resistance
whereas the venous (large vein) resistance represents a minimum for
postcapillary resistance. Under certain conditions the prevenous/-
venous resistance ratio provides a useful approximation of direct-
ional changes in the pre/postcapillary resistance ratio. If the
large veins constrict proportionately more than the small vessels
plus large arteries (decreased prevenous/venous resistance ratio)
then the pre/postcapillary resistance ratio will also be decreased,
providing the increase in small vessel resistance is uniformily
distributed within the pre- and postcapillary components of this
segment.

      All animals were bled either 25 (N = 10), 50 (N = 10), or 60
(N = 20) percent of their estimated blood volume (8% of body weight)
by arterial hemorrhage and remained hypovolemic for four hours. At
the end of the hypovolemic period all animals were transfused with
their shed blood warmed to 37°C and all responses were followed for
45 minutes. The average bleeding time required to remove 25, 50,
or 60 percent of the blood volume was 3, 45, and 120 minutes,
respectively.

      L-Norepinephrine bitartrate [1.5 mcg (N = 10) or 3.0 mcg (N = 10)
base/Kg/min] was infused (0.2 cc/min) for 3 hours I.V. All responses
were followed for up to 2 hours after cessation of the infusion.

HEMORRHAGIC SHOCK

25 (moderate) and 50 (severe) percent blood volume depletion.
Arterial hemorrhage produced steady-state reductions in all
measured arterial and venous pressures and forelimb blood flows
throughout a 4 hour hypovolemic period. These hymodynamic alterations were of a greater magnitude with the large bleeding stress.

Forelimb weight progressively decreased throughout the hypovolemic period with both bleeding stresses, the weight loss being
greater with severe hemorrhage. The initial rapid weigh loss
(0-10 min) is attributed to both a decreased intravascular blood
volume (vasoconstriction) and a net transcapillary absorption of
extravascular fluids. The slow persistent phase of weight loss
with moderate hemorrhage appeared to result primarily from transcapillary fluid reabsorption along with a small, further decrease
in intravascular blood volume. This blood volume loss is suggested since resistance in all vascular segments increased throughout the 25 percent hypovolemic period indicating a decline in mean
vessel caliber and, inferentially, in total vascular capacity. With
severe bleeding, vascular volume changes contributed little to the
slow component of weight loss since total forelimb small vessel
and venous resistances were relatively constant for the last 3
hours of the hypovolemic period. A constant resistance in these
segments (which together comprise about 90 percent of total vascular capacity) reflects a relatively constant mean vessel caliber
and consequently intravascular blood volume. In addition, the total
weight loss produced by severe hemorrhage exceeds both the total
forelimb intravascular blood volume and the weight loss produced
by maximum constriction of the forelimb vessels by local intra-
brachial arterial infusion of norepinephrine (10 mcg/min). Thus
the remainder of the weight loss must have represented continuous
fluid reabsorption.

The pressure-resistance data suggest a possible mechanism
responsible for the observed fluid influx. The decreased arterial
and venous pressures suggest that the fluid influx may be attributed to a sustained reduction in Pc. All segmental resistances
were markedly elevated relative to control during the hypovolemic
period. The large arteries and veins constricted proportionately
more than the small vessels in both muscle and skin. The large
vessel pre/postcapillary resistance ratio in both muscle and skin
was unchanged with moderate and increased with severe bleeding.
Thus with moderate bleeding the effects of the increased large
vein resistance on Pc were completely negated by a corresponding
increase in large artery resistance. With severe bleeding the
large arteries constricted proportionately more than the large
veins which would lower Pc. The prevenous/venous resistance
ratios in both muscle and skin were unchanged relative to control
with both bleeding stresses indicating that the large veins did

not constrict proportionately more than the combined large artery
plus small vessel resistances. Therefore, the continuous fluid
influx is attributed to a sustained reduction in Pc subsequent
to a fall in arterial and venous pressures. With severe bleeding
the increased large vessel pre/postcapillary resistance ratio would
also contribute to lower Pc. The effect of the small vessel pre/-
postcapillary resistance ratio on Pc cannot be determined. However,
since the forelimbs continuously lost weight it is assumed that
changes in this variable had no effect, augmented, or failed to
counteract the sustained reduction in Pc for fluid influx continued
throughout the hypovolemic period.

In the control period the large vessels contained 18 percent
(large artery 15%; large vein 3%) of total forelimb resistance,
after moderate bleeding and 4 hours of hypovolemia this increased
to 35 percent (large artery 28%, large vein 7%). With severe
bleeding the percentage of total forelimb resistance residing in
the large vessels increased from a control 29 percent (large
artery 24%, large vein 5%) to 44 percent(large artery 37%, large
vein 7%) after 4 hours of hypovolemia. Thus, it is evident that
the large artery constriction contributes significantly to the increased precapillary resistance in hemorrhagic hypotensive states,
and that the large vessels have an enhanced role in determining the
pre/postcapillary resistance ratio.

The initial constriction always developed more rapidly in the
muscle vascular segments with resistance being at or near maximum
during the first 15 min. Resistance in the skin segments showed
smaller initial elevation always followed by further increases
throughout most of the hypovolemic period. There was a partial
waning of total muscle resistance with severe bleeding with all segments participating in the decline. The waning of large artery resistance could be related to a changing level of baroreceptor activity
and to an increased transmural pressure since it occurred during the
time systemic pressure was increasing (15-60 min). During min 60-
240, when muscle large artery resistance was constant, baroreceptor
activity was also constant since systemic pressure was steady. Resistance in the muscle small vessels and large veins also decreased
during min 15-60. However, unlike the large arteries, these vessels
continued to display a slowly declining resistance during the last
3 hours of the hypovolemic period. This cannot be explained on the
basis of changes in baroreceptor activity, transmural pressure, or
viscosity (hematocrit), and therefore may represent active vasodilation by locally released metabolites. This possibility is supported by the arterial blood electrolyte and osmolarity data obtained
during severe bleeding. Increased plasma potassium and magnesium
concentrations and osmolarity were observed and have all been shown
to produce vasodilation [Haddy and Scott (1968)]. Thus, these
changes may be responsible for the partial waning of resistance
in the muscle small vessels and veins. Also, local tissue fluid

concentration of these and other "vasodilator metabolites" are
likely higher than those observed in systemic arterial blood.

Following the return of the shed blood all resistances
decreased and forelimb weight and blood flow increased, but all
variables failed to reach control levels 45 minutes after transfusion of the blood with both bleeding stresses. The weight gain
was probably due to an increased forelimb intravascular blood
volume (vascular resistance decreased) and fluid efflux to tissues.

60 Percent Blood Volume Depletion. The bleeding stress
caused sustained reductions in all measured arterial and venous
pressures and very marked steady-state reductions in forelimb
blood flows throughout a 4 hour hypovolemic period. This hemodynamic pattern is typically associated with bleeding stresses
sufficient to induce consistent irreversible shock in dogs. Indeed,
the bleedout volume was sufficient to cause death in a significant
number of animals (N = 8) during the latter part of the hypovolemic
period, further evidence of the severity of the bleeding stress.

Forelimb weight progressively decreased throughout the hypovolemic period in response to arterial hemorrhage. This weight loss
was accompanied by marked progressive increases in both total muscle
and skin resistances reflecting a decreasing mean vessel caliber and,
inferentially, intravascular blood volume. However, the weight loss
was much greater than could be accounted for by a decreased intravascular blood volume alone. Therefore a significant proportion of
the weight loss must be attributed to net continuous fluid movement
from tissue to blood (reabsorption). This weight loss pattern was
qualitatively similar in animals with an intact forelimb indicating
that the weight loss cannot be attributed to artifact induced by
surgical trauma and/or bypassing the downstream venous resistance
and the right atrial pressure influences on Pc.

The steady-state reductions in all measured arterial and
venous pressures suggests that the continuous fluid influx may be
due to a sustained reduction in Pc. Muscle and skin segmental
resistances increased progressively throughout the hypovolemic
period and were markedly increased relative to control after 4
hours of hypovolemia. In both muscle and skin the large artery
and vein resistances increased proportionately more than small
vessel resistances. The large vessel pre/postcapillary resistance
ratio was decreased in skin throughout most (0-210 min) of the
hypovolemic period indicating that the large veins constricted proportionately more than the large arteries. In muscle the large
vessel pre/postcapillary resistance ratio was unchanged relative
to control indicating that the large arteries and veins were constricting proportionately. In both muscle and skin the prevenous/-
venous resistance ratios were decreased suggesting that the pre/-
postcapillary resistance ratio was decreased which would increase

Pc. Therefore it is assumed that the continuous fluid influx is due to a sustained reduction in Pc subsequent to steady-state reductions in arterial and venous pressures despite a possible decreased pre/postcapillary resistance ratio in muscle and skin. This implys that the fall in arterial and venous pressure is more than sufficient to offset the effects of a decreased pre/postcapillary resistance ratio on Pc, for fluid influx continued throughout the hypovolemic period. In the control period the large vessels contained approximately 28 percent (large artery 24%, large vein 4%) of total forelimb resistance; after 4 hours of hypovolemia this increased to approximately 47 percent (large artery 39%, large vein 7.5%). It is apparent that the large artery constriction contributes significantly to the rise in precapillary resistance in hemorrhagic shock, and that the large vessels become increasingly important determinants of the pre/postcapillary resistance ratio.

Following the return of the shed blood all resistances fell The weight gain from min 5-90 was accompanied by further increases in forelimb resistances and, inferentially, further decreases in intravascular blood volume. This weight gain was associated with sustained increases in all arterial and skin small vein pressures which would increase Pc. In addition, the large vessel pre/postcapillary and prevenous/venous resistance ratios in skin were decreased suggesting that the pre/postcapillary resistance ratio was decreased which would also increase Pc. In muscle the large vessel pre/postcapillary resistance ratio was unchanged relative to control whereas the prevenous/venous resistance ratio was increased. Thus the influence of the two muscle large vessel segments on Pc in muscle would cancel. The effect of the muscle small vessel segment on Pc in muscle cannot be determined. Therefore, the weight gain must be attributed to a net movement of intravascular fluid to tissue (filtration) subsequent to an increased Pc. This weight gain may have been buffered to some extent by a declining intravascular blood volume. The weight loss from min 90-180 was accompanied by further increases in forelimb total and segmental resistances, and decreases in all arterial and muscle small vein pressures which fell below control. The fall in pressures suggests that Pc was decreased. Muscle large vessel pre/postcapillary and prevenous/venous resistance ratios were still increased relative to control. The former would decrease Pc whereas the influence of the latter on Pc cannot be determined. Both resistance ratios in skin were decreased suggesting that the pre/postcapillary resistance ratio was decreased which would increase Pc. Therefore the weight loss is attributed to both a decreasing intravascular blood volume and reabsorption of extravascular fluid subsequent to a decreased Pc despite a possible decreased pre/postcapillary resistance ratio in skin.

Upon cessation of the infusion forelimb weight increased (0.3 g/100g limb) within 3 min, remained relatively constant for

1 hour, and then slowly decreased during the remainder of the post-transfusion period (0.5 g/100g limb). Forelimb total and segmental resistances fell within 3 mins, but were still elevated relative to control and remained relatively steady throughout the post-transfusion period. This reflects a constant mean vessel caliber and, inferentially, intravascular blood volume from min 183-300. All arterial and small vein pressures fell below control suggesting that Pc was decreased. Muscle and skin prevenous/venous resistance ratios were at or near control indicating that the large veins did not constrict proportionately more than the combined large artery plus small vessel segments. The influence of the small vessel segments on Pc cannot be determined. The large vessel pre/postcapillary resistance ratio in both muscle and skin progressively increased which would also lower Pc. Since forelimb vascular capacity was relatively constant it is assumed that the weight loss during the latter part of the post-transfusion period largely represented continuous fluid influx subsequent to a fall and forelimb weight and blood flow increased, but all variables failed to reach control levels by the end of the post-transfusion period. The weight gain was probably due to an increased forelimb intravascular blood volume (vasodilation) and to fluid efflux to tissue.

These data are not in agreement with the studies of Lundgren et. al., (1964) in cats. These investigators reported filtration of intravascular fluid in skeletal muscle after only 20 min of hemorrhagic hypotension which was associated with complete dissipation of the resistance response at a time when the capacitance response was well maintained. The reason for such divergent results is not clear, but may be related to differences in vascular beds, species, anesthetics, or techniques. Nevertheless, these studies provide no evidence for forelimb transvascular fluid loss in canine hemorrhagic shock, but rather for continuous fluid influx from tissues to blood (reabsorption).

CATECHOLAMINE SHOCK

Norepinephrine (1.5 mcg base/Kg/min, I.V.). All arterial and small vein pressures increased abruptly in response to norepinephrine infusion, peaking at 2 min, and rapidly declined thereafter, falling to slightly below control by the end of the infusion period. Forelimb blood flows decreased rapidly within 2 min and continued to slowly decline during the remainder of the infusion period. Forelimb total and segmental resistances progressively increased throughout the infusion and were markedly elevated relative to control. In skin the large artery and small vessel resistances increased almost proportionately, but both increased proportionately less than large vein resistance. The large artery and small vessel resistances also

increased almost proportionately in muscle, and both increased proportionately more than large vein resistance. Total and segmental
resistances increased proportionately more in skin than in muscle.
The percent of the total resistance residing in the large vessels
was only slightly altered during norepinephrine infusion. This percentage in skin changed from a control of 23 percent (large artery
18%, large vein 5%) to 25.6 percent (large artery 18%, large vein
7.6%) at the end of the infusion period. In muscle this percentage
changed from a control of 26 percent (large artery 23%, large vein
3%) to 27 percent (large artery 25.5%, large vein 1.5%) at the end
of the infusion period.

Forelimb weight decreased rapidly (0-2 min) in response to norepinephrine infusion (1.2g/100g limb), increased slowly from min 5-90
(0.6g/100g limb), then slowly decreased during the remainder of the
infusion period (0.5g/100g limb). The initial weight loss (0-2 min)
was accompanied by increases in forelimb resistances reflecting decreases in vessel caliber and, inferentially, in vascular capacity.
in Pc. The percent of the total resistance residing in the large
vessels at the end of the post-transfusion period increased to
42 percent (large artery 34%, large vein 8%) in skin and 59 percent (large artery 57%, large vein 2.4%) in muscle.

Norepinephrine (3 mcg base/Kg/min, I.V.). Norepinephrine
infused for 3 hours produced progressive cardiovascular deterioration. Indeed all but two animals died shortly after cessation
of the infusion, evidence of the severity of the stress. All
arterial and small vein pressures increased markedly, peaking at
2 min, and rapidly declined thereafter. The arterial pressures
were well below control by the end of the infusion period whereas
small vein pressures were only slightly lower than control at
this time. Forelimb blood flows decreased markedly within 2
min and continued to slowly decline during the remainder of the
infusion period. Total forelimb resistance progressively increased
throughout the infusion period (except for min 5-15), with all vascular segments participating in the response. Segmental resistances
increased proportionately more in skin than muscle, but both were
markedly elevated relative to control at the end of the infusion
period. The large artery resistance in muscle and skin and the
large vein resistance in skin increased proportionately more than
small vessel resistance. In muscle the small vessel and large vein
resistances increased almost proportionately. The large veins constricted proportionately more than the large arteries in skin whereas in muscle the large arteries and veins constricted almost proportionately. The percent of the total resistance residing in the large
vessels increased during norepinephrine infusion. In the control
period the large vessels in both muscle and skin contained approximately 18 percent (large artery 14%, large vein 4%) of total resistance, by the end of the infusion period this increased to 28 percent

in muscle (large artery 24%, large vein 4%) and to 38 percent in skin (large artery 24%, large vein 14%).

Forelimb weight decreased rapidly within 2 min, increased slightly from min 5-15, and thereafter continued to slowly decline until cessation of the infusion. The initial (0-2 min) weight loss (1.6g/100g limb) was accompanied by abrupt increases in forelimb total and segmental resistance reflecting a decreased mean vessel caliber and, inferentially, vascular capacity. From min 5-15 forelimb weight increased slightly (0.4g/100g limb). This weight gain was associated with a fall in forelimb total and segmental vascular resistances reflecting an increasing mean vessel caliber and consequently intravascular blood volume. All forelimb arterial and skin small vein pressures were increased well above control suggesting that Pc was increased. The large vessel pre/postcapillary and prevenous/venous resistance ratios were decreased markedly in skin and slightly in muscle suggesting that the forelimb pre/postcapillary resistance ratio was decreased (particularly in skin) which would also increase Pc. Thus the weight gain is attributed to an increased intravascular blood volume and net movement of fluid from blood to tissue (filtration) subsequent to an increased Pc. There was a slow weight loss (0.6 g/100g limb) from min 15-75 which was accompanied by further increases in forelimb total and segmental resistances and, inferentially, a decreasing intravascular blood volume. All arterial and small skin vein pressures were falling but still elevated relative to control suggesting that Pc was still increased. The resistance ratios were still decreased in skin suggesting that the pre/postcapillary resistance ratio was decreased which would increase Pc. In muscle both resistance ratios were unchanged relative to control. The effect of the increased muscle large vein resistance on Pc was negated by a corresponding increase in muscle large artery resistance. The effect of the muscle small vessel segment on Pc cannot be determined. Therefore the weight loss is attributed to a decreased intravascular blood volume which may have been buffered to some extent by filtration of vascular fluid to tissue in skin owing to an increased Pc. Forelimb weight continued to decline slowly from min 75-180 (1.3 g/100g limb). This weight loss was accompanied by relatively constant forelimb small vessel and large vein resistances reflecting a reasonably constant mean vessel caliber in these segments. Since these segments together compromise approximately 90 percent of total vascular capacity it is assumed that forelimb blood volume was reasonably constant during this time. All pressures continued to decline with arterial pressures dropping well below control and small vein pressures to slightly below control suggesting that Pc was decreased. The resistance ratios in muscle were unchanged relative to control. The effects of the muscle large vessel resistances on Pc canceled each other while that of the muscle small vessels cannot be determined. The resistance ratios in skin were still

decreased suggesting that the pre/postcapillary resistance ratio
was decreased which would increase Pc. Thus it is concluded that
the weight loss during this period is largely due to continuous
fluid influx and to a small extent a further decrease in vascular
capacity. The reabsorption of extravascular fluid is attributed
to a decreased Pc despite a possible decreased pre/postcapillary
resistance ratio in skin.

Three minutes after cessation of the infusion muscle and skin
large vein resistances were still at maximum values while large
artery and small vessel resistances fell, but were still significantly elevated relative to control. Most animals died 5-30
min after cessation of the infusion.

These experiments provide no evidence to support the concept
that extensive transvascular fluid loss in skeletal muscle and
skin is an important determinant of irreversibility in catecholamine shock.

BIBLIOGRAPHY

1. Abboud, F.M.: Vascular responses to norepinephrine, antio-
    tensin, vasopressin and serotonin. Federation Proceedings,
    Vol. 27, p1391, 1968.

2. Abboud, F.M., and J.W. Eckstein: Comparative changes in seg-
    mental vascular resistance in response to nerve stimulation
    and norepinephrine. Circulation Research, Vol. 18, p263, 1966.

3. Bloch, J.H., C.L. Pierce, and R.C. Lillehei: Adrenergic block-
    ing agents in the treatment of shock. Annual Review of Medi-
    cine, Vol. 17, p483, 1966.

4. Chien, S.: Role of the sympathetic nervous system in hemorr-
    hage. Physiological Reviews, Vol. 47, p214-288, 1967.

5. Daugherty, R.M., J.B. Scott, T.E. Emerson, and F.J. Haddy: Com-
    parison of iv and ia infusion of vasoactive agents in dog fore-
    limb blood flow. American Journal of Physiology, Vol. 214,
    p611, 1968.

6. Haddy, F.J., H.W. Overbeck, and R.M. Daugherty, Jr.: Peri-
    pheral vascular resistance. Annual Review of Medicine, Vol.
    19, p167, 1968.

7. Haddy, F.J., and J.B. Scott: Metabolically linked vasoactive
    chemicals in local regulation of blood flow. Physiological
    Reviews, Vol. 48, p688, 1968.

8. Lundgren, O., J. Lundwall, and S. Mellander: Range of sym-
    pathetic discharge and reflex vascular adjustments in skeletal
    muscle during hemorrhagic hypotension. Acta Physiological
    Scandanavia, Vol. 62, p380, 1964.

9. Mellander, S. and D.H. Lewis: Effects of hemorrhagic shock
    on the reactivity of resistance and capacitance vessels and
    on capillary filtration transfer in cat skeletal muscle.
    Circulation Research, Vol. 23, p105, 1963.

10. Miller, M.E.: Anatomy of the dog. W.B. Saunders Co., p337,
    1964, Philadelphia, Pennsylvania.

11. Porciuncula, C., and Crowell, J.W.: Quantitative study of
    intestinal fluid loss in irreversible hemorrhagic shock.
    American Journal of Physiology, Vol. 205, p261, 1963.

12. Smith, E.E., J.W. Crowell, C.J. Moran, and R.A. Smith: Intesti-
    nal fluid loss during irreversible hemorrhagic shock. Surgery,
    Gynecology and Obstetrics. Vol. 125, p1, 1967.

ACKNOWLEDGEMENTS

    The authors are indebted to Mr. Sim Swindall, Mr. W. Jeffrey
Weidner, Mr. Ed Gersabeck, Jr., Miss Janice Homann, and Mr. Ber-
nard Walulik for their very capable surgical assistance throughout
the course of these studies, and to Miss Sylvia Krieger for her
invaluable assistance in the preparation of manuscripts.

RENAL FAILURE IN HEMORRHAGIC SHOCK

Kurt Kramer

PHYSIOLOGISCHES INSTITUT DER UNIVERSITÄT MUENCHEN

MUENCHEN - GERMANY

In 1961, at the Symposium on shock in Stockholm, we presented evidence of persistent renal vasocon- striction in and following hemorrhagic shock which was suggested to take place on the preglomerular level (1). However, total renal blood flow was not so much reduced that hypoxia resulted. This was con- cluded from measurements of oxygen saturations of cortical blood in the low pressure phase of shock (2).

There was, however, an obvious disagreement con- cerning intrarenal vascular flow pattern. Since the work of TRUETA in 1941, it was generally accepted that, at least in traumatic shock, a diversion of blood from cortical to medullary areas occurred. By means of clearance techniques, SELKURT came to a si- milar conclusion. It was suggested that there is a closure of the cortical circulation but some persis- tence of the medullary circulation. In a more direct approach to the problem - the use of red sensitive photometers applied to the surface of cortex and inner medulla and the evaluation of dye dilution curves within these tissues - DEETJEN has shown that cortical and medullary vessels constrict to the same extent when a hemorrhagic shock is induced. It can even happen that dye passages of medullary vessels are even more reduced than those through cortical areas. This is demonstrated in a representative ex- periment (Fig. 1). According to these results, there seems to be no doubt that in hemorrhagic shock shun- ting of blood through medullary vessels does not

15

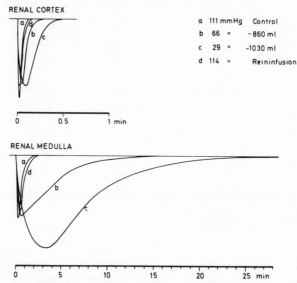

CARDIOGREEN DILUTION CURVES FOLLOWING HEMORRHAGIC SHOCK

RENAL CORTEX

a	111 mmHg	Control
b	66 "	- 860 ml
c	29 "	-1030 ml
d	114 "	Reininfusion

RENAL MEDULLA

Fig. 1a. Cardiogreen dilution curves obtained by a
microphotoelectric technique applied on the
surface of renal cortex and inner medulla in
a nembutalized dog.

occur. If the reduction of renal perfusion pressure is
only due to partial aortic clamping, the reduction of
blood flow is much less pronounced than in shock experiments. It could, therefore, be concluded that the
general vasoconstriction in shock was also present in
the whole kidney, in cortex and medulla as well
(DEETJEN, 1962).

In the experiments reported here, a modification
of the tissue dye dilution technique was introduced
to the effect that changes of secretory processes in
the cortical areas could be measured. This was achieved
by simultaneous injection of cardiogreen and indigocarmine into the renal artery. The latter dye is known
since the days of HEIDENHAIN (1880) to be secreted in
proximal tubules. It could be expected that the photometric recordings would indicate intensity and duration
of dye secretion in the cortical nephrons.

Fig. 2 demonstrates 3 functional states of the
kidney in dogs under nembutal anaesthesia, i.e. in
antidiuresis, in NaCl-diuresis and under Furosemide-
Polyuria. First of all it is evident that all dye

MEAN PASSAGE TIME OF CARDIOGREEN DILUTION CURVES
IN RENAL CORTEX AND MEDULLA DURING HEMORRHAGIC SHOCK

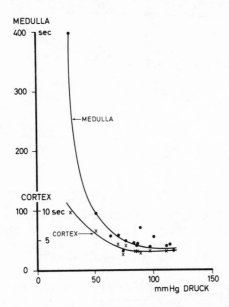

Fig. 1b. Mean passage times taken before hemorrhage
amount to 3 sec and about 1 min in cortex and
medulla respectively. During hemorrhage, duration of passage times increase considerably,
more in medulla than in cortex, indicating
vasoconstriction in both renal regions. After
reinfusion of blood, control values are obtained.

curves cortical and medullary exhibit a much longer
time to return to the control level than the dye curves
derived from cardiogreen injections only (see Fig. 1).
This was expected because of the outlasting secretory
process and the slower flow rate of tubular fluid than
blood flow. Secondly, it is shown that depending on the
state of diuresis, the passage of dye through the distal
part of the nephron is accelerated with urine flow. This
is more pronounced in the inner medulla than in the
cortex. Thirdly, in the inner medulla there appear two
distinct waves following the first vasa recta wave of
mixed cardiogreen and indigocarmine passages. The two
waves demonstrate the urine passage through Henle's
loop and collecting ducts successively.

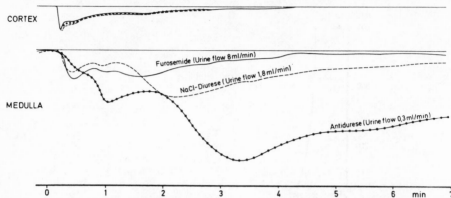

DILUTION CURVES OF CARDIOGREEN- INDIGOCARMINE MIXTURES IN RENAL CORTEX AND MEDULLA

Fig. 2. Dye dilution curves obtained by using the same
technique as in Fig. 1, but with combined injections of a secretable dye (indigocarmine)
and a non-filtrable and non-secretable dye
(cardiogreen).
Cortical curves. The first sudden decline of
all cortical curves indicates the appearance of
the non-filtrable dye followed by the secreted
dye. While, as shown in Fig. 1, the non-filtrable dye rushes in a few seconds through the
cortical region, the secreted dye is slowly
passing the proximal tubules. After a period of
about 4 min, it has left the cortical region.
Medullary curves. With a short delay (not seen
in the Figure), the non-filtrable dye appears
in the medullary blood vessels indicated by a
decline of the photoelectric records. Their
return is interrupted by two further waves
which followed each other; the faster the urine
flow, the earlier the appearance of the second
wave. It seems probable that the first of these
two waves indicates the passage of the secreted
dye through Henle's loops, whereas the second
reflects the passage through collecting ducts.
The extreme acceleration of tubular fluid may
be noticed, especially in Henle's loops with
increased diuresis.

The faster the inflow into the medullary nephron, as
can be expected in NaCl and Furosemide diuresis, the
earlier the appearance of the waves and also their disappearance.

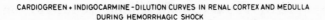

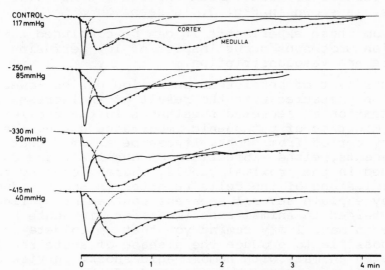

Fig. 3. Nembutalized dog, 20 kg. Cardiogreen-indigo-
         carmine dilution curves in renal cortex and
         inner medulla in hemorrhagic shock. It may be
         noticed that after blood losses of 330 and 415
         ml, corresponding to arterial pressure of 50
         and 40 mm Hg, the secreted dye appears only in
         cortical region showing almost no change of
         concentration, indicating stagnation in proxi-
         mal tubules. At this stage of shock medullary
         curves indicate dye passage through vasa recta
         vessels only.

     These results can be used as controls in the ex-
periments of hemorrhagic shock.

     Fig. 3 shows records taken in different stages of
shock due to progressive hemorrhage. The functional
state of the kidney before hemorrhage is diuretic
(urine flow 1 ml/min) following a small isotonic NaCl
infusion. With the first blood loss of 250 ml, arterial
blood pressure decreases to 85 mm Hg. Extrapolated cardiogreen curves show already a definite lengthening,
indicating slowing of blood flow through cortical and
medullary tissue as well. After continuing blood loss
the indigocarmine curves indicate at the pressure
level of 50 mm Hg that in the cortical nephrons, i.e.
mainly in proximal tubules, the dye is still secreted
and appears to be stagnant with little indication of
leaving the area. At 40 mm Hg this phenomenon is even
more pronounced and combined with complete cessation

of tubular fluid flow to the inner medulla. Only a
slower passage of cardiogreen through the medullary
vessels, as shown in Fig. 1, is seen.

From these experiments it can be concluded that
secretion processes occur inspite of low perfusion
pressure and vasoconstriction.

This fact of persistent secretion during lowest
perfusion pressures with the result of an increase in
concentration of secreted substances in the proximal
tubule might be of pathogenic importance during the
recovery period from shock. It can be assumed that
toxic agents, either infectious or chemical, are concentrated in the proximal tubule, thereby causing the
typical lesions of the cells reported in shock kidneys.
This may explain several apparent contradictory findings obtained in animal experiments and in acute renal
failure in man. I may remind you that up to date it
was impossible to produce the disease of acute renal
failure in animals with hemorrhagic shock. In view of
the absence of toxic substances and of the shortness of
the hypotonic period of the experimental shock, we are
inclined to believe that lesions of tubular cells, if
occurring at all, may be repaired within a reasonable
time.

The manifestation of such reversible lesions, however, may be recognized a few hours during the recovery
period when the hemorrhagic blood is reinfused. The impairment is related to three fundamental functions of
the kidney:

1) Reabsorption of filtered sodium along the entire
   nephron

2) Maintenance of permeability properties which enable
   the cells to reabsorb water, which takes place in
   the proximal as well as the distal nephron

3) Control of glomerular filtration rate

ad 1) Na-reabsorption along the entire nephron may
      easily be checked by clearance techniques.
      Fig. 4a shows the Na-excretion pattern after a
      3 hours hypotonic period due to hemorrhage. The
      experiment has been performed on a dog being on
      a salt poor diet, so that control urinary Na-
      excretion is almost zero. After reinfusion of
      the blood, Na-excretion is immensely increased,
      but only for a few hours. At this period, Na-
      rejection amounts to about 4 - 8% of filtered
      Na. This may be considered as a definite impair-

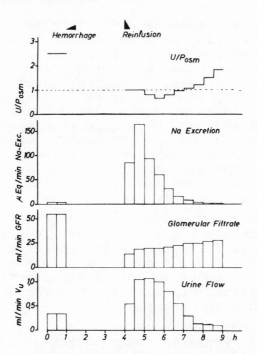

Fig. 4a. Hemorrhagic hypotension in a dog of 34 kg over
a period of 3 hours with an arterial blood
pressure of 50 mm Hg. After reinfusion, complete recovery of arterial pressure up to 120
mm Hg. Note polyuric phase with high Na-output,
low glomerular filtration rate (GFR) and hypo-
tonicity of urine (U/P$_{osmol}$). After a recovery
period of 5 hours, GFR and U/P$_{osmol}$ did not
reach normal values.

ment of the active Na-transport mechanism of the
tubular cells (Fig. 4b), being due to functional
lesions of the early distal nephron, particularly
at the level of Henle's loop (THURAU and
SCHNERMANN).

ad 2) The response of the medullary concentrating mechanism to ADH can be used to test the permeability
properties of the nephron. Over a period of 2 - 3
hours after reinfusion of the blood the concentrating mechanism is definitely impaired (Fig. 5).
The urine osmolar concentration is almost isotonic
or even slightly hypotonic and urine flow is very
high. This means that H_2O-reabsorption mainly in
the distal nephron is insufficient. Infusions of

antidiuretic hormone which is supposed to increase membrane permeability to water at the
distal nephron site, have no effect on urine flow
nor on osmolar concentrating power of the medullary system. We may, therefore, conclude that the
permeability function of the distal nephron cells
has been impaired during the hypotonic period.
GRANTHAM and BURG have furnished evidence for an
exhaustion of cyclic AMP possibly due to regional
hypoxia in medullary areas. This theory would be
in agreement with our finding of an extreme
lowering of blood flow rate through the vasa
recta (see Fig. 1).

ad 3) Although blood pressure is quickly restored when
the circulatory system is refilled with blood,
glomerular filtration rate remains markedly reduced. Its final recovery may last over periods
of several hours in animal experiments and in
the classical disease of acute renal failure
days and even months.

THURAU and SCHNERMANN have proposed a feedback
mechanism that regulates renin output of the juxtaglo-
merular apparatus and thereby angiotensin production
around the afferent arteriole. The stimulus is the Na-
concentration of the tubular fluid passing the macula

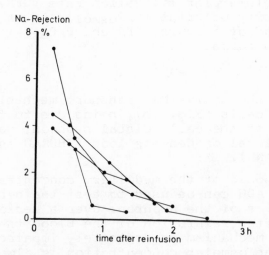

<u>Fig. 4b.</u> High Na-rejection after hemorrhagic shock in-
dicating impairment of Na-reabsorption along
the nephron.

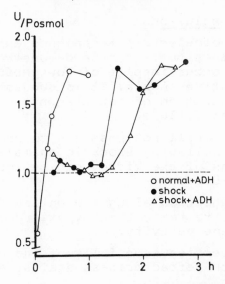

Concentrating Ability of Normal
and Shock Kidneys and their
Response to ADH.

Fig. 5. Refractoriness of antidiuretic hormone in hemorrhagic shock in nembutalized dogs.
Control is taken from an experiment of water
diuresis with prompt response to ADH. In the
two shock experiments, U/P$_{osmol}$ does not rise
1 1/2 hours after reinfusion of the blood. Infusions of different concentrations of ADH have
no influence on recovery of the concentrating
mechanism.

densa area and the latter is regarded as the receptor
zone.

In their micropuncture experiments on rats an
increase in Na-concentration in the macula densa region
was followed by an immediate decrease of filtration
rate. The authors believe to have found a triggering
mechanism whereby glomerular Na-filtration can be adjusted to the reabsorption capacity of the tubule.

In our particular problem the low glomerular filtration rate could be explained by an action of high
Na-concentration at the macula densa due to an impairment of Na-reabsorption proximally to it. Also the long
term processes of recovery of GFR, as observed in man's
disease, could be caused by such a feedback mechanism

since many reabsorptive functions, especially the
active Na-transport through tubular cell membranes,
show a pronounced delay of recovery.

Conclusions

By means of photoelectric techniques applied to
the kidney of dogs in situ it can be demonstrated that
secretory processes occur inspite of low perfusion
pressure and consecutive anuria. It is suggested that
secretion and concentration of toxic agents due to
shock may cause renal failure.

Although it is still not possible to produce
acute renal failure following shock in animals, several
fundamental functions of the kidney can be shown to
play a role in this disease:

1) Impaired Na-reabsorption along the entire nephron
   possibly due more to toxic than hypoxic destructions
   of tubular membrane activity.

2) Permeability properties especially of the distal
   nephron cells with refractoriness against ADH
   causing polyuria.

3) Persistent vasoconstriction at the preglomerular
   level as a result of a Na-triggering mechanism of
   the renin-angiotensin liberation.

References

1) Deetjen, P. (1962):
        Intrarenale Hämodynamik im hämorrhagischen
        Schock.
        1. Symposion der Ges. Nephrologie, Freiburg/Br.,
        Stuttgart 1962.

2) Grantham, J.J., and M.B. Burg (1966):
        Effect of vasopressin and cyclic AMP on per-
        meability of isolated collecting ducts.
        Amer.J.Physiol. 211, 225.

3) Heidenhain, R. (1880):
        Physiologie der Absonderungsvorgänge.
        In Hermanns Handbuch der Physiologie, Vol. 5.

4) Kramer, K. (1962):
        Renal failure in shock, pathogenesis and
        therapy.
        Symposion edited by K.D. Bock, Heidelberg,
        Göttingen, Berlin, page 134.

5) Kramer, K., and P. Deetjen (1964):
   Physiological aspects of acute renal failure.
   14th Biennal International Congress of the
   International College of Surgeons, page 79.

6) Munck, O., N.A. Lassen, P. Deetjen and K. Kramer
   (1962):
   Evidence against renal hypoxia in acute hemorrhagic shock.
   Pflügers Arch.ges.Physiol. 274, 356.

7) Schnermann, J., W. Nagel und K. Thurau (1966):
   Die frühdistale Na-Konzentration in Rattennie-
   ren nach renaler Ischämie und hämorrhagischer
   Hypotension.
   Pflügers Arch.ges.Physiol. 287, 296.

8) Selkurt, E.E. (1962):
   Renal blood flow and renal clearance during
   hemorrhage and hemorrhagic shock.
   In "Shock Pathogenesis and Therapy", Heidelberg,
   Göttingen, Berlin, page 145.

9) Trueta, J., A.E. Barcley, P.M. Daniel, K.J. Franklin
   and M.M.L. Prichard (1947):
   Studies of renal circulation, Oxford.

A CONSIDERATION OF THE ROLE OF THE RETICULOENDOTHELIAL SYSTEM

(RES) IN ENDOTOXIN SHOCK

N. R. Di Luzio and Clifford G. Crafton

Tulane University School of Medicine

University of Tennessee Medical Units

A recent hypothesis concerning host susceptibility to shock postulates that the basic etiology of shock phenomena centers on vascular smooth muscle injuries (Palmerio and Fine, 1969). Palmerio and Fine (1969) presented evidence that resistance to shock is dependent upon the antibacterial and detoxification potential of the RES. A shock model in which the critical nature of the RES has been implicated is endotoxin-induced shock (Beeson, 1947 a,b). Beeson in 1947 first demonstrated the importance of RES function in host defense against endotoxin-induced pathology (Beeson, 1947 a,b). Rabbits, previously tolerant to the febrile effects of endotoxin and subsequently treated with a large dose of colloidal materials which were known to temporarily depress RES activity, responded to the pyrogenic effects of endotoxin (Beeson, 1947a). In addition, an RES "blockading" dose of colloidal material resensitized tolerant rabbits to the Shwartzman reaction and enhanced lethality when endotoxin was subsequently administered (Beeson, 1947b). Passive plasma transfer studies indicated that RES blockade retarded the clearance of circulating endotoxin (Beeson, 1947a). Beeson speculated that diminution in phagocytosis of endotoxin enabled the endotoxin to injure various tissues as reflected by fever (Beeson, 1947a).

Studies with radioactively labeled endotoxin stressed the localization of intravenously administered endotoxin in the RES, particularly the liver (Braude, Carey and Zalesky, 1955, and Noyes, McInturf and Blahuta, 1959). In addition to clearing the vascular compartment of endotoxin, the liver and spleen are important in endotoxin detoxification (Rutenburg, Skarnes, Palmerio and Fine, 1967). While Greisman, Carozza and Hills (1963)

and Wharton and Creech (1949) have demonstrated the importance of
humoral factors in preventing the pyrogenic and lethal effects of
endotoxin, recent studies have focused attention on splenic detoxification mechanisms as a factor in endotoxemia (Rutenburg,
et al., 1967). The endotoxin macrophage interaction has been
speculated to be of significance not only in detoxification of
endotoxin, but also in inducing some of the injurious effects of
endotoxin via alterations in lysosomal stability (Lemperle, 1966).
Indeed, in vitro release of hepatic lysosomal enzymes from rabbits
treated with endotoxin occurs at an accelerated level relative to
saline-treated control rabbits (Weissmann and Thomas, 1962).
Based upon the multipotential nature of RES involvement in host-
defense, the population and status of the RES may well be the
basis of host response to endotoxin as well as a major determinant
in endotoxin lethality.

The development of highly purified chemical agents which
possess the ability to accelerate (Riggi and Di Luzio, 1961) or
depress (Di Luzio and Blickens, 1966) RES activity provided the
foundation for a more definitive evaluation of the role of RES
function and status on host defense against endotoxemia. Earlier
studies, utilizing the RES stimulants, BCG (Suter, Ullman and
Hoffman, 1958), zymosan (Benacerraf, Thorbecke and Jacoby, 1959),
and triolein (Stuart and Cooper, 1962) indicated that these RES
stimulants induced endotoxin hyper-reactivity in mice. Our
studies in rats using glucan, a selective RES stimulant (Riggi
and Di Luzio, 1961) and methyl palmitate (Di Luzio and Blickens,
1966), a phagocytic and immune depressant, demonstrated that
alteration of RES functional activity is associated with striking
modulations in host reactivity to intravenously administered
endotoxins.

MATERIALS AND METHODS

Sprague-Dawley rats weighing approximately 200-320 g. were
maintained on commercially available laboratory chow and water
ad libitum. The reticuloendothelial stimulant, glucan, (Riggi
and Di Luzio, 1961) was injected intravenously for 2 or 5 days at
a dose of 1 mg/100 g. In another group of rats, methyl palmitate
(Di Luzio and Blickens, 1966) purity 99.8% (Applied Sciences
Laboratories, State College, Pa.) was administered intravenously
in a dose of 100 mg/100 g for 2 consecutive days to induce RE
depression. Since methyl palmitate was sonified in a 0.1% Tween 20
and 5% dextrose aqueous solution, the Tween 20 and dextrose solution was given isovolumetrically. Saline was administered as a
control for glucan treatment. In an evaluation of the presence
of humoral factors in altered endotoxin sensitivity, blood from
control groups of rats and those treated with the RE depressant or

stimulant was obtained by cardiac puncture using Mepesulfate
(Hoffman-LaRoche, Inc., Nutley, N. J.) as anticoagulant. The
plasma from experimental or control groups was injected intravenously into normal rats in a dose of 1 ml/100 g. One hour after
plasma administration S. enteritidis endotoxin (0.75 mg/100 g) was
administered and mortality subsequently observed. Control rats
received saline isovolumetrically prior to endotoxin injection.

In an effort to evaluate the influence of RES functional modification on plasma lysosomal enzyme activity, blood from the vena
cava was collected with Mepesulfate 3 hours after S. enteritidis
endotoxin administration. The plasma activity of β-glucuronidase
was assayed according to the technique of Plaice (1961) and expressed in terms of mg of phenolphthalein released per 100 ml plasma
per hour at 37°C per ml of incubation media. The activity of acid
phosphatase was measured by a modification of the procedure of
Berthet and DeDuve (1951). The activity of the enzyme is determined
by cleavage of β-glycerophosphate and the analysis of the free inorganic phosphate by the technique of Fiske and Subbarow (1925).
The unit of activity of acid phosphatase was mg of inorganic phos-
phous released per 100 ml plasma at 37°C per ml of incubation media.

In an attempt to dissociate the hyperphagocytic phase and the
RE hypertrophy state as mediators of the glucan-induced endotoxin
hyper-reactivity, rats were treated with glucan for 5 days and 24
and 48 hours later received methyl palmitate to abolish the hyperfunctional state of the RES. Twenty-four hours after the final
methyl palmitate injection, or three days following the final glucan
injection, S. enteritidis endotoxin, suspended in pyrogen-free
saline, was injected into the dorsal vein of the penis of control
and experimental rats. Uninjected, normal rats also received the
dose of endotoxin and the mortality of the 24 hour period determined.

In all experiments, the endotoxin preparations were administered in the volume of 0.5 ml/100 g. Although in all cases mortality occurred within the first 24 hours following endotoxin administration, rats were observed for a 7 day period for possible
latent mortality. The following endotoxins were used: Salmonella
enteritidis (Difco, LPS, B, Control 172145 and Control 500998),
Escherichia coli (Difco, LPS, B, Control 490943) and Salmonella
typhi-murium (Difco, LPS, B, Control 188427).

The effect of altered RES function on vascular clearance and
tissue localization of endotoxin was studied using S. enteritidis
endotoxin. The labeling procedure of Braude, Carey, Sutherland and
Zalesky (1955) utilizing hexavelent Na_2 $^{51}CrO_4$ has been demonstrated to provide a stable, firm endotoxin label (Braude, et al., 1955;
Chedid, Skarnes and Parant, 1963). The LD_{70} dose of endotoxin in
normal rats was administered in clearance studies; for the endotoxin preparation employed the LD_{70} was 4.0 mg/100g.

Phagocytic activity of the RES was measured by the employ-
ment of the gelatinized "RE test lipid" emulsion (Saba and Di Luzio
1968). An anhydrous base was prepared utilizing glycerol, alcohol soluble soya lecithin, and I^{131} triolein (Raolein, Abbott
Laboratories) diluted with peanut oil in a ratio of 10:1:10 by
weight. The base was used to make a 10% emulsion in aqueous
solution of 5% dextrose and 0.3% gelatin, the pH of which was
adjusted to approximately 8.4 before the base was added. The
emulsion was given in a dose of 0.5 ml/100 g equivalent to 50 mg/
100 g. The average particle diameter of the gelatinized "RE test
lipid" emulsion upon microscopic examination was 1-3u.

The rate of clearance of the "RE test lipid" emulsion and
^{51}Cr-labeled endotoxin, as well as their tissue distribution,
was determined by previously described techniques (Saba and
Di Luzio, 1968). After the colloids were injected intravenously,
0.1 ml aliquots of blood were collected from the tail vein at
frequent intervals and hemolyzed in 1 ml of 0.1% $NaCO_3$ solution.
At least five blood samples were collected during the measurement
of phagocytic activity and the duration of the collecting period
and times of collection were modified to insure accurate assessment of vascular clearance of the test colloid in view of the
vastly different clearance rates observed in rats with altered RE
function. The blood activity, as per cent of the injected dose,
was plotted semi-logarithmically against time in minutes, and the
intravascular half-time determined.

Tissue distribution of the gelatinized "RE test lipid" emulsion was measured 5 and 20 minutes after its injection in glucan
and methyl palmitate-treated rats respectively. The fate of
^{51}Cr-labeled endotoxin was measured 30 minutes after administration in both groups. In the glucan-methyl palmitate combination
study rats were sacrificed 10 minutes after injection of colloid.
Radioactivity of liver, lung and spleen was determined in both RE
stimulated and depressed groups by previously described procedures
(Saba and Di Luzio, 1968). The tissue localization of the radioactive emulsion was expressed on a weight and total organ basis.

Student's "t" test and chi square test, utilized with
Yate's correction factor, were employed where appropriate to
determine significance which was set at the 95% confidence level.

RESULTS

In accordance with past observations (Ashworth, Di Luzio and
Riggi 1963; Di Luzio and Riggi, 1964; Morrow and Di Luzio, 1965;
Riggi and Di Luzio, 1961; Wooles and Di Luzio, 1963), glucan
administration induced profound RES hyperfunction as indicated by

a 1.4 minute half-time for the vascular removal of the gelatinized
"RE test lipid" emulsion as contrasted to a saline control group
half time of 9.0 minutes (Table 1). A significant 119% increase
in hepatic uptake of the emulsion was associated with the approximate six-fold enhancement in emulsion clearance. Pulmonary
localization of the lipid emulsion on an organ basis was normal;
however, uptake by spleen was significantly reduced. Uptake of the
test colloid by spleen and lung on a weight basis, was significantly
reduced due in part to glucan-induced hypertrophy of these organs
which was also observed.

Glucan treatment, in addition to inducing RES hyperplasia,
hypertrophy, and hyperfunction, also induced hyper-reactivity of
rats to lethal effects of S. enteritidis and E. coli endotoxins
(Table 2). The striking enhancement in host sensitivity to
endotoxin after glucan treatment was indicated by 100% mortality
in this group as compared to the low mortality manifested in both
control groups when S. enteritidis endotoxin was administered in
the dose of 0.5 mg/100 g. In addition, the lower endotoxin doses
employed in the study, i.e., 0.063, 0.031 and 0.01 mg/100 g,
resulted in significant mortality in glucan groups, in contrast to
the absence of mortality in control and normal rats at these
reduced endotoxin levels. Moreover, the LD_{50} of normal rats was
0.67 mg/100 g (Table 3), while an endotoxin dose of 0.017 mg/100 g
approximated the LD50 after glucan treatment. The glucan hyper-
reactivity was not specific for S. enteritidis endotoxin as
significantly enhanced susceptibility to E. coli endotoxin was
also observed (Table 2). At all doses and for both endotoxin
preparations the glucan-injected rats demonstrated a significantly
greater mortality than that observed in the control or normal groups.

The effects of methyl palmitate administration on endotoxin
lethality and RES function were studied concomitantly. In basic
agreement with past findings (Di Luzio and Blickens, 1966;
Di Luzio and Wooles, 1964; Saba and Di Luzio, 1968; Wooles and
Di Luzio, 1963), methyl palmitate treatment led to significant
impairment of RES function as measured in this study by the
clearance of gelatinized "RE test lipid" emulsion (Table 1). The
mean intravascular half-time for the removal of the test colloid
in 10 methyl palmitate-treated rats was 23 minutes which was
significantly prolonged relative to the 10 minute control half-
time observed in Tween-treated rats. Commensurate with the
approximate two-fold impairment in vascular removal rates observed after methyl palmitate treatment, hepatic and splenic
uptake were significantly reduced on an organ and weight basis.
Pulmonary localization of the emulsion, however, was not significantly altered.

TABLE 1

VASCULAR CLEARANCE AND TISSUE DISTRIBUTION OF GELATINIZED
"RE TEST LIPID" EMULSION IN METHYL PALMITATE AND GLUCAN-TREATED RATS

Group	Number of Rats	t/2 (min)	TISSUE DISTRIBUTION					
			Liver		Lung		Spleen	
			%ID/g	%ID/TO	%ID/g	%ID/TO	%ID/g	%ID/TO
Tween	8	9.8 ±1.3	4.3 ±0.5	51.2 ±5.5	1.2 ±0.2	1.7 ±0.3	7.7 ±0.8	5.5 ±0.4
Methyl Palmitate	10	21.9* ±2.0	1.7 ±0.2	17.9* ±0.9	1.8 ±0.4	2.5 ±0.5	3.7* ±0.6	3.2* ±0.6
Saline	8	9.0 ±0.8	3.0 ±0.2	35.9 ±2.8	1.1 ±0.1	1.5 ±0.2	4.2 ±0.2	3.3 ±0.2
Glucan	8	1.4* ±0.1	5.9* ±0.3	78.6* ±1.8	0.3* ±0.1	1.2 ±0.1	0.7* ±0.1	2.1* ±0.1

All rats were injected with 50 mg "RE test lipid" emulsion per 100 g. Five minutes after the injection, saline and glucan rats were killed. The methyl palmitate and Tween-treated rats were killed 20 minutes after the injection. Tissue distribution of the emulsion is expressed as per cent of the injected dose (%ID) per gram wet weight (g) or total organ (TO). The data are expressed as mean ± standard error.

*The significance of the difference between the mean values of the experimental and respective control group has a P value less than 0.01.

TABLE 2

EFFECT OF GLUCAN ADMINISTRATION
ON ENDOTOXIN MORTALITY

Group and Treatment	Endotoxin Dose, mg/100 g	Number of Rats	Per Cent Mortality
S. enteritidis			
Normal	0.5	8	25
	0.25	8	0
	0.125	6	17
	0.063	10	0
	0.031	5	0
	0.010	5	0
Control (Saline)	0.5	13	15
	0.25	10	10
	0.125	10	0
	0.063	5	0
	0.031	5	0
	0.010	5	0
Glucan*	0.5	10	100
	0.25	10	100
	0.125	10	100
	0.063	16	81
	0.031	10	90
	0.010	9	33
E. coli			
Normal	0.25	6	0
Control (Saline)	0.25	10	0
Glucan	0.25	10	100

Glucan was injected intravenously for five days at a dose of 1 mg/100 g. The endotoxin was suspended in saline and administered via the dorsal vein of the penis 72 hr. after the final glucan injection. *At all doses of both endotoxins, the glucan rats possessed a significantly (P value less than 0.025) higher mortality than either the saline or normal rats receiving the same dose. (To be published in American Journal of Physiology, vol. 217, 1969, in the article "Relationship of Reticuloendothelial Functional Activity to Endotoxin Lethality").

TABLE 3

MODIFICATION OF LETHALITY TO INTRAVENOUSLY ADMINISTERED
S. ENTERITIDIS ENDOTOXIN IN METHYL PALMITATE-INDUCED
RE-DEPRESSED RATS

Group	Endotoxin Dose, mg/100 g	Number of Rats	Per Cent Mortality
Normal	0.5	8	38
Control (Tween)	0.5	12	0
Methyl Palmitate	0.5	12	0
Normal	0.75	10	60*
Control (Tween)	0.75	11	0
Methyl Palmitate	0.75	13	0
Normal	1.00	10	70*
Control (Tween)	1.00	10	30
Methyl Palmitate	1.00	12	0
Normal	1.50	11	100*
Control (Tween)	1.50	11	91*
Methyl Palmitate	1.50	11	9
Normal	2.00	10	100*
Control (Tween)	2.00	30	74*
Methyl Palmitate	2.00	21	14
Normal	3.00	9	100*
Control (Tween)	3.00	10	80*
Methyl Palmitate	3.00	10	0

S. enteritidis endotoxin was suspended in pyrogen-free saline
and administered via the dorsal vein of the penis. Methyl palmitate
was suspended in Tween 20 and dextrose in water solution and injected 48 and 24 hr. prior to endotoxin. *The per cent mortality
in these groups is significantly (P value less than 0.025) greater
than the death rate in the methyl palmitate group which received
the same dose of endotoxin. (To be published in American Journal
of Physiology, vol. 217, 1969, in the article "Relationship of
Reticuloendothelial Functional Activity to Endotoxin Lethality").

In direct contrast to the deleterious consequences of glucan-induced RE stimulation on endotoxin lethality, methyl palmitate-induced RE depression significantly enhanced survival after S. enteritidis endotoxin administration at endotoxin dose levels ranging from 0.75 to 3.0 mg/100 g (Table 3). The protective effect of methyl palmitate treatment was demonstrated by the observation that 0.5 mg/100 g of endotoxin caused 39% mortality in normal rats, but a six-fold increase of this endotoxin dose resulted in no deaths in the methyl palmitate group. Tween, the suspending agent of methyl palmitate, did exert a significant protective. effect relative to normal rats at the 0.75 mg/100 g dose. The protective influence was not observed at endotoxin doses of 1.50 mg/100 g and above.

In accord with the loss of the protective effect of Tween with the higher doses of S. enteritidis endotoxin, no protection was conferred with Tween treatment with S. typhi-murium and E. coli endotoxins (Table 4). The mortality of normal rats which received E. coli and S. typhi-murium endotoxins (1 mg/100 g) was 70 and 100 per cent respectively. In marked contrast, 0 and 10 per cent mortality were observed in the methyl palmitate group treated with E. coli and S. typhi-murium endotoxins, indicating the methyl palmitate protection effect is not specific for one endotoxin species.

The influence of glucan and methyl palmitate treatment on clearance of intravenously administered ^{51}Cr-labeled endotoxin was undertaken in an effort to correlate mortality alterations with clearance patterns after RES functional modification. The clearance of the endotoxin was demonstrated to be biphasic, possessing both an initial, fast component and a secondary, slow component (Fig. 1). RE hyperactivity induced by glucan treatment was associated with a significant enhancement of both the initial and secondary clearance rates (Table 5). The enhanced vascular disappearance of the endotoxin after glucan treatment was cor-related with a 53% and 85% increment in hepatic phagocytosis of the endotoxin expressed on a gram and organ basis respectively. In the glucan group, pulmonary radioactivity, 30 minutes post endotoxin injection, was reduced but not significantly. Splenic uptake was significantly diminished by 55% on a weight basis, reflecting a glucan-induced splenomegaly and significantly increased by 30% on a total organ basis. The glucan-induced hypertrophy of the lung and spleen which were increased 22% and 193% respectively, account for the observed reduction of endotoxin uptake expressed on a weight basis.

In contrast to the striking modification in endotoxin clear-ance and fate induced by glucan treatment, methyl palmitate altered neither the initial nor the secondary phase of endotoxin

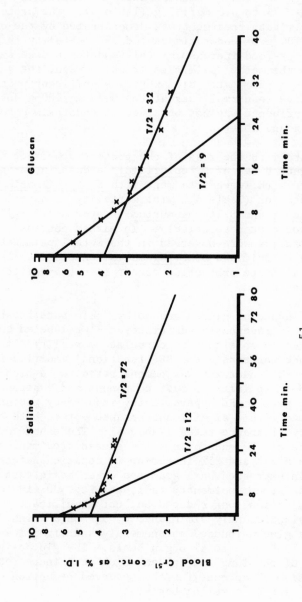

Fig. 1. Typical semilogarithmic plot of Cr^{51}-labeled S. enteritidis endotoxin radioactivity in blood of a representative rat previously treated with either saline or the RES stimulant, glucan. The decrease in blood endotoxin concentration as a function of time, indicates the existence of a bimodal clearance rate in both control and RE-hyperfunctional rats.

TABLE 4

INHIBITION OF S. TYPHI-MURIUM AND E. COLI ENDOTOXIN-INDUCED
MORTALITY IN METHYL PALMITATE-TREATED RATS

Group	Endotoxin	Per Cent Mortality
Normal	E. coli	70*
Normal	S. typhi-murium	100*
Control (Tween)	E. coli	55*
Control (Tween)	S. typhi-murium	70*
Methyl Palmitate	E. coli	0
Methyl Palmitate	S. typhi-murium	10

The endotoxins were administered intravenously via the dorsal vein of the penis in a dose of 1 mg/100 g. *The per cent mortality in these groups is significantly (P value less than 0.05) greater than that of the methyl palmitate group which received the same dose of endotoxin. Each group contained 9-10 rats. (To be published in American Journal of Physiology, vol. 217, 1969, in the article "Relationship of Reticuloendothelial Functional Activity to Endotoxin Lethality").

TABLE 5

VASCULAR CLEARANCE AND TISSUE DISTRIBUTION OF ^{51}Cr-LABELED
S. ENTERITIDIS ENDOTOXIN IN SALINE AND GLUCAN-TREATED RATS

Treatment	Intravascular t/2 (min)		TISSUE ACTIVITY					
			Liver		Lung		Spleen	
	Fast	Slow	%ID/g	%ID/T.O.	%ID/g	%ID/T.O.	%ID/g	%ID/T.O.
Saline	15.3 ±2.6	55.3 ±4.8	3.0 ±0.21	22.8 ±1.37	2.0 ±0.14	3.1 ±0.25	7.0 ±0.49	4.1 ±0.33
Glucan	6.2 ±1.5	35.1 ±3.4	4.6 ±0.36	44.1 ±2.61	1.6 ±0.14	3.1 ±0.30	3.2 ±0.28	5.3 ±0.40

Glucan and saline were injected for two days at the dose of 1 mg/100 g. S. enteritidis endotoxin was administered intravenously in a dose of 4.0 mg/100 g and its tissue distribution was measured 30 minutes after injection. The tissue distribution data are expressed as per cent injected dose (%ID) per gram wet weight (g) and total organ (T.O.). Mean values of seven or eight rats per group are expressed as mean ± standard error. (To be published in the Proceedings of the Society for Experimental Biology and Medicine in the article, "Influence of Altered Reticuloendothelial Function on Vascular Clearance and Tissue Distribution of S. enteritidis endotoxin.")

removal from the vascular compartment (Table 6). Relative to
Tween-treated controls, the methyl palmitate group demonstrated
unaltered hepatic and pulmonary radioactivity 30 minutes after
endotoxin injection. In contrast, splenic localization of endotoxin was diminished significantly relative to its control on
both an organ and weight basis as denoted by an approximate 85%
reduction in splenic radioactivity.

A combination regimen of glucan administration followed by
methyl palmitate treatment was employed to dissociate glucan-
induced RE hyperfunction from RE hypertrophy and hyperplasia;
this experimental model would distinguish RE hyperfunction from
RE hypertrophy relative to their contributions to the glucan-
induced enhancement in endotoxin lethality. In this study, ran-
domly chosen control and experimental rats were utilized either
for the assessment of S. enteritidis endotoxin mortality or for
the evaluation of RE hypertrophy and RE function.

Glucan treatment (Group D), resulted in RES hypertrophy
(Table 7) and hyperfunction (Table 8) as compared to normal rats
(Group A). The administration of Tween (Group E), the suspending
medium for methyl palmitate, subsequent to glucan treatment had
no influence on RES hypertrophy (Table 7), hyperactivity (Table 8),
or body weights demonstrated (Table 7) in the glucan group.

In striking contrast, the administration of methyl palmitate
to glucan-injected rats (Group F) resulted in a significant loss
in body weight, as well as a decrease in lung and spleen (D,E)
(Table 7). As compared to the various control groups (A,B,C)
significant RE hypertrophy of the glucan-methyl palmitate group
(Group F) was maintained, as denoted by an approximate 20%
increase in liver weight and nearly two and three-fold increase in
lung and spleen weight, respectively.

In agreement with previous data, glucan treatment (Groups D,
E) (Table 8) resulted in enhanced RES function as denoted by the
increased vascular clearance and elevated hepatic uptake of the
gelatinized "RE test lipid" emulsion relative to values obtained
in normal rats (Group A). Methyl palmitate-treated rats (Group C)
showed a significant depression in vascular clearance and hepatic
as well as splenic uptake, relative to either the Tween control
group (B) or the normal group (A).

The administration of methyl palmitate to glucan-treated rats
(Group F) was associated with normal (Group A and B) vascular
clearance rate of gelatinized "RE test lipid" emulsion. The
elimination of the classical glucan-induced hyperfunctional state
was related to reduction in hepatic phagocytosis (Table 8).

TABLE 6

VASCULAR CLEARANCE AND TISSUE DISTRIBUTION OF ^{51}Cr-LABELED S. ENTERITIDIS
ENDOTOXIN IN TWEEN AND METHYL PALMITATE-TREATED RATS

Treatment	Intravascular t/2 (min)		TISSUE ACTIVITY					
			Liver		Lung		Spleen	
	Fast	Slow	%ID/g	%ID/T.O.	%ID/g	%ID/T.O.	%ID/g	%ID/T.O.
Tween	18.3 ±0.7	85.2 ±7.5	3.9 ±0.57	28.7 ±4.42	2.1 ±0.14	3.7 ±0.34	5.6 ±0.73	3.5 ±0.25
Methyl Palmitate	21.3 ±2.0	67.0 ±3.3	2.7 ±0.15	24.4 ±1.70	2.4 ±0.23	4.1 ±0.30	0.8 ±0.22	0.6 ±0.13

S. enteritidis endotoxin was administered intravenously in a dose of 4.0 mg/100 g, and its tissue distribution measured 30 minutes after injection. Six rats were analyzed in the Tween treated group, whereas eight rats were utilized in the methyl palmitate-treated group which received two injections (100 mg/100 g) 48 and 24 hrs. prior to endotoxin. Data are reported as mean ± standard error. Tissue activity is expressed as per cent of the injected (%ID) per gram (g) and total organ (T.O.). (To be published in the Proceedings of the Society of Experimental Medicine and Biology in the article "Influence of Altered Reticuloendothelial Function on Vascular Clearance and Tissue Distribution of S. enteritidis endotoxin").

TABLE 7

BODY AND TISSUE WEIGHTS AFTER COMBINED GLUCAN AND METHYL PALMITATE TREATMENT

Group	Initial Treatment	Final Treatment	Initial Body Weight, g	Final Body Weight, g	Liver, g	Lung, g	Spleen, g
A	Uninjected	Uninjected	253 ± 7	304 ± 7	11.9 ±0.44	1.3 ±0.03	0.7 ±0.02
B	Uninjected	Tween	285 ±14	320 ± 8	12.4 ±0.44	1.4 ±0.03	0.8 ±0.02
C	Uninjected	Methyl Palmitate	279 ±12	300 ± 7	13.1 ±0.46	1.6 ±0.04	0.7 ±0.04
D	Glucan	Uninjected	287 ± 8	295 ±12	14.2 ±0.44	3.1 ±0.18	2.9 ±0.18
E	Glucan	Tween	280 ±10	287 ± 8	14.1 ±0.46	3.3 ±0.33	2.8 ±0.13
F	Glucan	Methyl Palmitate	281 ±14	271 ± 6	14.4 ±0.69	2.5 ±0.23	2.0 ±0.14

All values are expressed as mean ± standard error and are derived from 5-8 rats/group. The initial treatment consisted of five daily injections of glucan 1 mg/100 g. The final treatment consisted of two daily intravenous injections of methyl palmitate 100 mg/100 g or isovolumetric Tween on days 6 and 7 of the experiment. (To be published in American Journal of Physiology, vol. 217, 1969 in the article, "Relationship of Reticuloendothelial Functional Activity to Endotoxin Lethality.")

TABLE 8

VASCULAR CLEARANCE AND TISSUE DISTRIBUTION OF GELATINIZED "RE TEST LIPID" EMULSION IN RATS TREATED WITH GLUCAN AND METHYL PALMITATE

Group	Initial Treatment	Final Treatment	T 1/2 (min)	Liver %ID/g	Liver %ID/TO	Lung %ID/g	Lung %ID/TO	Spleen %ID/g	Spleen %ID/TO
A(7)+	Uninjected	Uninjected	17.5 ±2.3	3.1 ±0.3	36.6 ±2.7	0.7 ±0.02	0.9 ±0.1	6.9 ±0.5	4.5 ±0.4
B(5)	Uninjected	Tween	13.0 ±2.5	3.6 ±0.5	45.4 ±1.8	0.6 ±0.03	0.9 ±0.03	5.7 ±0.2	4.4 ±0.2
C(4)	Uninjected	Methyl Palmitate	23.6 ±3.0	0.9 ±0.2	12.4 ±2.3	1.3 ±0.2	2.1 ±0.3	0.9 ±0.1	0.6 ±0.1
D(6)	Glucan	Uninjected	1.2 ±0.1	5.7 ±0.2	80.3 ±2.3	0.3 ±1.0	0.8 ±0.2	0.6 ±0.1	1.8 ±0.2
E(8)	Glucan	Tween	1.0 ±0.1	5.6 ±0.6	78.8 ±7.0	0.3 ±0.1	1.0 ±0.4	0.6 ±0.1	1.8 ±0.3
F(6)	Glucan	Methyl Palmitate	12.9 ±4.2	3.0 ±0.6	44.6 ±9.1	1.0 ±0.2	2.4 ±0.5	1.0 ±0.2	2.2 ±0.5

+Number in parentheses represents number of rats per group. Data are expressed as mean ± standard error. All rats were injected with 50 mg of "RE test lipid" emulsion per 100 g. Ten minutes after injection the rats were killed. Tissue distribution of the emulsion is expressed as per cent of the injected dose (%ID) per gram wet weight (g) or total organ (TO). (To be published in American Journal of Physiology, 217, 1969, in the article "Relationship of Reticuloendothelial Functional Activity to Endotoxin Lethality.")

In agreement with previous data (Table 2), glucan administration (Group D) induced the characteristic enhancement in endotoxin lethality (Table 9). To test glucan-induced endotoxin
hyper-reactivity, a low endotoxin dose (0.063 mg/100 g) was
employed which did not induce mortality in the normal group (Group
A). For unknown reasons, one methyl palmitate-treated rat died
after the small dose of endotoxin.

The administration of methyl palmitate, which restored the
glucan-induced hyperphagocytic state to normal, did not significantly modify the glucan-induced hypersensitivity to S. enteritidis endotoxin, clearly disassociating enhanced phagocytic
function, as reflected by vascular clearance of the gelatinized
"RE test lipid" emulsion from endotoxin lethality.

To determine whether the glucan or methyl palmitate plasma
possess an endotoxin sensitizing or protective factor, passive
plasma transfer studies were also undertaken. The administration
of saline, or plasma obtained from either saline or Tween-injected
rats (Table 10), did not modify endotoxin response, when compared
to that manifested by normal rats (Table 3). Likewise, the administration of plasma from glucan-injected rats or methyl palmitate-
injected rats did not alter the mortality to endotoxin, suggesting
the absence of a plasma factor as the mediator of endotoxin sensitivity alterations.

To evaluate the role of lysosomal enzyme activity in altered
sensitivity to endotoxin, plasma lysosomal enzyme activities were
determined in glucan or methyl palmitate treated rats 3 hours
following endotoxin administration. Five daily injections of
glucan exerted no significant influence on plasma acid phosphatase
or β-glucuronidase activity as compared to normal or saline-treated
rats (Table 11). S. enteritidis endotoxin in a dose of 0.01 mg/
100 g resulted in 33% mortality in glucan-treated rats but was not
lethal in normal and saline-treated controls (Table 1). Plasma
β-glucuronidase and acid phosphatase activity were significantly
elevated 219% and 76%, respectively, relative to saline-treated
controls 3 hours after the 0.01 mg/100 g dose of endotoxin was
given (Table 11). The normal and saline treated groups maintained
normal plasma lysosomal enzyme activity after receiving this low
dose of endotoxin. Thus, elevated plasma lysosomal enzyme activity
was manifested in the glucan-treated rats which were extremely
susceptible to the injurious effect of endotoxin.

The administration of methyl palmitate did not alter plasma
lysosomal activity (Table 12). Three hours after the administration of endotoxin in the dose of 1.0 mg/100 g, plasma acid phosphatase activity was not significantly elevated in either control
or experimental groups. This endotoxin dose induced a 70%

TABLE 9

EFFECT OF METHYL PALMITATE ADMINISTRATION ON GLUCAN-INDUCED
HYPERSENSITIVITY TO S. ENTERITIDIS ENDOTOXIN

Group	First Treatment	Second Treatment	Number of Rats	Per Cent Mortality
A	Uninjected	Uninjected	9	0
B	Uninjected	Tween	7	0
C	Uninjected	Methyl Palmitate	7	14
D	Glucan	Uninjected	9	100*
E	Glucan	Tween	10	90
F	Glucan	Methyl Palmitate	10	90*

S. enteritidis endotoxin in a dose of 0.063 mg/100 g was injected into the dorsal vein of the penis on day 8 of the experimental procedure. The first treatment consisted of 5 daily intravenous injections of glucan in a dose of 1 mg/100 g. The second treatment consisted of 2 daily intravenous injections on days 6 and 7 of the experiment of methyl palmitate emulsion in a dose of 100mg/100g or isovolumetric Tween. *The mortality in these groups is increased significantly (P value less than 0.01) as compared to all groups not pretreated with glucan. (To be published in American Journal of Physiology, 217, 1969, in the article "Relationship of Reticuloendothelial Functional Activity to Endotoxin Lethality").

TABLE 10

EFFECT OF PLASMA OBTAINED FROM GLUCAN OR METHYL PALMITATE-
TREATED RATS ON S. ENTERITIDIS ENDOTOXIN LETHALITY
IN NORMAL RATS

Donor Treatment (Plasma Source)	Endotoxin Lethality (%)
Toxicity Control	50
Saline	58
Glucan	50
Tween	92
Methyl Palmitate	67

S. enteritidis endotoxin suspended in pyrogen-free saline was
administered intravenously in a dose of 0.75 mg/100 g. Donor rats
were treated with glucan (1 mg/100 g) or saline for 5 days or
methyl palmitate (100 mg/100 g) or Tween for 2 days. Rats were
exsanguinated by cardiac puncture using Mepesulfate as anticoagulant
72 hrs. after final glucan or 24 hrs. after final methyl palmitate
injection. Plasma was injected (1 ml/100 g) into the dorsal vein
of the penis 1 hr. prior to endotoxin injection. A toxicity control group was treated with saline (1 mg/100 g) 1 hr. prior to
endotoxin injection. Each type of plasma or saline was given to
12 recipient rats in which endotoxin mortality was observed.
(To be published in American Journal of Physiology, vol. 217,
1969 in the article, "Relationship of Reticuloendothelial
Functional Activity to Endotoxin Lethality").

TABLE 11

EFFECT OF GLUCAN ON PLASMA β-GLUCURONIDASE AND ACID PHOSPHATASE ACTIVITY
THREE HOURS AFTER <u>S</u>. ENTERITIDIS ENDOTOXIN

Group	Treatment	β-glucuronidase Activity	Acid Phosphatase Activity
Uninjected	Saline	0.33 ± 0.07 (9)*	0.84 ± 0.04 (9)*
Saline	Saline	0.28 ± 0.06 (8)	0.89 ± 0.09 (9)
Glucan	Saline	0.36 ± 0.05 (8)	1.09 ± 0.09 (8)
Uninjected	Endotoxin	0.36 ± 0.05 (8)	0.93 ± 0.07 (8)
Saline	Endotoxin	0.38 ± 0.08 (9)	0.84 ± 0.04 (9)
Glucan	Endotoxin	1.14 ± 0.13 (9)	1.92 ± 0.32 (9)

Rats received five daily glucan injections (1 mg/100 g). After 72 hours respite
<u>S</u>. enteritidis endotoxin, which was suspended in saline, was administered in a dose of 0.01 mg/
100 g. One unit of β-glucuronidase activity equals 1 mg of phenolphthalein released per 100 ml
plasma per hour at 37°C per ml incubation mediu. One unit of acid phosphatase activity equals
1 mg of inorganic phosphorus released per 100 ml plasma per hour at 37°C per ml incubation
medium. *Number of rats per group.

TABLE 12

EFFECT OF METHYL PALMITATE ON PLASMA β-GLUCURONIDASE AND ACID PHOSPHATASE
ACTIVITY THREE HOURS AFTER S. ENTERITIDIS ENDOTOXIN

Group	Treatment	β-Glucuronidase Activity	Acid Phosphatase Activity
Uninjected	Saline	0.37 ± 0.08 (10)*	1.07 ± 0.13 (8)*
Tween	Saline	0.42 ± 0.09 (10)	0.90 ± 0.14 (8)
Methyl Palmitate	Saline	0.39 ± 0.04 (9)	1.02 ± 0.13 (8)
Uninjected	Endotoxin	0.75 ± 0.15 (9)	1.65 ± 0.66 (7)
Tween	Endotoxin	0.66 ± 0.19 (9)	1.01 ± 0.11 (6)
Methyl Palmitate	Endotoxin	1.40 ± 0.19 (9)	1.16 ± 0.18 (8)

Methyl palmitate was administered intravenously in a dose of 100 mg/100 g for 2 days.
Twenty-four hours after the second methyl palmitate injection, S. enteritidis endotoxin was
administered intravenously in a dose of 1 mg/100 g. One unit of β-glucuronidase activity equals
1 mg of phenolphthalein released per 100 ml plasma per hour at 37°C per ml incubation medium.
One unit of acid phosphatase activity equals 1 mg of inorganic phosphorus released per 100 ml
plasma per hour at 37°C per ml incubation media. *Number of rats per group.

mortality in normal rats and a 30% mortality in Tween-injected
controls, but methyl palmitate-treated rats were characterized by
the absence of mortality (Table 2). Plasma β-glucuronidase activity, however, was significantly elevated 259% in the methyl palmitate group receiving endotoxin. The control groups treated with
endotoxin did not demonstrate any alterations in plasma β-glucuroni-
dase activity (Table 12), thus, the methyl palmitate-induced
resistance to endotoxin occurred in the presence of either normal
or elevated plasma lysosomal enzyme activity.

Discussion

In confirmation of past findings, the administration of
glucan and methyl palmitate exerted their chemical RES altering
effects. Glucan administration resulted in hepatic, splenic,
and pulmonary hypertrophy, in addition to RES hyperfunction, as
measured by gelatinized "RE test lipid" emulsion clearances
(Ashworth, et al., 1963; Di Luzio and Riggi, 1964; Riggi and
Di Luzio, 1961; Wooles and Di Luzio, 1963). Methyl palmitate
administered intravenously resulted in significantly impaired RES
function as assayed by the vascular clearance of "RE test lipid"
emulsion or other colloidal agents (Di Luzio and Blickens, 1966;
Di Luzio and Wooles, 1964; Saba and Di Luzio, 1968; Wooles and
Di Luzio, 1963).

The present studies also corroborate previous observations
that the RES, particularly the liver, exerts a predominant
influence on the vascular clearance of endotoxin (Braude, Carey
and Zalesky, 1955; Rowley, Howard, and Jenkin, 1956; Golub,
Groschel and Nowotny, 1968; Barnes, Lupfer, and Henry, 1952;
Noyes, McInturf, and Blahuta, 1959). In agreement with the
observations of Stuart and Cooper (1962), however, that little
correlation between endotoxin susceptibility and phagocytic
capacity of the RES exists, the present studies indicate that
alterations in endotoxin susceptibility are not readily explained
on the rate of vascular clearance of endotoxin. Methyl palmitate
which is a selective RES depressant agent (Di Luzio and Blickens,
1966) does not alter the vascular clearance of endotoxin from
the blood while inducing a profound resistance to endotoxin
lethality. The accelerated clearance of endotoxin induced by
glucan treatment appears not to be related to the profound enhancement of endotoxin lethality which characterized the glucan-
treated group, since glucan-methyl palmitate treated rats demonstrated normal phagocytic clearance of gelatinized "RE test lipid"
emulsion in the presence of an enhanced susceptibility to endotoxin.

Beeson (1947a), observed that impairment of RES activity by
the administration of so called "RE blocking" agents enhanced
the pathologic effects of endotoxin and speculated that the RES

was a determinant in host response to endotoxin. Furthermore, this investigator hypothesized that the impaired clearance of endotoxins induced by RE blocking agents promoted the deleterious effects of endotoxin (Beeson, 1947b).

Recent work by Fisher (1967) challenge the speculations of Beeson regarding prolonged endotoxemia subsequent to RES blockade. Fisher reported that $\underline{E}$. $\underline{coli}$ endotoxin labeled with ^{131}I was phagocytized more rapidly in RES blockaded rabbits and mice than in normal animals. Fisher hypothesized that the sensitivity of RES blockaded animals to endotoxin was a function of delayed hepatic and splenic disposal, rather than reduced vascular clearance of endotoxin. Noyes, McInturf and Blahuta (1959) demonstrated that mice which were treated with the RE blocking agent, trypan blue, which enhances endotoxin susceptibility, maintained an appreciable elevation of blood endotoxin levels after intravenous or intramuscular endotoxin administration but demonstrated no alteration in the hepatic localization of ^{51}Cr-labeled endotoxin. The lethality of endotoxin in mice could not be related to alterations in tissue distribution of the endotoxin. Additional data relative to effect of RES blockade and endotoxin pathology was presented by Greisman, Carozza, and Hills (1963) who investigated the effect of thorium dioxide-induced RES blockade on both RES activity as measured by phagocytosis of colloidal carbon as well as the pyrogenic effects of endotoxin in both normal and endotoxin tolerant rabbits. After RES block-ade, both normal and endotoxin tolerant hosts manifested the same degree of RES depression; however, the endotoxin tolerant group demonstrated a significantly reduced fever index indicating an estrangment of the febrile response from RE functional status.

In contrast to the varied reports of the influence of RES depression on endotoxin clearance and pathology, RES stimulation induced by a variety of agents, i.e., zymosan (Benacerraf, $\underline{et}$ $\underline{al}$., 1959), BCG (Suter, $\underline{et}$ $\underline{al}$., 1958), triolein (Stuart and Cooper, 1962), or glucan (Lemperle, 1966) clearly enhanced endotoxin lethality in mice. The present studies dramatically demonstrate the hyper-reactivity of glucan injected rats to intravenously administered endotoxins. Although glucan induces enhanced vascular clearance of endotoxin, endotoxin hyper-reactivity does not appear to be caused by a hyperphagocytic RES, since glucan injected rats treated with methyl palmitate demonstrated normal RES function as measured by clearance of "RE test lipid" emulsion. The locus of glucan-induced sensitivity to endotoxin is, therefore, not phagocytosis $\underline{per}$ $\underline{se}$ but most probably some other alteration, either cytological, enzymatic, or functional which is possibly related to the massive RE cell population which characterize the glucan-treated rats (Ashworth $\underline{et}$ $\underline{al}$., 1963; Filkins, Lubitz, and Smith, 1964; Riggi and Di Luzio, 1961; Wooles and Di Luzio, 1963).

Lysosomal membrane permeability alterations have been speculated as possible etiologic factors in glucan-induced endotoxin
hyper-reactivity (Lemperle, 1966). Lysosomes have been hypothesized as an intracellular target for endotoxin (Weissmann and
Thomas, 1964) since endotoxins induce lysosomal instability and
cause a release of lysosomal enzymes into the cell sap and plasma
(Janoff, Weissmann, Zweifach, and Thomas, 1962; Weissmann and
Thomas, 1962). In addition, Saito and Suter demonstrated that
treatment of mice with the RES stimulant BCG, not only elevated
lysosomal hydrolase activity in liver, peritoneal macrophages, and
plasma (Saito and Suter, 1965a) but also resulted in endotoxin
hyper-reactivity which was fairly well correlated with endotoxin
induced elevations in plasma β-glucuronidase activity (Saito and
Suter (1965b). Our results basically corroborate the findings of
Saito and Suter (1965b), in that glucan-treatment resulted in hyper-
reactivity to endotoxin which was associated with significant
elevations of plasma lysosomal enzyme activity subsequent to
endotoxin treatment.

A speculated mechanism of lysosomal involvement in endotoxin
injury centers on the formation of phagosomes or their pathologic
counterpart, autophagic vacuoles (Weissmann and Thomas, 1964).
Host treatment with RES stimulants or RES blockading agents have
been speculated to induce formation of numerous phagosomes filled
with acid hydrolases which upon interacting with endotoxin become
labilized into autophagic vacuoles (Weissmann and Thomas, 1964)
as evidenced by enhanced lysosomal activity released from liver
lysosomes (Janoff and Zwiefach, 1963) or enhanced plasma lysosomal
enzyme activity (Saito and Suter, 1965b). Endotoxin tolerance or
treatment with cortisone, both of which enhance survival to
endotoxemia (Stuart and Cooper, 1962; Spink and Anderson, 1954)
result in a population of lysosomes which are resistant to the
effects of endotoxins (Weissmann and Thomas, 1964) resulting in a
retardation in the release of acid hydrolase activity (Janoff and
Thomas, 1963).

Results of the methyl palmitate portion of this study tend to
de-emphasize the role of lysosomes as causative agents in endotoxin
lethality, and suggest that lysosomal breakdown may be a result of
endotoxin injury rather than its cause. An LD_{100} dose of S. enteritidis endotoxin in normal rats did not result in significant elevation of plasma β-glucuronidase or acid phosphatase activity,
whereas, this same dose, which is non-lethal in methyl palmitate-
treated rats caused either the same or greater elevation of plasma
acid hydrolase activity. The delineation of the temporal sequence
of plasma lysosomal enzyme activity after endotoxin is clearly
necessary to precisely understand the contribution of lysosomal
enzymes to the altered states of endotoxin susceptibility noted
in glucan and methyl palmitate treated rats.

Since the RES is responsible not only for the vascular clearance of endotoxin but also its detoxification (Palmerio and Fine, 1969; Rutenburg, Skarnes, Palmerio, and Fine, 1967), RES functional modification resulting in alterations in endotoxin reactivity may center on the metabolism of the phagocytized endotoxin particle. Cremer and Watson (1957) using a labeled antibody technique to localize endotoxin, found that treatments affecting endotoxin lethality affect not only clearance of endotoxin from the vascular compartment but also its subsequent elimination from liver, lung and spleen. In addition, Fisher (1967) found that blockade of the RES altered both vascular clearance of ^{131}I-labeled E. coli endotoxin as well as its hepatic and pulmonary disposal. Since Rutenburg et al. (1967) have reported the ability of liver and spleen to rapidly detoxify bacterial endotoxins, it remains to be established whether RES altering agents such as glucan and methyl palmitate modify the detoxification capability of liver and spleen. It is possible that altered endotoxin catabolism within phagosomes of RE cells in rats treated with glucan or methyl palmitate may contribute to the observed changes in endotoxin sensitivity seen after treatment with these agents. These data suggest that RES involvement in host defense against endotoxin may reside in the endotoxin detoxification phase as proposed by Palmerio and Fine (1969).

An alteration created by glucan or methyl palmitate treatment which may affect endotoxin reactivity focuses on the immunologic status of the host. The clearance and distribution of foreign red blood cells (Morrow and Di Luzio,1965) as well as antibody response to sheep erythrocytes (Wooles and Di Luzio, 1963) varied profoundly in mice with altered RE function. The analogy between endotoxin shock and anaphylactoid shock (Gilbert and Braude, 1962; Weil and Spink, 1957) suggest that glucan hyperreactivity to endotoxin may represent a modified hypersensitivity reaction and the methyl palmitate refractoriness may reflect a diminished immunologic response to endotoxin.

The observation that prior administration of plasma from methyl palmitate or glucan-treated rats to normal rats which received endotoxin exerted no significant effect on mortality suggests that no stable, circulating plasma factor is involved in the altered sensitivity to endotoxin induced by methyl palmitate or glucan treatment.

The disassociation of RES hyperactivity and hypertrophy of organs containing RE cells induced by glucan-methyl palmitate treatment is an interesting phenomenon because RES hyperfunction is usually associated with an increase of the organs containing large populations of RE cells. With BCG (Halpern, 1959), endotoxin (Benacerraf and Sebestyen, 1957), zymosan (Benacerraf et al., 1959), glucan (Ashworth et al., 1963; Riggi and Di Luzio, 1961),

triolein treatments (Stuart and Cooper, 1962) and graft versus
host disease (Di Luzio, 1967; Di Luzio, 1968), RES hyperactivity is associated with hypertrophy of the liver, spleen and,
in some cases, lung. The loss of RE hyperfunction in glucan-
injected rats subsequently treated with methyl palmitate denote
an impaired ability of Kupffer cells to phagocytize.

The present studies indicate that purified chemical agents
which induce striking alterations in RES structure and function
exert profound influences on endotoxin lethality. Indeed, rats
treated with the RE stimulant, glucan, are exquisitely sensitive
to endotoxin; whereas, a three-fold increase of the LD_{70} dose of
endotoxin is non-lethal in methyl palmitate-induced RE depressed
rats.

The locus of influence of the glucan-induced hyper-reactivity
or methyl palmitate-induced resistance to endotoxin does not
appear to be the phagocytic event. Since the RES has a determinant influence not only on the vascular removal but also the
endotoxin detoxification mechanisms, an intracellular interaction
between endotoxin and macrophage seems to be the critical factor
governing the lethality of endotoxins. Although the precise
definition of altered host sensitivity to endotoxin is not
presently known when specific RE modifying agents are employed,
the mechanism may well involve endotoxin detoxification potential
of RE cells or an altered immunologic response to endotoxins.
The ability of glucan and methyl palmitate to profoundly modify
host response to endotoxemia suggest the utility of employing
these agents in the elucidation of the sequela of endotoxemia.

Summary

Glucan and methyl palmitate, agents which significantly alter
RES activity, as measured by the clearance of various colloids,
profoundly influence endotoxin shock in rats. Glucan-treated rats,
which manifest profound hyperphagocytosis and hypertrophy of
liver, lung, and spleen, were extremely sensitive to intravenously
administered S. enteritidis and E. coli endotoxins. In marked
contrast, methyl palmitate administration, which resulted in
impaired phagocytosis due to depression of Kupffer cell activity,
produced almost complete refractoriness to S. enteritidis, E. coli,
or S. typhi-murium endotoxins at lethal and also supralethal
doses.

In an effort to define the influence of RES activity on endotoxin lethality, vascular clearance and tissue distribution of
Cr^{51}-S. enteritidis endotoxin were determined in rats pretreated
with either glucan or methyl palmitate. The data indicate these

agents do not exert their modifying effect on endotoxin lethality by altering the vascular clearance or initial tissue localization of endotoxin. Moreover, the restoration of phagocytic activity to normal values in glucan-treated rats by means of methyl palmitate administration was associated with maintenance of the hyper-reactive state to endotoxin, denoting that glucan induced hyper-reactivity to endotoxin is not mediated by hyper-phagocytosis. Absence of a humoral factor in mediation of glucan-induced hyper-reactivity or methyl palmitate-induced endotoxin resistance was demonstrated by the finding that passive plasma transfer from experimental animals into normal recipients prior to endotoxin treatment had no significant effect on endotoxin lethality.

In an effort to evaluate the role of lysosomal enzymes in the modification of endotoxin lethality, plasma β-glucuronidase and acid phosphatase activity were measured in glucan and methyl palmitate-treated rats. Alterations in plasma β-glucuronidase and acid phosphatase activity observed in glucan or methyl palmitate-treated rats which received endotoxin did not correlate with observed mortality patterns. The mechanisms by which functional alterations of the RES profoundly influence host susceptibility to endotoxin shock appears to be associated neither with the vascular clearance of endotoxin, nor existence of plasma factors. These composite studies stress the prime importance of a macrophage-endotoxin interaction, as yet to be defined, as a major determinant in the sequela of endotoxemia.

References

Ashworth, C. T., Di Luzio, N. R., and Riggi, S. J. (1963): A morphologic study of the effect of reticuloendothelial stimulation upon hepatic removal of minute particles from the blood of rats. Experimental Molecular Pathology Supplement, 1, 83.

Barnes F. W., Jr., Lupfer, H., and Henry, S. S. (1952): The biochemical target of Flexner dysentery somatic antigen. Yale Journal of Biology and Medicine, 24, 384.

Beeson, P. B. (1947a): Tolerance to bacterial pyrogens. Journal of Experimental Medicine, 86, 39.

Beeson, P. B. (1947b): Effect of reticulo-endothelial blockade on immunity to the Shwartzman phenomenon. Proceedings of the Society for Experimental Biology and Medicine, 64, 146.

Benacerraf, B., and Sebestyen, M. (1957): Effect of bacterial endotoxins on the reticuloendothelial system. Federation Proceedings, 16, 860.

Benacerraf, B., Thorbecke, G. J. and Jacoby, D. (1959): Effect
of zymosan on endotoxin toxicity in mice. Proceedings of the
Society for Experimental Biology and Medicine, 100, 796.

Berthet, J. and De Duve, C. (1951): Tissue fractionation studies.
Biochemical Journal, 50, 174.

Braude, A. I., Carey, F. J., and Zalesky, M. (1955): Studies
with radioactive endotoxin. Journal of Clinical Investigation,
34, 858.

Braude, A. I., Carey, F. J., Sutherland, D. and Zalesky, M. (1955):
Studies with radioactive endotoxin. Journal of Clinical
Investigation, 34, 850.

Chedid, L., Skarnes, R. C., Parant, M. (1963): Characterization
of Cr^{51}-labeled endotoxin and its identification in plasma
and urine after parenteral administration. Journal of
Experimental Medicine, 117, 561.

Cremer, N., and Watson, D. W. (1957): Influence of stress on
distribution of endotoxin in RES determined by fluorescein
antibody technic. Proceedings of the Society for Experimental
Biology and Medicine, 95, 510.

Di Luzio, N. R. (1967): Evaluation by the graft-versus-host
reaction of the immune competence of lymphoid cells of mice
with altered reticuloendothelial function. Journal of the
Reticuloendothelial Society, 4, 459.

Di Luzio, N. R. (1968): Evaluation of reticuloendothelial activity
in the graft-versus-host reaction. Journal of the Reticuloendothelial Society, 5, 368.

Di Luzio, N. R. and Blickens, D. A. (1966): Influence of intravenously administered lipids on reticuloendothelial function.
Journal of the Reticuloendothelial Society, 3, 250.

Di Luzio, N. R. and Riggi, S. J. (1964): The development of a
lipid emulsion for the measurement of reticuloendothelial
function. Journal of the Reticuloendothelial Society, 1, 136.

Di Luzio, N. R. and Wooles, W. R (1964): Depression of phagocytic activity and immune response by methyl palmitate.
American Journal of Physiology, 206, 939.

Filkins, J. P., Lubitz, J. M. and Smith, J. J (1964): The
effect of zymosan and glucan on the reticuloendothelial system
and on resistance to traumatic shock. Angiology, 15, 465.

Fisher, S. (1967): Localization of radioiodinated endotoxin in organs of mice and rabbits; Effect of throtrast, trypan blue, endotoxin and carbon administered intravenously. Nature, 213, 511.

Fiske, C. H. and Subbarow, T. (1925): The colorimetric determination of phosphorous. Journal of Biological Chemistry, 66, 375.

Gilbert, V. E. and Braude, A. I. (1962): Reduction of serum complement in rabbits after injection of endotoxin. Journal of Experimental Medicine, 116, 477.

Golub, S., Groschel, D. and Nowotny, A. (1968): Factors which affect the reticuloendothelial system uptake of bacterial endotoxins. Journal of the Reticuloendothelial Society, 5, 324.

Greisman, S. E., Carozza, F. A., Jr., and Hills, J. D. (1963): Mechanisms of endotoxin tolerance. Journal of Experimental Medicine, 117, 663.

Halpern, B. N. (1959): The role and function of the reticuloendothelial system in immunological processes. Journal of Pharmacy and Pharmacology, 11, 321.

Janoff, A., Weissmann, G., Zwiefach, B. W., and Thomas, L. (1962): Pathogenesis of experimental shock. Journal of Experimental Medicine, 116, 451.

Janoff, A. and Zwiefach, B. W. (1963): Effect of endotoxin-tolerance, cortisone, and thorotrast on release of enzymes from subcellular particles of mouse liver. Proceedings of the Society for Experimental Biology and Medicine, 114, 695.

Lemperle, G. (1966): Effect of RES stimulation on endotoxin shock in mice. Proceedings of the Society for Experimental Biology and Medicine, 122, 1012.

Morrow, S. N. and Di Luzio, N. R. (1965): The fate of foreign red cells in mice with altered reticuloendothelial function. Proceedings of the Society for Experimental Biology and Medicine, 119, 647.

Noyes, H. E., McInturf, C. R., Blahuta, G. J. (1959): Studies on distribution of Escherichia coli endotoxin in mice. Proceedings of the Society for Experimental Biology and Medicine. 100, 65.

Palmerio, C. and Fine, J. (1969): The nature of resistance to shock. Archives of Surgery, 98, 679.

Plaice, C. H. (1961): A note on the determination of serum
   beta-glucuronidase activity. Journal of Clinical Pathology,
   14, 661.

Riggi, S. J. and Di Luzio, N. R. (1961): Identification of
   reticuloendothelial stimulating agent in zymosan. American
   Journal of Physiology, 200, 297.

Rowley, D., Howard, J. G., and Jenkin, C. R. (1956): The fate
   of 32P-labeled bacterial lipopolysaccharide in laboratory
   animals. Lancet, 1, 366.

Rutenburg, S., Skarnes, R., Palmerio, C., and Fine, J. (1967):
   Detoxification of endotoxin by perfusion of liver and spleen.
   Proceedings of the Society for Experimental Biology and
   Medicine, 125, 455.

Saba, T. M. and Di Luzio, N. R. (1968): Evaluation of humoral
   and cellular mechanisms of methyl palmitate induced reticuloendothelial depression. Life Sciences, 7, 337.

Saito, K. and Suter, E. (1965a): Lysosomal acid hydrolases in mice
   infected with BCG. Journal of Experimental Medicine, 121, 727.

Saito, K. and Suter, E. (1965b): Lysosomal acid hydrolases and
   hyper-reactivity to endotoxin in mice infected with BCG.
   Journal of Experimental Medicine, 121, 739.

Spink, W. W. and Anderson, D. (1954): Experimental studies on
   the significance of endotoxin in the pathogenesis of brucellosis.
   Journal of Clinical Investigation, 33, 540.

Stuart, A. E. and Cooper, G. N. (1962): Susceptibility of mice
   to bacterial endotoxin after modification of reticuloendothelial
   function by simple lipids. Journal of Pathology and Bacteriology, 83, 245.

Suter, E., Ullman, E G. and Hoffman, R. G. (1958): Sensitivity
   of mice to endotoxin after vaccination with Bacillus Calmette-
   Guerin. Proceedings of the Society for Experimental Biology
   and Medicine, 99, 167.

Weil, M. H., and Spink, W. W. (1957): A comparison of shock
   due to endotoxin with anaphylactic shock. Journal of
   Laboratory and Clinical Medicine, 50, 501.

Weissmann, G. and Thomas, L. (1964): Bacterial Endotoxins,
   p. 602, Rutgers University Press, New Brunswick, N. J.

Weissmann, G. and Thomas, L. (1962): Studies on lysosomes.
   I. The effect of endotoxin, endotoxin tolerance and cortisone
   on the release of acid hydrolases from a granular fraction of
   rabbit liver. Journal of Experimental Medicine, 116, 433.

Wharton, D. R. A. and Creech, H. J. (1949): Further studies of
   the immunological properties of polysaccharides from Sarratia
   Marcescens (Bacillus prodigiosus) II. Journal of Immunology,
   62, 135.

Wooles, W. R. and Di Luzio, N. R. (1963): Reticuloendothelial
   function and the immune response. Science, 142, 1078.

BEHAVIOUR OF HISTIDINE DECARBOXYLASE (HDC)

IN VARIOUS FORMS OF SHOCK*

A. Schauer, L. Gielow and G. Geissl

Department of Pathology

University of Munich, West-Germany

The liberation of deposit histamine from mast cells and the role of histamine in immunological (anaphylactic) shock reactions is well established. Concerning endotoxin shock and various other forms of shock, however, the significance of histamine is still subject to discussion, although the histamine liberating effect of endotoxins from mast cells has been proved by Hinshaw et al. (1960).

Since the endotoxin shock is an useful model of biochemical mechanism of shock and its morphological alterations we endeavoured to clarify behaviour and significance of histidine decarboxylase (HDC) activity in this type of shock (Schauer et al. 1966, 1967).

MATERIAL AND METHODS

Female Sprague Dawley rats of 200-250 g bodyweight and LAF$_1$ resp. NMRI mice of both sexes of 20-30 g bodyweight were used under the same conditions (air conditioning, altromin-feeding).

E. coli endotoxin (E. coli O 111 B4 lipopolysaccharide W Difco laboratories Detroit, U.S.A., resp. E. coli O 111 endotoxin, Dr. Metz, Max von Pettenkofer Inst., University of Munich), resp. S. anatum endotoxin or S. abortus equi endotoxin (Dr. Metz), were used. E. coli endotoxin was applicated at rats intraperitoneally in a dosage of 8 mg/kg bodyweight, to mice in a dosage of 10-30 mg/kg bodyweight. The dosage of S. anatum, applicated at rats, were 8 resp. 12 mg/kg, the dosage of S. abortus equi was 15 mg/kg bodyweight.

* Supported by Deutsche Forschungsgemeinschaft and Volkswagen-Stiftung

The animals were sacrificed routinously 6 hours after endotoxin application.

The organs were taken for enzyme determinations under sterile
conditions and homogenized with m/15 phosphate buffer, (1:20)
pH 7,2. The homogenate was centrifuged at 100 000 g. To inhibit bacterial growth 50 ug tetracyclin/ml incubate were
added. For inhibition of amineoxidases aminoguanidin was
added in a final concentration of 3.10^{-4}molar.

1,25 µg ring labeled 2 C^{14} histamine were added as substrate,
pyridoxal-5' phosphate was added in $1,5.10^{-5}$ molar final concentration. Incubation time 30 minutes, at 37°C, nitrogen at-
mosphere.

For determination of enzyme activity we have used an isotopic
dilution method similar to that of Schayer (1959) and a micromethod for the determination of radioactive C^{14} O_2 similar to
that of Aures and Clark (1964).

RESULTS

With both methods a significant increase in histidine decarboxylase activity could be demonstrated in tissue of mice
of various strains (NMRI, LAF_1) two hours after application
of E. coli endotoxin (figure 1).

Fig. 1

Controls	Endotoxin treated animals	Glucocorticooid pre- treatment and endotoxin application
0	15500	3700
0	18300	3000
0	17000	4680
0	17500	3350
	18580	7100
av. 0	17378	4365

Results in Counts / min. / 100 mg BSH

===

Increase in histidine decarboxylase activity of mice lung
in endotoxin shock; inhibitory effect of glucocorticoid
pretreatment.

Control animals died in endotoxin shock, in the average after 18 to 20 hours, at most 30 hours after i.p. endotoxin application.

In parallel experiments with Sprague-Dawley- and Wistar-rats a significant increase in histidine decarboxylase activity has been found after E. coli endotoxin applications, although not all of the control animals died (figure 2).

Fig. 2.

Controls	Endotoxin treated animals	Glucocorticoid pretreatment and endotoxin application
900	3.900	500
0	8.000	0
1.100	3.200	0
1.500	1.400	1.300
0	3.800	0
1.400	2.500	0
900	5.500	
2.000	3.700	
4.700	(3.000 - 5.000)	
av. 1.388	4.000	300

==

Results in counts / min. / 100 mg
benzenesulfonylhistamine (BSH)

Increase in histidine decarboxylase activity of rat lung following endotoxin application; inhibitory effect of glucocortidoid pretreatment.

Endotoxins of Salmonella anatum (8-12 mg/kg) i.p. and Salmonella abortus equi (15 mg/kg)i.p. at rats also produced an
increase in HDC-activity (figure 3).

Fig. 3.

Controls	S. anatum - Endotoxin 8 mg/kg i.p.
350	2.300
1.100	6.400
3.000	6.600
800	4.300
av. 1.320	4.900

Controls	S. anatum - Endotoxin 12 mg/kg i.p.
850	12.000
1.400	10.200
3.700	7.800
600	9.500
750	9.100
av. 1.460	9.720

Controls	S. abortus equi - Endotoxin 15 mg/kg i.p.
950	11.400
1.100	6.990
2.000	7.200
1.400	0
av. 1.360	6.370

Results in c.p.m. / 100 mg BSH

Increase in histidine decarboxylase activity of rat lung
following Salmonella endotoxin dependent of dosage.

The effect of these endotoxins was stronger than that of E. coli endotoxin, this may possibly depend upon the degree of purification.

Using again rats and mice of the same strains, increased enzyme activity was also found in kidney, liver and spleen after endotoxin administration. Here it is of interest that increased enzyme level was especially distinct in kidney and liver, although these organs showed no or very little enzyme activity under normal conditions.

Since HDC-activity could be demonstrated in each investigated organ of shocked animals we had to consider the possibility of transport of the enzyme from organs with high activity to other organs by serum component. Experiments with rats showed no measurable HDC-activity of the serum after endotoxin application although these experiments showed a regular increase of HDC-activity of various organs in different species. From this we conclude that histidine decarboxylase is not transferred by way of the serum. In this state of experiments we had to consider whether an increasing formation of histamine could be responsible for the fatal outcome of shock and whether histidine decarboxylase plays an important role in the microcirculation disorder of shock. Our results, however, show peak levels of lung-HDC-activity in mice from 6 to 12 hours and a progressive decrease during the next 8 hours (figure 4).

<u>Fig. 4.</u>

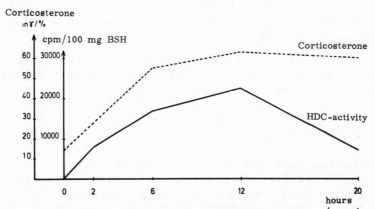

Temporal behaviour of histidine decarboxylase (HDC) activity of mice lung during endotoxin shock and of plasma corticosterone concentration in mice.

An eventual therapeutic effect of glucocorticoids especially
in endotoxin shock could depend whether there is an effect
of these substances on adaptive histamine formation in endotoxin shock.

Pretreatment of rats and mice with glucocorticoids two days
before endotoxin application as depot in a dosage of 30 - 40
mg/kg/day and application as soluble glucocorticoid (predni-
solon, Soludecortin H)at the day of endotoxin application)
resulted in a definite or total decrease in HDC activity in
the lungs of these species (figure 1 and 2).

However, this marked suppression of HDC activity is far from
being competitive. In vitro addition of glucocorticoids
had a distinct inhibitory effect up to 30 to 50 %, only in
high final concentration (5×10^{-3}m). In tissues those concentrations were reached not even approximately.

Measurements of the endogenous plasma concentration of corticosterone as the main part of total glucocorticoids in
rats and mice, indicated a marked increase up to 6 hours
after endotoxin application. This high level continued until death.

Furthermore, a high percentage of endotoxin-treated mice
(about 90 %) survived after injection of glucocorticoids,
while all untreated animals died.

The effect of glucocorticoids might be explained as a suppression of enzyme proteinsynthesis. Conversely, growth
hormone eventual should increase HDC activity by means of
increased RNA and protein synthesis (Di Stefano, Bass,
Dierheimer and Teppermann, 1952).

5 days pretreatment with growth hormone (0.5mg i.m./day)
produced a tenfold increase of HDC activity in rat lung.
Two days pretreatment with growth hormone (2 mg i.m./day)
and additional endotoxin (E. coli O 111 B_4 lipopolysaccharid
Difco) application (8 mg/kg i.p.) at the day of investigation produced a still higher activity of HDC (figure 5).

To examine the question of de novo-synthesis of HDC-enzyme
protein Actinomycin C (Sanamycin Bayer Leverkusen) was applicated to mice in a dosage of 500 µg/kg i.p. and cycloheximide
(Actidion, Upjohn, Kalamazoo, Michigan) in a dosage of 25 -
35 µg/kg i.p. for three following days.

Fig. 5.

	Controls	Endotoxin treated animals	Growth hormone pretreatment and endotoxin application
		Method of Schayer Results in cpm/100 mg BSH	
	850	10.000	28.000
	1.400	7.400	11.200
	3.700	7.900	11.000
	600	3.900	18.000
	750	8.000	
av.	1.460	7.440	17.050
		Method of Aures and Clark Results in cpm/mg protein	
	660	1.560	8.600
	620	1.900	11.400
	630	1.330	15.200
av.	635	1.570	11.700

Increase in histidine decarboxylase activity of rat lung after endotoxin application and additional effect of growth hormone.

There was no suppressive influence of actinomycin C or Cycloheximide on the HDC activity in mice lungs in our experiments, although these substances block RNA- and/or protein synthesis.

Early vasoconstriction in shock is due to liberation of epinephrine (Zweifach et al. 1956). Schayer (1959) suggested that catecholamines are the chemical mediators of stress-induced increase in HDC activity.

As a test of this working hypothesis, 0,6 mg norepinephrine
resp. 1 mg epinephrine per kg bodyweight were applied three
times with an interval of two hours. No increase in HDC activity could be demonstrated.

Plasma kinins appear early in shock and are predominant factors in hypotension. So, we injected two doses of 20 mg/kg
bodyweight bradykinin or 50 mg/kg bodyweight kallidin intravenously per animal 4 hours resp. 2 hours before sacrificing.
In our experiments the problem remained unresolved whether
plasma kinins are triggers of increased HDC activity. To
elucidate the role of endogenous plasma kinins and the significance of these substances with regard to histidine decarboxylase we have tried Trasylol^R. This strong inhibitor
of plasma kallikrein was applied in increasing dosages of
5000 to 15000 units/kg bodyweight together with or 60 minutes
after S. anatum resp. E. coli endotoxin doses of 12 to 16 mg/kg
bodyweight. In one experiment using Salmonella endotoxin the
HDC activity was suppressed, while in another one using coli
endotoxin no effect could be demonstrated (figure 6).

Fig. 6.

Salmonella endotoxin treatment (12 mg/kg)	S. endotoxin treatment 12 mg/kg + kallikrein inhibitor (10.000 units/kg)
12.000	5.800
10.200	4.850
7.000	4.400
7.000	7.300
9.100	3.600
9.000	3.000
av. 8.900	4.800

Coli endotoxin treatment (12 mg/kg)	C. endotoxin treatment (12 mg/kg) + kallikrein inhibitor (10.000 units/kg)
9.200	10.000
7.600	7.400
3.650	7.900
8.000	
6.850	
av. 7.000	8.400

Results in cpm/100 mg BSH

Histidine decarboxylase activity of rat lung following
treatment with various endotoxins and the influence of
plasma kallikrein inhibitor.

In survival studies we used LAF_1 mice and MMRI mice. The survival rate of endotoxin shock after S. anatum application was 29 of 30 animals after simultaneous i.v. injection of 1000 units Trasylol^R per animal, whereas with Coli endotoxin the survival rate was only about 20 %.

The effect of different endotoxins on HDC activity is well established now at about 100 animals.

In order to clarify the eventual significance of histidine decarboxylase in other types of shock, rats were subjected to blood loss and skin burns. Shock due to haemorrhage was produced by withdrawing 3 ml of blood from the femoral vein under sterile conditions. This procedure was lethal for about 30 % of the animals.

Determination of HDC activity at various time intervals of 3 to 16 hours after blood loss yielded no increase in HDC activity (figure7).

Fig. 7.

Hours after treatment	Treated animals	Controls (sham operation)
3	1.200	1.300
3	2.320	800
3	3.250	2.570
3	3.200	400
av.	2.300	1.540
6	2.000	1.350
6	4.000	2.350
6	0	2.200
6	1.700	
av.	1.920	1.960
24	1.750	1.300
24	550	900
av.	1.150	1.100

Results in cpm / 100 mg BSH

Histidine decarboxylase activity of rat lung various times after haemorrhage (3 ml per animal).

Large and severe skin burns were produced on the back of
anesthesized Sprague-Dawley-rats; from this procedure about
50 % of the animals died. The lungs were examined for HDC
activity 6 hours after burning. Again, the rate of histamine formation was nearly the same as in the controls.
These latter types of shock will need further research.

DISCUSSION

If continuous adaptive histamine production is an important
factor in defective microcirculation, this assumption requires that histamine should act "intrinsically" as it has
been discussed for the first time by Schayer, for the amount
of histamine production is relatively small.

Where could adaptive histamine production be involved in the
mechanism of shock?

Direct observation of the microcirculation (Zweifach et al.
1956) has shown that after a short phase of vasodilatation
there is a vasocontriction with a hyperreactivity to catecholamines.

If this vasoconstriction alone induces total stasis and hyp-
oxidosis, the therapeutic use of alpha-adrenergic blocking
agents should prevent the fatal course of shock. Experiments
of Lillehei and coworkers (1963) have shown that usually this
does not occur.

After three hours the vasoconstriction is followed by a progressive and irreversible vasodilatation. This phase of defective microcirculation might be enhanced by adaptive histamine formation. Subsequent steps as e.g. hypercoagulability
followed by consumption of thrombocytes and blood clotting
factors with the development of microthrombi, severe hypoxia
and cell necroses could be of secondary although decisive
order (figure 8 and 9).

In our experiments the triggering mechanism of HDC activity
increase has remained obscure.

The next question would be, whether histamine acts directly
or is its action mediated through other substances?

From the well known effects of histamine on blood vessels a
direct action is possible and cannot be ruled out. However,
Brocklehurst and Lahiri (1962) have pointed out that preceding
histamine release is necessary for kinin formation. One might
presume that final vasodilatation in shock is produced by the

Fig. 8.

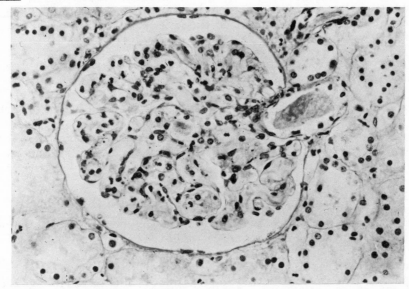

Glomerulum of human kidney in endotoxin shock with an obturating thrombus in the Vas afferens. (Ladewig-Stain).

Fig. 9.

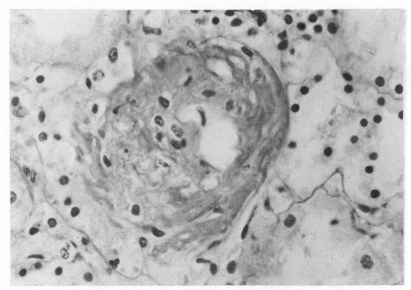

Necrosis of a little artery of the human kidney in endotoxin shock.

still more vasoactive kinins, the kinin formation again being
dependent on adaptive histamine formation. On the other hand,
the two substances could act without any mutual dependence.
(figure 10).

A further point of discussion would be if histamine is important in each type of shock?

Several types of shock, especially shock caused by haemorrhage
might be accompanied by severe hypoxia due to loss of erythrocytes. In this state, the histamine mechanism might be
unimportant or even absent as indicated by our preliminary
results.

This point, however, needs further investigation.

The next question might be: is there any conceivable therapeutic use of glucocorticoids in endotoxin shock?

Although our experiments with glucocorticoid pretreatment
yielded an almost complete protection of the animals against

Fig. 10.

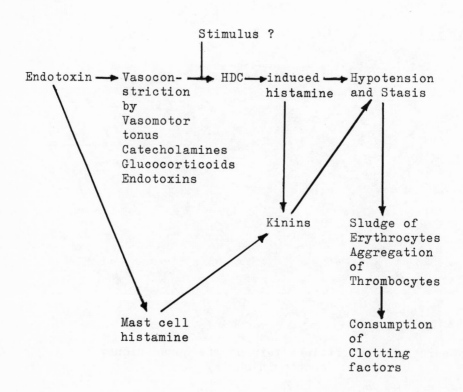

the fatal consequences of shock, administration of these hormons in a completely developed shock syndrome might be of doubtful use. In most clinical cases application of glucocorticoid in shock might be too late; for when hypoxia has reached a certain degree, sometimes very early, the process can probably not be stopped anymore. At this time application of glucocorticoids might even be dangerous, because of their influence on blood coagulation.

This reflection, however, needs further investigations, too.

CONCLUSION

Concluding, it should be pointed out that the true significance of adaptive histamine formation is still uncertain. However, the role of histamine has been neglected for a long time in the discussion of different forms of shock.

The proof of adaptive histamine formation in endotoxin shock demonstrated in our experiments should reinstate histamine into its proper place among the different factors of certain forms of shock.

REFERENCES

AURES D., and
W.G. CLARK:

A Rotating Diffusion Chamber for $C^{14}O_2$. Determination as Applied to Inhibitor Studies on Mouse Mast Cell Tumor Histidine Decarboxylase. Analytical Biochem. 2, 35 (1964).

BROCKLEHURST W.E. and
S.C. LAHIRI:

J. Physiol. 160, 15 (1962).

DI STEFANO H.S.,
A.D. BASS,
H.F. DIERMEIER and
J. TEPPERMANN:

Nucleic acid patterns in rat liver following hypophysectomy and growth hormone administration. Endocrinology 51, 386, 1952.

HINSHAW L.B.,
J.A. VICK,
C.H. CARLSON and
Y.L. FAN:

Role of histamine in endotoxin shock. Proc. Soc. exp. Biol. Med. 104, 379 (1960).

LILLEHEI R.C.,
J.K. LONGERBEAM,
J.H. BLOCH and
W.G. MANAX:

Hemo dynamic changes in endotoxin shock. In: Shock and Hypotension, The XII. Hahnemann Symposium. Ed. L.C. Millis and J.H. Moye Grune and Stretton, New York-London, P. 442, 1965.

SCHAUER A.,
I. MENZINGER AND
L. GIELOW:

Increased histidine decarboxylase
activity of rat lung in endotoxin
shock. Nature (Lond.) 212, 1249,
(1966).

SCHAUER A.,
L. GIELOW:

Beeinflussung der "induzierbaren"
Histidindecarboxylase durch Gluco-
corticoide nach Endotoxingabe.
Naturwissenschaften, 54, 589/90
(1967).

SCHAUER, A., und
L. GIELOW:

Steigerung der Histidindecarboxy-
laseaktivität während des Endo-
toxinschocks. Verh. Dt. Gesch. Path.
51, 271 (1967).

SCHAUER A.,
L. GIELOW und
R. CALVOER:

Zur Pathogenese des Endotoxin-
schocks. Klin. Wo. 65, 593 (1967).

SCHAUER A.,
L. GIELOW und
G. GEISSL:

Das Verhalten der Histidindecarboxylase und der Plasmakinine in Endo-
toxinschock. Ref. Peptidsymp. anläß-
lich des 65. Geburtstags von Prof.
Werle.

SCHAYER R.W.,
Z. ROTHSCHILD and
P. BIZONY:

Increase in histidine decarboxylase
activity of rat skin following
treatment with compound 48/80. Am.
J. Physiol. 196, 295 (1959).

SCHAYER R.W. and
O.H. GANLEY:

Adaptive increase in mammalian
histidine decarboxylase activity
in response to nonspecific stress.
Am. J. Physiol. 197, 721 (1959).

SCHAYER R.W.:

Evidence that induced histamine is
an intrinsic regulator of the microcirculatory system. Am. J. Physiol.
202, 66 (1962).

ZWEIFACH B.W.,
A.L. NAGLER and
L. THOMAS:

The role of epinephrine in the reactions produced by the endotoxins
of gram negative bacteria II. The
changes produced by endotoxin in
the vascular reactivity to epinephrine in the rat mesoappendix
and the isolated perfused rabbit
ear. J. exp. Med. 104, 881 (1956).

EXTRINSIC VERSUS INTRINSIC, COAGULATION-FIBRINOLYSIS: IN

THE PATHOPHYSIOLOGY OF SHOCK AND EXSANGUINATING DIATHESES

Charles L. Schneider, Ph.D., M.D.

University of Michigan, Obstetrics & Gynecology

Wayne County General Hospital, Eloise, Michigan
U.S.A.   48132

Disseminated intravascular coagulation (DIC) can cause circulatory failure and/or depletion of hemostasis. "Reactive" fibrinolysis removes fibrin from vital circulations, occlusions, of which otherwise could be fatal. Inhibitors released during the fibrinolysis (the ICF, or intravascular coagulation-fibrinolysis) can cause anticoagulation, adequate in itself to cause total incoagulability and exsanguinating hemorrhagic diathesis. DICs without, or with lysis (ICF), can be initiated in diverse ways and conditions.

A direct mechanism of production of extreme DIC or ICF, with circulatory obstruction and failure is <u>fibrination</u>: "The hyperacute coagulation of fibrinogen to fibrin, within and of, the circulating blood". There can be deposition of circulating fibrin, predominantly in the pulmonary arterial tree. This can cause not only hyperacute cor pulmonale, by obstruction of the lesser circulation, but failure of the greater circulation, which is connected "in series." Experimental animals undergo syncope, convulsions and coma. Following such fibrination-fibrinolysis (FF or ICF) dogs, rats, mice and monkeys, recover in a few minutes. Rabbits develop fibrination without reactive fibrinolysis (fibrination but not FF or ICF); they die promptly following doses of tissue thromboplastin (or other coagulants) that would be, at most, transiently convulsant to animals that are capable of spontaneous activation of their circulating fibrinolysin systems; i.e., capable of ICF.

If such "reactive fibrinolysis" fails (or is inhibited), some or all of these species can become as susceptible, as is the rabbit, to another kind (in timing, distribution and composition) of "DIC", mediated by the "provoking" dose of a gram-negative bacterial endotoxin in the Sanarelli-Shwartzman phenomenon (SSP).

73

AMNIOTIC EMBOLISM

As a control disorder to fibrination, disseminated embolism of bland particulate debris (provided by nature in the form of maternal, amniotic embolism) can also cause circulatory failures of variable severity, including instant death.[64] In experimental animal meconium embolism (and in the maternal disorder) the actual duration of shock before death can be too brief to cause stasis metabolic acidosis and activation of ICF. But less massive doses of amniotic embolism are sometimes sufficient to cause progressive pulmonary edema, shock and death (or recovery) within some hours.

When of sufficient intensity, that shock causes activation of peripheral stasis coagulation-fibrinolysis of unusual severity, similar to an ICF mechanism suggested postmortem (and during preceding antemortem shock) by Mole, long ago. I conclude that release of fibrin degradation products (FDP or "fibrin derivatives" in the hyperfibrinogenemic gravida) can develop so potently as to produce total anticoagulation, while still leaving a relatively normal level of fibrinogen. A probable mechanism (Fig. 1) is suggested in the accompanying outline (IIA 1), whereby the circulatory shock from bland amniotic embolism (without primary activation of coagulation) can cause a secondary ICF productive of an agonal exsanguinating diathesis (anticoagulation diathesis). Other cases of amniotic embolism are reported in which the total incoagulability is interpreted to be the result of "afibrinogenemia". Definitive confirmatory assays would be required to measure (or exclude) the presence of fibrinogen or of FDP anticoagulation. While, in some obstetric accidents, that distinction could be important for a therapeutic decision (to administer pharmaceutical fibrinogen, or not), in amniotic embolism the primary disseminated emboli persist and if extensive enough to have caused shock, are likely to cause death (irrespective of coagulation diatheses) before their ultimate removal by phagocytosis. In lesser degrees of amniotic embolism the foreign debris is removed apparently without a remaining trace within several days.

FIBRINATION-FIBRINOLYSIS OF ABRUPTIO

By contrast, from comparison of observations in obstetrics, with experimental inductions of fibrinations (and from contrast with meconium embolisms in animals), I conclude that autoextraction of tissue thromboplastin and resultant hyperacute fibrination, does indeed sometimes act as a pathophysiologic process during abruptio placentae (and, during the "concealed accidental haemorrhage" which is the equivalent English nomenclature of Sheehan and Moore). By contrast, a similar, but chronic fibrination of threshold level of intensity, probably occurs during toxemia of pregnancy.

The human organism has among other safeguards against the fibrination of abruptio and against diverse other DICs, a considerable
"reactive" fibrinolysis such that despite immediate circulatory

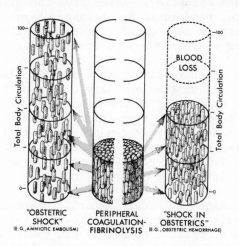

"OBSTETRIC   PERIPHERAL   "SHOCK IN
SHOCK"   COAGULATION-   OBSTETRICS"
(E.G.,AMNIOTIC EMBOLISM)   FIBRINOLYSIS   (E.G.,OBSTETRIC HEMORRHAGE)

Fig. 1. Effect of final, circulating volume, on hemostatic failure
from intravascular coagulation-fibrinolysis (ICF).
Center of diagram: During shock of increasing duration, peripheral
stasis acidosis can initiate threshold, efficient "pooling and feedback" coagulation-fibrinolysis with release of anticoagulant fibrin
degradation products. With focal perfusion, the stasis pools return
to the circulation and this can cause profound incoagulabilities of
the circulating blood, differing, as functions of the volumes into
which the "exchange perfusion" occurs.
Left: "Obstetric shock" anticoagulation. The exchange perfusion becomes diluted into a normovolemic circulation of amniotic embolism.
At the onset there is no external blood loss, but instead, splanchnic
and venous pooling as a result of the obstruction of the pulmonary
arterial tree. The exchange perfused "early phase" FDP can cause
total anticoagulation but with a remaining essentially normal fibrinogen level (diluted only fractionally from the pre-existing hyperfibrinogenemic level of late pregnancy). Resultant blood with 200-
250 mg per cent of fibrinogen[2,3,50] may be so totally anticoagulated
as to inhibit the coagulation of normal blood with which it is mixed
in a test tube.[50]
Right: "Shock in Obstetrics." Pools of peripheral stasis are incre-
mentally exchange perfused into a hypovolemic circulation and the
depletions of the substrate fibrinogen and of other hemostatic and
fibrinolytic agents, become significant, and can approach afibrinogenemia. When the shock continues for many hours there may be
progression from early stage FDP to the late stage FDP which are less
effective anticoagulants.[25] The final state, in hemorrhagic shock,
while still having anticoagulation, may include a major deficit of
the platelet and plasma hemostatic and fibrinolysin mechanisms.

failure at the level of the pulmonary arterial tree, syncope or death from fibrination in abruptio (Fig. 2) is rare. Coma, shock, defibrination, hemiplegia and recovery[17] can occur (with anatomically subsequently proven abruptio). Aside from the clinical triad of constant uterine pain, tenderness and tetany, diagnostic of abruptio, an asymptomatic course is more usual than complications; marked fibrinogenopenia occurs once in 500-1000 live births.

Such production of acute fibrination and circulatory failure is consistent with reversal of the legendary case report, that: A pregnant woman may fall, strike her abdomen (and uterus) thereby causing abruptio placentae (presumably, traumatically from the fall), to a sequence of events, that: A mother can develop abruptio placentae spontaneously, causing autoextraction, fibrination and syncope, during which she may fall. Of course, neither sequence of events excludes the possibility of the other.

Subtotal disseminated pulmonary arterial obstruction from fibrination (or similarly disseminated obstruction, of greater duration, from particulate amniotic embolism) can cause non-perfused "alveolar dead space" of the respiratory tree. Like physiologic arteriovenous shunting, this can lead to one kind of inadequate exchange of carbon dioxide and can be added to the list of causes of "acute respiratory (i.e., pulmonary) failure."[18,68]

MICROANGIOPATHY

In contrast to fibrination, there can occur, a disseminated thrombosis (another kind of DIC) in which the stimulus for platelet and/or fibrin deposition is released, not into the circulating blood but externally to the blood stream, on the vessel wall or within the wall itself. Examples occur 1. in "microangiopathic hemolytic anemia"[6] and probably 2. in the SSP (endotoxin DIC), in which disseminated injury to the endothelial or to the intimal linings of vessel walls provides a widespread stimulus for disseminated thrombosis. The obstructions in some organs in some species (unlike those in the lung) are not necessarily subject to reactive fibrinolysis; hence, focal infarction necrosis may follow in a vital region such as the renal cortex.

Glomerular "Fibrin Thrombi"

Just as there are not enough symptoms for every disease to have unique symptoms, so also there are clinical signs and/or pathological lesions in common, to more than one disorder. One such lesion at consideration is renal glomerular "fibrin" thrombosis. Not only can "fibrin thrombi" be the final common end result of diverse pathogenetic mechanisms, but the thrombi can be structurally different.

Fibrin deposits from fibrination. I have noted a characteristic fibrin obstruction during abruptio (in a fatal case of Bartholomew, Colvin, Grimes and Fish) in many organs, including the renal

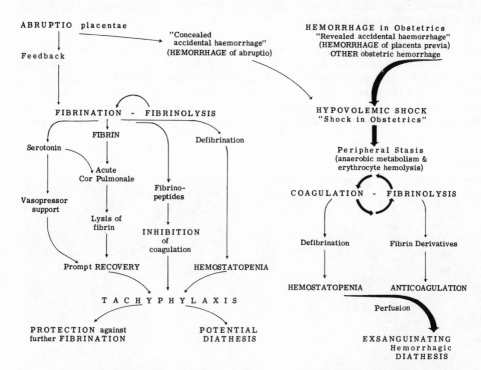

Fig. 2. Flow diagrams of fibrination- and thrombosis- fibrinolysis, abruptio placentae versus hemorrhagic shock. Abruptio placentae may cause depletions and anticoagulation of hemostatic mechanisms by two pathologic processes: (1) fibrination and (2) hypovolemic shock. The fibrination is mediated by an autoextraction peculiar to the arterial hematoma of abruptio placentae. The hypovolemic shock can be caused by the "concealed accidental haemorrhage" and/or other hemorrhage, whether or not associated with abruptio or with pregnancy. The fibrination can cause pulmonary arterial fibrin deposition and circulatory failure (rarely lethal, and more often relieved by spontaneous plasminogenolysis of the fibrin). Anticoagulant fibrin derivatives (FDP) tend to reinforce a tachyphylaxis that tends to prevent further fibrination and thereby to limit depletion of fibrinogen to a level of approximately 100 mg per cent. By contrast, the coagulation-fibrinolysis of hypovolemic shock can "exchange perfuse" incremental pools of hemostatically and fibrinolitically deficient blood (erythrocytes in "serum"). This is analogous to the postmortem defibrination of Mole. The two processes may be interrelated as in the diagram, and either may develop alone. Modified from: Thrombosis[54] and from Disseminated Intravascular Coagulation,[55] with permissions of the publishers.

glomeruli (Fig. 3). As in the characteristic fibrin deposits produced by fibrination in animals, there is no reason to assume primary or pre-existing microangiopathy. I interpret the fibrin to
have been formed within, and deposited out of, the circulating blood
within intact normal vessels.

From the clinical circumstances and from the linear deposition
of the fibrin filaments in the lines of flow, these fibrin deposits
appear to be different than SSP (Sanarelli-Shwartzman phenomenon)
thrombi. I interpret than to be the product of a primary fibrination of abruptio, probably produced by autoextraction of tissue
thromboplastin from the laceration of the decidua during the premature

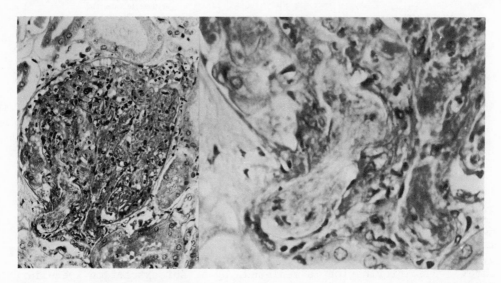

Fig. 3. Fibrin deposits from "fibrination." Low and high magnifica-
tion. Glomerular capillaries, afferent and efferent arterioles of
renal glomerulus. Insufficient antemortem duration for "incubated"
renal cortical necrosis. Fatal fibrination, abruptio placentae. The
fibrillae of fibrin are arranged in the lines of flow through the
vessels (as in experimental animals into which tissue thromboplastin
or thrombin has been infused intravascularly) and is not laminated
as in the classic vessel wall thrombus, nor dense as is the fibrin
of the GSR and of the specific (endotoxin) SSP "thrombi" of the renal
cortex. I interpret this fibrin to have been deposited within
vessels with intact endothelial linings, i.e., in the sense of fibrination (deposited from hyperacute coagulation of fibrinogen to fibrin,
within and of, the circulating blood) and not in the sense of thrombosis onto vessel walls injured or conditioned by a preceeding endotoxin or other provoking agent, or by degeneration from anoxia as in
the Sheehan and Moore "reflow thrombosis." (H & E stain.)

separation of the placenta. Unlike the persistent dense "reflow" or "GSR" thrombi that can develop 18 hours later[60] in the same glomeruli, these hyperacute intravascular fibrin deposits are so susceptible to removal by reactive fibrinolysis that if the gravida survives the interval of the acute episode of the abruptio itself, which she usually does, the fibrin disappears without leaving a visible trace.

Random focal endothelial fibrination. From comparison with the experiments of Winternitz, Mylon and Katzenstein of repeated daily infusions of tissue thromboplastin into dogs, it seems probable that the transient fibrin obstructions can tend to predispose to scattered classic thrombosis and infarction or hemorrhage, during subsequent episodes of fibrination. I have not found such thrombi following single injections. Since abruptio is an acute (usually self-limiting) accident, such random infarcts (and/or hemorrhages) including central nervous system accidents (secondarily to a repeated bout of fibrination after an interval of a day or more) are the exception (but perhaps do occur[66]).

A localized predispostion to secondary "reflow thrombosis" occurs in the (portal) circulations of the renal cortex, and the stalk of the pituitary gland. (Curiously, these persistent thrombi seem to develop as a local phenomenon, after recovery from abruptio placentae and hemorrhagic shock.) By contrast, the great filtering vascular beds of the hepatic portal system (but especially of the pulmonary circulation) are noted for fibrinolytic activation, and thrombi in them are not usually persistent under the same conditions. Sheehan and Moore interpreted their renal cortical "reflow thrombi" to be a response to focal ischemic injury.

Renal glomerular "reflow thrombi". These are also called GSR "fibrin thrombi"[26]. They form in the renal glomeruli independently of (a day later than) the fibrination and fibrinogenopenia of the fibrination-fibrinolysis (FF or ICF) of abruptio; i.e., formation of this fibrin is not contemporaneous with fibrination-defibrination (defibrinogenation) but occurs many hours later, when the fibrinogen level is largely restored toward its hyperfibrinogenemic level; these secondary reflow "fibrin thrombi" are dense and/or fibrinoid, and (in one and the same abruptio subject) are paradoxically not readily subject to, indeed are resistant to, fibrinolysis. These thrombi remain so well preserved as to be found at autopsy within their "incubated" infarcts (renal cortical necrosis) at maternal death from secondary or tertiary complications (e.g., from renal failure) one or more days postabruptio, notably in those cases with severe hemorrhage and hypovolemic shock postabruptio.

There is no necessary contradiction between the interpretations of renal "reflow thrombosis"[60] and the GSR "fibrin thrombi" of McKay. Indeed, since apparently similar dense fibrin glomerular thrombi, are

found by Sheehan and Moore and by McKay beginning at an interval of
nearly one day after the abruptio (and hemorrhage) in late pregnancy
(indeed, within apparently identical postabruptio women), it seems
probable that these investigators are describing the same thrombi
and symmetrical renal cortical (infarction) necrosis.

It is pertinent that McKay does not require bacterial endotoxin
as a pathogenetic mediator, thereby distinguishing his generalized
Shwartzman reaction ("GSR"), as a broad generic category of renal
cortical necrosis, mediated by any DIC. The renal cortical necrosis
of the classic Sanarelli-Shwartzman phenomenon (SSP, as defined by
Selye) is then a specific (endotoxin) etiologic and pathogenetic example of a GSR (or of a thrombohemorrhagic phenomena, THP[58]).

Anticoagulation prophylaxis. For an interval after abruptio
placentae with fibrination-fibrinolysis, the mother is anticoagulated
by her own FDP. Perhaps this natural anticoagulation prevents reflow or GSR thrombosis (renal and/or pituitary) during a predictable
interval before onset of the thrombosis, of up to 18 hours (after
abruptio complicated by hypovolemic hemorrhagic shock, as described
by Sheehan and Moore[60]).

It follows that there is time for a clinical decision for prophylactic anticoagulant management, to extend that interval, and
thereby to prevent or minimize, the renal cortical thrombosis and
its irreversible infarction necrosis.

SUMMARY

Intravascular coagulation-fibrinolysis can cause, or be caused by,
circulatory shock. In obstetrics, 1. bland foreign particulate debris (in amniotic embolism) and 2. disseminated activation of coagulation (in abruptio placentae), can cause circulatory failures and
hemostatic failures. Anticoagulations from fibrin degradation products can cause or aggravate a depletion hemorrhagic diathesis until
the hemorrhage, diathesis and shock become all but irreversible.
Thus, in obstetrics and elsewhere in medicine, "hemorrhage can beget
an exsanguinating diathesis." Heroic management, including massive
support of circulating blood volume saves lives of military personnel
"who would previously have been listed as 'killed in action." The
patient with a medical, surgical, obstetric, traumatic or military
accident is not always able to present himself for diagnostic and
prophylactic management, in time to prevent nearly lethal shock.
Heroic management with recovery (e.g., following abruptio placentae)
carries with it more or less severe degrees of continuing disability
from such vital organ degenerations as 1. anterior pituitary necrosis
which may require lifelong corticosteroid replacement therapy and/or
2. varying degrees of lower nephron nephrosis or renal cortical necrosis, which for survival may require replacement dialysis and/or
renal transplant, to prevent death from the renal failure.

PATHOGENESIS, DISSEMINATED INTRAVASCULAR COAGULATION (DICs):
Fibrination- versus disseminated thrombosis- fibrinolysis

I. Primary mechanisms
  A. Intermediary mechanisms of blood plasma coagulation (Fig. 1)
    (i.e., via autocatalytic activation of prothrombin to thrombin)
    1. By extrinsic activation (tissue thromboplastin) mechanism[41]
      a. Normally acts externally to circulation[41]
        1) With total conversion of fibrinogen to fibrin
          a) within a hematoma (in tissues) or in a vessel wall[6]
      b. Intravascularly: "toxic"[40,41] fibrination:[49] "Coagulates
      fibrinogen to fibrin, within and of, the circulating blood"[50]
        1) Natural model: abruptio placentae of late pregnancy[43]
          a) not total coagulation (some fibrinogen remains)[53]
        2) Large dose rapid fibrination (animal): promptly lethal[44]
          a) especially in hyperfibrinogenemia[15]
            1. i.e., fibrinogen level sensitive
          b) primarily arterial, pulmonary, fibrin deposition[42]
            1. causes systemic circulatory failure ("in series")[56]
        3) Slow, prolonged infusion: less fibrin deposition[21,40]
          a) intravascular fibrin, viscera, glomeruli (Fig. 3)
        4) Depletions of agents of coagulation, coagulopenia,[34,43]
        (hemostatopenia, or "Verbrauchskoagulopathie")[23]
          a) thromboplastin dose dependent[41]
          b) defibrinogenation (defibrination) from "fibrination"
            1. proportionate fibrinogenopenia[12]
            2. and thrombocytopenia[10]
            3. organism tends to limit fibrinogenopenia,[54,55] and
            4. to prevent propagation to "afibrinogenemia"[53,55]
          c) F. V, VIII deficiencies, plasminogenopenia: also
          d) prothrombin- antithrombin- antiplasmin- openia[37]
        5) Fibrinolysis: secondary "reactive" activation, hence:
        6) Fibrination-fibrinolysis[44] (FF) feedback autocatalysis:
          a) pooling and feedback (of thrombin and of plasmin)[54,55]
          b) increases efficiency of clotting and lysis[28] (C 2b, F)
          c) release of fibrin degradation products (FDP)[25,64]
            1. FDP are now sometimes proposed as proof:[8]
              a. of coagulation-fibrinolysis; thereby:
              b. of intravascular coagulation, "FF" or "DIC"
            2. some FDP are potent inhibitors of coagulation:[25,65]
          d) anticoagulation: progressive in abruptio placentae
            1. thereby: tachyphylaxis against fibrination[54,55]
        7) Tachyphylaxis, feedback protection of the organism:
          a) FDP anticoagulation limits initial fibrination
            1. during initial placental separation (abruptio)[54]
          b) minimize FF during subsequent extensions of abruptio
            1. tends to preserve some hemostatic capability[54,55]
              a. fibrinogen remains above 100 mg per cent[53]
              b. surgery usually permissible (e.g. cesarean)[44]

              c. (but, prevent hypovolemic shock: C2, below)
2. By thrombin infusion:[21]
   This model uses the enzymatic "final common pathway"
   (But: thrombin causes autocatalytic "intrinsic" activation)
   a. Coagulation, within and of, the plasma; i.e., fibrination:
      1) Rapid infusion promptly fatal; circulatory failure:
         a) fibrin deposition, primarily pulmonary intra-arterial
      2) Slow infusion, is not fatal[22]
         a) fibrin in glomeruli, viscera (Jürgens and Studer)[22]
      3) Approach afibrinogenemia with large (secondary) doses[14]
3. By coagulase infusion
   (Bacterial staphylocoagulase, Smith and Johnstone)[61]
   a. Mediation by direct activation, prothrombin to thrombin
      1) promptly fatal fibrination (rabbits, but not mice)
   b. Staphylocoagulase fibrination, pathogenetically:
      1) No human cases reported, but
      2) Search among septicemia cases may not be complete
      3) Antistaphylocoagulase (antigenically induced)[61]
         a) human resistance to staphylococcus infection
         b) rabbits resistant to fibrination by coagulase
4. By intrinsic complex
   (Platelet, erythrocyte, "partial", or "blood" thromboplastin)
   a. Model to circumvent defense against dissemination:
      1) Laboratory "generation" of intrinsic complex:
         a) incubate platelet f. 3 with plasma co-factors (C 1a2)
         b) at moment of maximum activation,
         c) infuse activated complex (Spaet and Kropatkin)[62]
      2) Thereby can cause intrinsic "fibrination", any degree,
         a) as potently lethal, as extrinsic fibrination
   b. In Sanarelli-Shwartzman phenomenon (endotoxin SSP)[58]
      1) Intrinsic and/or endothelial activator? (6c below)
      2) Glomerular thrombi versus "fibrination" (1b 3 above):
         a) "reflow thrombi" occur one day after abruptio
            (Sheehan and Moore)[60] or renal ischemia[59]
         b) identical to the abruptio "GSR" (of McKay)[28]
            (glomerular fibrin thrombi, renal cortical necrosis)
         c) a and b, both occur in postabruptio patients
      3) Therefore "reflow" and "GSR" thrombosis mechanisms
      are probably identical and of non-endotoxin origin
         a) i.e., not necessarily bacterial dependent
         b) not Sanarelli-Shwartzman phenomenon (endotoxin SSP)
         c) not necessarily imply septicemia, nor antibiotic
   c. Postulated, within placental intervillous lake stasis
      (via platelet agglutination, McKay)[26]
      1) Toxemia of pregnancy: experimental rat,[26,31] rabbit[1]
         a) and human (Schmorl)[39] (see III A1 below)
      2) Dead fetus syndrome: placental trophoblast degeneration[26]
   d. Shock (peripheral stasis activations[15,16] (see C below)
5. By intrinsic activation secondarily to extrinsic initiation
   (Autocatalytic intrinsic- by extrinsic- activation)

     a. Thrombin, activated by tissue thromboplastin, promotes:
       1) Platelet f. 3 release; F. II, V activations, hence:
     b. Tends to activate "blood" thromboplastin (see 4a above)
       1) However: this secondary activation is dose dependent
         a) upon (causative dose of) extrinsic thromboplastin
       2) Circulating propagation is "forbidden"; all or none:
         a) coagulation goes to completion, at stasis
         b) but propagation in circulation; i.e., fibrination,
         c) is usually prevented by dynamics of circulation[49]
     c. Secondarily to vascular wall tissue thromboplastin,
       1) Released during stasis anoxia (compare 4b above)
       2) Contrast with direct "vasculokinase"[32] (see IV C below)
6. By primary intrinsic "generation" (activation at stasis)[28]
   (see C below; e.g., peripheral activation during shock)
     a. Organism tends to prevent[54] propagation of DICs
       (otherwise, dissemination to death or "afibrinogenemia")
       1) Sequestration, phagocytosis, remove foreign particles
         a) removal (tissue) initiators, halts fibrination:
           1. tissue thromboplastin is sedimentable
         b) partial thromboplastin is a phospholipid micelle
           1. platelet f. 3 is sedimentable
       2) Removal of particulate components of initiators
         a) by entrappment (in the clot) and/or perhaps by:
         b) blood protein coating, phagocytosis (Knisely)
       3) Metabolic removal of fibrin (and FDP)
         a) by reticuloendothelial system (RES)
         b) and/or by catabolism of FDP
         c) by filtration (renal glomerular membrane, McKay)[26]
     b. Organism tends to prevent propagation of thrombosis
       (otherwise any thrombus could propagate to catastrophy)
       1) Platelet and/or fibrin emboli, removed from circulation
       2) By deportation (embolization) to vascular beds, and/or
       3) By thrombolysis by plasmin (fibrinolysin) and RES
     c. Overwhelm protective mechanisms: propagate fibrination
       1) Test tube, intrinsic activation (see 4 above)
       2) Provoking phenomenon: SSP, or "GSR" (of McKay)
         a) endothelium and/or intima injured by endotoxin
         b) exposes endothelial "thromboplastin" (Williams)[67]
           1. chemical injury and/or actual desquamation
             a. platelet agglutination, thrombosis
             b. and/or fibrin thrombosis in situ (SSP)
         c) hyperfibrinogenemia (at provoking dose)[26] supports:
         d) massive fibrination (is fibrinogen level sensitive)
         e) i.e., SSP is substrate concentration, responsive
       3) Lability of coagulation system: "reactive" fibrinolysis
         a) species with labile fibrinolysis to DIC, e.g., dog:
           1. are not susceptible to SSP thrombosis,
           2. can withstand endotoxemia (up to direct toxicity)
         b) species without reactive fibrinolysis, e.g. rabbit:
           1. are susceptible to SSP (and to "GSR")

        c) fibrinolysis is prevented by exogenous inhibition:
           1. epsilon amino caproic acid (EACA) promotes SSP[26]
B. Lag phase for extrinsic, and for intrinsic thromboplastin:[49]
   1. Appreciable lag, intrinsic prothrombin activation complex
   2. Short lag, for extrinsic tissue thromboplastin with F. VII
      a. Minimal delay until initiation of coagulation
         1) Can activate within circulating blood (fibrination)
C. Activation, intrinsic: "blood thromboplastin generation"
   1. Classic test tube coagulation:
      a. Essential components, incubation mixture: Phospholipid:
         1) Platelet f. 3, or other "partial thromboplastin"
         2) Plus plasma Factors V (AcG), VIII, IX, X, XI, XII
      b. Normally progresses to completion; e.g., in test tube,
         1) At stasis (within physiologic hemostatic thrombi)
         2) Blind circulation pathogenetic (cavernous hemangioma)
         3) Pathogenetic activation at peripheral stasis (shock):
           a) ICF can approach afibrinogenemia
   2. Peripheral stasis[28]
      a. Can mediate coagulation-fibrinolysis, efficiently[28]
         1) At low pH from anaerobic metabolic (lactic) acidoses[28]
         2) No blood flow to remove fibrin or enzyme activators
      b. "Pooling" (adsorption onto fibrin), and:
        "Feedback" (release by fibrinolysis)
         1) Of thrombin and plasmin, in concert, produce (see F):
         2) Efficient peripheral coagulation-fibrinolysis
      c. "Exchange perfusion" from peripheral pools, disseminates:
         1) Hemostatopenia, and anticoagulation (by FDP)[54,55]
      d. Erythrocytes enmeshed (lysed 36) in thrombi or at stasis
         1) Can contribute energy, adenosine diphosphate (ADP):
           a) ADP supports platelet adhesion and agglutination
           b) thereby, release of intrinsic platelet f. 3
         2) Erythrocyte hemolysis releases partial thromboplastin
          (phospholipid micelles) "erythrocyte erythroplastin":
           a) phosphatidylethanol amine and phosphatidyl serine
           b) "generation" of prothrombin conversion complex
   3. Incompatible transfusion reactions
      a. Erythrocyte antibodies: agglutination and hemolysis
         1) Supports stasis intrinsic initiation (see 2d above)
         2) Erythrocytes agglutinated, lysed: emboli and thrombi
           a) disseminated pulmonary, other vascular obstructions
           b) circulatory shock and/or peripheral stasis
           c) aggravation during surgery (parturition, cesarean)
         3) Anaerobic activation intrinsic coagulation (2 above)
   4. Antigen-antibody reactions can activate intrinsic mechanism
      a. Bacterial and allergic antigens
      b. Incompatible transfusions (3, above) maternal,
         1) Or fetal intra-uterine (for erythroblastasis fetalis)
      c. Autotransfusions (feto-maternal, transplacental)[9]
      d. Transplacental maternal antibodies (Rh, ABO)
         1) Erythroblastosis fetalis

          a) hydrops, anemia, kern icterus
            1. mother tolerates (the fetal) hemolysis well
            2. but mother can develop "dead fetus syndrome"
            3. increased incidence of abruptio? (Betts)[3]
          b) jaundice, hemorrhagic diathesis in the newborn
       e. Incompatible (renal, other) transplant, tissue rejections
         1) Fetus is usually successful parasite (not rejected)
    5. Toxins, GSR agents, venoms (but see "Reptilase", IV below)
    6. Exogenous endothelial sclerosing, or surface active agents
       a. Morrhuate, e.g., for sclerosing varicosities
         1) Escape of morrhuate into general circulation
           a) pathogenetic endothelial, platelet activation, DICs
       b. Intrauterine abortificants (infusion, attempted abortion)
D. Conditions productive of peripheral stasis intrinsic activations
    1. Peripheral cyclus vitiosus: postmortem model (Mole)[28]
      (Efficient stasis autocatalytic coagulation-fibrinolysis)
       a. Perhaps activations begin during antemortem shock (Mole)[28]
         1) Postulated hyperactivation, fibrinolysin (acidic pH)[28]
       b. Cardiac circulatory failure (myocardial failure)
       c. Embolism, lesser circulation (amniotic[64], or gross)
       d. Hypovolemic shock, versus splanchnic or venous pooling
         1) Hemorrhagic stage, abruptio placentae (postabruptio)[53]
         2) Placenta previa, obstetric, postpartum hemorrhages[28]
       e. Other shock (electrical, clostridial or neurotoxin)
    2. Incompatible transfusion reaction, maternal, fetal (C 2,3)
    3. Erythrocyte hemolysis, tolerated alone (Hardaway)[15,12] but:
       a. With hypovolemia, trauma: coagulation-fibrinolysis
       b. Clinical conditions productive of hemolysis
         1) Water infusion (not benign in shock or trauma)
         2) Soaps, caustics other infusions (attempted abortion)
         3) Hemolysis (mechanism unknown) secondarily to FF, DICs
           a) in: eclampsia[45], abruptio[52], SSP, trauma[15,16]
    4. Blood sludging, diverse origins (Knisely), any of above
E. Feedback, from the organism or from coagulation
    1. Vaso-active and cardiotonic agents released by coagulation
       a. Interrelations, catechol amines (endocrine, neurogenic)
         1) Arterial vaso-activation postulated to predispose to:
         2) Renal cortical thromboses and/or necrosis of (GSR)[26]
       b. Serotonin (released from platelets during coagulation)
         1) "Amphibaric" and inotropic responses
         2) Specific pulmonary arterial constriction[57]
           a) influence pulmonary fibrination-fibrinolysis
         3) High dosage: renal cortical necrosis, rat (E. Page)[35]
       c. Histamine, kinins, prostaglandins, others
    2. Some organisms can anticoagulate themselves, in shock
       a. Dogs release heparin[48] (just as in peptone shock)[47]
         1) Meconium embolism (experimental "amniotic embolism")[48]
         2) Not during comparable syncope from "fibrination"[48]
       b. But, the human has no heparin, and releases none[18,30]
       c. Nevertheless, human can become auto-anticoagulated,

       1) To any degree by circulating FDP (amniotic embolism[2,3])
         a) potent early phase FDP inhibit thrombin,
           and fibrin polymerization (Latallo, et al)[25]
         b) less potent late phase FDP
           1. inhibit fibrin polymerization (Latallo, et al)[25]
   3. Peripheral stasis, pooling-feedback, autocatalytic ICF:
F. Pooling and feedback (cyclus vitiosus) thrombin and plasmin[54,55]
Threshold coagulation-fibrinolysis, markedly synergistic[27,28]
   1. Thrombin is accumulated by adsorption onto fibrin, there
     a. Protected against circulating plasma antithrombin
   2. Plasminogen (and plasmin) pooled by adsorption onto fibrin
     a. Plasminogen adsorbs onto fibrin, activates to plasmin
       1) Molecular proximity to its substrate, fibrin,
       2) Substrate proximity permits efficient fibrinolysis
   3. Feedback from adsorption onto fibrin, by fibrinolysis:
     a. Thrombin is released into the plasma again
       1) Causes more fibrinogen to coagulate to fibrin
         a) and can be adsorbed on more fibrin
     b. Plasmin is released during fibrinolysis, into plasma
       1) Adsorbs onto more fibrin; lyses more fibrin; thus:
     c. Thrombin and plasmin can act repeatedly, efficiently
       1) Promote intense (anaerobiosis) peripheral stasis ICF
   4. Intermittant perfusion returns stasis pools to circulation
     a. Incremental "exchange perfusions" can disseminate:
     b. Progressive circulating "anticoagulation"
     c. Progressive hemostatopenia
     d. And cause corresponding diatheses (see II, below)
G. Threshold coagulation-fibrinolysis
  (e.g., amniotic embolism; peripheral stasis)[53]
   1. Fibrinolysis can be markedly activated (II A 1,2)
     a. Coagulation activation (alone) may be minimal
       1) Tissue thromboplastin, trace only in amniotic fluid[43]
     b. But, FDP anticoagulation can be extreme (II A 1a)[2,3]
   2. Interpretation: feedback, marked autocatalytic ICF[53]
    (Cyclus vitiosus stasis coagulation-fibrinolysis)
H. Plasmin: Aggravates coagulopenia and anticoagulation
   1. Organism tends to forbid primary fibrinogenolysis:
     a. Circulating antiplasmin, inactivates plasmin,
       1) Pharmaceutical plasmin therapy, not yet successful
     b. Pathogenetic fibrinogenolysis, postulated[29,38] but:
       1) Remains to be demonstrated,
         a) cases in obstetrics are "reactive" fibrinolysis
     c. Therapeutic activations (streptokinase or urokinase)
       1) Produce coagulopenia, similar to that from ICF:
         a) with reactive fibrinolysis: F. I, V, VIII -openias
           1. depletions which are indistinguishable from ICF
           2. (Platelets are postulated not to be consumed)
       2) Competetive anticoagulation by FDP
         a) potential exsanguinating diathesis, becomes:
           1. overt, if trauma or laceration supervenes

   I. Prophylactic anticoagulation against FF, ICF, SSP[58], GSR[26]
      1. Heparin therapy inhibits blood clotting: Stages I and II:
         a. Inhibits activation of prothrombin to thrombin,
         b. Inhibits coagulation of fibrinogen to fibrin
            1) To prevent: fatal coagulation, hemostatic failure
         c. Heparin overdosage antidote: protamine sulfate
      2. Coumadins, decrease production of prothrombin, and of:
         a. Prothrombin dependent (P and P) plasma Factors VII, IX, X
         b. Antidote: vitamin K (plasma for acute source prothrombin)
      3. Therapeutic activation of fibrinogenolysis (to release FDP)
         a. Profound anticoagulation: but Factors V, VIII depleted
      4. Therapeutic activation of ICF
         a. Thrombin activations hazardous, but Reptilase (IV below)
   J. Gram-negative bacterial endotoxin (E. coli, other septicemia)
      1. Disseminated thrombosis (DIC) without reactive fibrinolysis
         a. SSP with renal cortical and/or other thrombosis, necrosis
      2. Nonspecific (anamnestic) antibody stimulations;
         a. By typhoid antigen, unacceptable (endotoxin toxicity)
      3. SSP- and GSR- resistant species: endotoxin toxicity kills
   K. Gram-positive bacterial (septicemia) fibrinogenolysis (or ICF)
      1. Pyogenic strepto- or staphylo- kinase, can,
         a. Activate circulating activator of plasminogen to plasmin
            1) Lysis of (hemostatic) thrombi, hemorrhagic diathesis
               a) hemostatic failure (e.g., at pulmonary surgery)
   L. Gram-positive coagulation, with or without reactive fibrinolysis
      1. Coagulase fibrination (see A 3 above); no cases recognized
 II. Variables that lead to different clinical coagulation disorders
   A. Differential: Diatheses[53] by "exchange perfusions" (Fig. 2)
      1. Normovolemic "obstetric shock" (amniotic embolism)
         a. Potent fibrinolysis, inhibiting "early phase" FDP
         b. FDP anticoagulation cause hemorrhagic diathesis[2,3,47,48]
            1) Circulation totally anticoagulated[48], despite:
               a) persistence adequate hemostatic system[50], e.g.,
                  1. 200-250 mg per cent fibrinogen (cases)[2,3,50]
                  2. from above 300 in late pregnancy)
               b) afibrinogenemia also reported (other cases)
               c) no diathesis if prompt death (i.e., if no shock)[47,48]
      2. Hypovolemic (hemorrhagic) "shock in obstetrics"[53] (Fig. 2)
         a. Relatively massive effect of back perfusion, into:
            1) Small remaining (hypovolemic) blood volume (Fig. 2)
         b. Final profound hemostatopenia and anticoagulation
            1) May respond to heroic replacement blood volume
               a) blood, fluids (tissue perfusion, Hardaway)[16,17]
            2) Hemostatic support from large blood replacement,
               a) pharmaceutical blood products: fibrinogen
               b) contains Factors VIII and V, as well
   B. Differential: Coagulation versus fibrinolysis
      1. Coagulation: "fibrin" thrombosis, inadequate fibrinolysis
         (Endotoxin SSP: infected abortion, amnionitis and non-
         bacterial, postabruptio reflow thrombosis or "GSR")

    a. Intra-arterial, glomerular, fibrin tends to persist[26],[58]
        1) Platelet antifibrinolysin[20] (plasminogen depletion by FF)
    2. Fibrination-fibrinolysis: tachyphylaxis (e.g., abruptio)[53],[55]
        a. Fibrination-defibrination (coagulopenia)[20],[23],[43],[44]
        b. Reactive fibrinolysis, restores circulation
        c. FDP (late phase) partial anticoagulation
        d. Thereby, tachyphylaxis, against total FF or ICF and:
        e. Some hemostatic capability is preserved (in abruptio),
            1) Unless, hypovolemic shock is superimposed[53]
    3. Fibrinolysis potent, early and late phase FDP (Fig. 2)
        (pooling and feedback, peripheral stasis ICF, see A above)
        a. Both normovolemic and hypovolemic diatheses, severe
            1) Amniotic embolism: anticoagulation diathesis[48],[49],[50]
            2) Hypovolemic shock: coagulopenia and anticoagulation[15],[53]
                a) "hemorrhage begets exsanguinating diathesis"
III. Mechanisms, autoextraction of tissue thromboplastin into circulation
    A. Chronic intravascular coagulation and reactive fibrinolysis[8],[11],[45]
        1. Release of trophoblast emboli, from placenta
            a. Postulated etiology of toxemia of pregnancy (Schmorl)[40]
            b. Occurs in uncomplicated gestation, FDP demonstrated (Cash)[8]
        2. Malignancy, mechanism unknown (intravascular emboli?)[11]
            a. Heparin can restore hemostasis (but does not suppress the
                malignancy) Didisheim, Bowie and Owen[11]
        3. Recurring fibrination: animals[69], abruptio[17],[66]
    B. Acute fibrination[42]-[57]
        1. Prostatic resection, isotonic irrigating fluid
            a. Vehicle for autoextraction of tissue thromboplastin
                1) ICF and hemostatopenia-anticoagulation (FDP)
            b. But, hypotonic irrigating fluid (e.g., distilled water):
                1) Also: erythrocyte hemolysis (intrinsic activations)
            c. In presence of surgical shock: hemorrhagic diathesis,
                1) Hemolysis plus shock (see I D 3 above)
        2. Abruptio placentae, hydraulic pump, arterial actuation:[46]
            (Autoextraction, tissue thromboplastin, maternal circulation)
            a. Macro-extraction from decidua via intervillous lake[46]
            b. Micro-extraction via decidual arteriovenous shunt[46]
                1) Rabbit (both experimental[42], and spontaneous[1])
                2) Human, spontaneous (early, or micro- abruptio)
IV. Direct fibrin coagulation (no thromboplastin, thrombin activation)
    A. Reptilase:
        (Direct enzymatic conversion, fibrinogen to fibrin, Latallo et al[25])
        1. Prolonged action; no circulating antireptilase exists
            a. Not inhibited by heparin
        2. Little or no thrombocytopenia (no thrombin production), but
        3. Reactive fibrinolysis; thereby FDP anticoagulation via
            a. Efficient threshold fibrination-fibrinolysis, its:
        4. Suggest antithrombosis therapy: fibrinogenopenia and FDP
        5. While preserving hemostatic thrombosis by preserving,
        6. Platelets, plasma coagulation factors for thrombus formation
    B. Theoretically could achieve also with plasmin activation

1. But activators (F. V, VIII) are reported to be depleted[37]
C. "Vasculokinase" (like reptilase) coagulates directly (Murray)[32]

BIBLIOGRAPHY

1. Anderson, J.R. and Johnstone, J.M. (1956): Fatal intravascular fibrin formation during labour in an iso-immunised doe rabbit. Scottish Medical Journal, 1, 363.
2. Baker, S.J. and Jacob, E. (1960): A haemorrhagic disorder in pregnancy due to an "anticoagulant" preventing the conversion of fibrinogen to fibrin. Journal of Clinical Pathology, 13, 214.
3. ___, ___ and Attwood, H.D. (1964): "Hypofibrinogenaemia in pregnancy. The Lancet, 1, 438.
4. Betts, J.S. (1966): Hypofibrinogenemia: Its diagnosis and treatment in the obstetric patient. Michigan Medicine, 65, 725.
5. Boyd, J.F. (1967): Disseminated fibrin thromboembolism among neonates dying within 48 hours of birth. Archives of Disease in Childhood, 42, 401.
6. Brain, M.C., Dacie, J.V. and Hourihane, D.O. (1962): Microangiopathic haemolytic anaemia: The possible role of vascular lesions in pathogenesis. British Journal of Haematology, 8, 358.
7. Brown, L.J. and Stalker, A.L. (1965): The maternal and foetal microcirculations following placental separation or trauma. Journal of Pathology and Bacteriology, 90, 53.
8. Cash, J.D. (1969): Serum factors associated with probable pulmonary thrombosis and infarction. Presented at: J.F. Mitchell Foundation Symposium on: Blood Coagulation and Lung Pathology. Washington.
9. Chown, B. (1955): The fetus can bleed. American Journal of Obstetrics and Gynecology, 70, 1298.
10. Dam, H., Larsen, H. and Plum P. (1941): Om fibrinopeni ved for tidlig løsning af placenta. Ugeskrift for Laeger, 103, 257.
11. Didisheim, P., Bowie, E.J.W. and Owen, C.A. (1969): Intravascular coagulation-fibrinolysis (ICF) syndrome and malignancy: Historical review and report of two cases with metastatic carcinoid and with acute myelomonocytic leukemia. In: Disseminated Intravascular Coagulation. (E.F. Mammen, G.F. Anderson and M.I. Barnhart, Eds.). Thrombosis et Diathesis Haemorrhagica, Friedrich-Karl Schattauer, Stuttgart, Supplement 36, 215.
12. Dieckmann, W.J. (1941): The Toxemias of Pregnancy, 1st edition, C.V. Mosby, St. Louis, Missouri. (1952) 2nd edition.
13. Ferreira, H.C., Murat, L.G. and Ferri, R.G. (1964): Rapid test for fibrinolysis in vivo. Transfusion, 1, 21.
14. Fulton, L.D. and Page, E.W. (1948): Nature of refractory state following sublethal dose of human placental thromboplastin. Proceedings of the Society for Experimental Biology and Medicine, 68, 594.
15. Hardaway, R.M. (1966): Syndromes of Disseminated Intravascular Coagulation With Special Reference to Shock and Hemorrhage. Charles C Thomas, Springfield, Illinois.
16. ___, (1968): Clinical Management of Shock: Surgical and Medical.

Charles C Thomas, Springfield, Illinois.

17. Hartmann, R.C. and McGanity, W.J. (1957): Fibrinogen deficiency in pregnancy. Report of an unusual case. Obstetrics and Gynecology, 9, 466.

18. Jaques, L.B. (1968): Personal communication.

19. Johnson, S.A. and Schneider, C.L. (1953): The existence of anti-fibrinolysin activity in platelets. Science, 117, 229.

20. Johnstone, J.M. and McCallum, H.M. (1956): Hypofibrinogenaemia in pregnancy. Report of a case. Scottish Medical Journal, 1, 360.

21. Jürgens, R. and Studer, A. (1948): Zur Wirkung des Thrombins. Helvetica Physiologica et Pharmacologica. Acta. 6, 130.

22. Käser, O. (1952): Über Blutgerinnungsstörungen bei Fällen von schwerer vorzeitiger Lösung der Plazenta. Geburtshilfe und Frauenheilkunde, 12, 10.

23. Lasch, H.G., Heene, D.L., Huth, K. and Sandritter, W. (1967): Pathophysiology, clinical manifestations and therapy of consumption-coagulopathy ("Verbrauchskoagulopathie"). American Journal of Cardiology, 20, 381.

24. Lee, L. (1962): Reticuloendothelial clearance of circulating fibrin in the pathogenesis of the generalized Shwartzman reaction. Journal of Experimental Medicine, 115, 1065.

25. Latallo, Z.S., Budzynski, A.Z., Lipinski, B. and Kowalski, E. (1964): Inhibition of thrombin and of fibrin polymerization; two activities derived from plasmin-digested fibrinogen. Nature 203, 1184.

26. McKay, D.G. (1965): Disseminated Intravascular Coagulation. An Intermediary Mechanism of Disease. Harper and Row, New York.

27. ___, Kliman, A. and Alexander, B. (1959): Experimental production of afibrinogenemia and hemorrhagic pheonomena by combined fibrinolysis and disseminated intravascular coagulation. New England Journal of Medicine, 261, 1150.

28. Mole, R.H. (1948): Fibrinolysis and the fluidity of the blood postmortem. Journal of Pathology and Bacteriology, 60, 413.

29. Moloney, W.C., Egan, W.J. and Gorman, A.J. (1949): Acquired afibrinogenemia in pregnancy. New England Journal of Medicine, 240, 596.

30. Monkhouse, F.C. (1953): Personal communication.

31. Moore, H.C. (1962): The renal lesions associated with intrauterine haemorrhage and foetal death in pregnant rats given progesterone and an experimental diet. Journal of Pathology and Bacteriology 84, 137.

32. Murray, M. (1962): Terminal amino-acid analysis of vasculokinase-activated fibrin. Nature 194, 681.

33. Niewiarowski, S. and Kowalski, E. (1958): Un nouvel anticoagulant derive du fibrinogene. Revue d'hematologie 13, 320.

34. Page, E.W., Fulton, L.D. and Glendening, M.B. (1951): The cause of the blood coagulation defect following abruptio placentae. American Journal of Obstetrics and Gynecology 61, 1116.

35. ___ and Glendening, M.B. (1955): Production of renal cortical necrosis with serotonin (5-hydroxy-tryptamine); theoretical relationship to abruptio placentae. Obstetrics and Gynecology 5, 781.

36. Pederson, H.J., Tebo, T.H. and Johnson, S.A. (1967): Evidence of hemolysis in the initiation of hemostasis. American Journal of Clini-

cal Pathology 48, 62.

37. Phillips, L.L., Skrodelis, V. and Taylor, H.C. (1962): Hemorrhage due to fibrinolysis in abruptio placentae. American Journal of Obstetrics and Gynecology, 84, 1447.

38. Pritchard, J.A. and Brekken, A.L. (1967): Clinical and laboratory studies on severe abruptio placentae. American Journal of Obstetrics and Gynecology, 97, 681.

39. Schmorl, G. (1893): Pathologisch-Anatomische Untersuchungen über Puerperal-Eklampsie. F.C.W. Vogel, Leipzig.

40. Schneider, C.L. (1946): Placental toxin: Inactivation and tolerance during pregnancy. American Journal of Physiology, 147, 255.

41. ___, (1947): The active principal of placental toxin: Thromboplastin; its inactivator in blood: antithromboplastin. American Journal of Physiology, 149, 123.

42. ___, (1950): Complications of late pregnancy in rabbits induced by experimental placental trauma. Surgery, Gynecology & Obstetrics, 90, 613.

43. ___, (1950): Thromboplastin complications of late pregnancy. Toxaemias of Pregnancy, Human and Veterinary. (J. Hammond, F.J. Browne, and G.E.W. Wolstenholme, Eds.) J.&A. Churchill, London, p. 163.

44. ___, (1951): "Fibrin embolism" (disseminated intravascular coagulation) with defibrination as one of the end results during placenta abruptio. Surgery, Gynecology & Obstetrics, 92, 27.

45. ___, (1951): Fibrin embolism (disseminated intravascular coagulation) and the aetiology of eclampsia. Journal of Obstetrics and Gynaecology of the British Empire, 58, 538.

46. ___, (1952): Rupture of the basal (decidual) plate in abruptio placentae: A pathway of autoextraction from the decidua into the maternal circulation. American journal of Obstetrics and Gynecology, 63, 1078.

47. ___, (1953): Release of anticoagulant during shock of experimental meconium embolism. American Journal of Obstetrics and Gynecology, 65, 245.

48. ___, (1955): Coagulation defects in obstetric shock: Meconium embolism and heparin; fibrin embolism and defibrination. American Journal of Obstetrics and Gynecology, 69, 758.

49. ___, (1956): Mechanism of production of acute fibrinogen deficiencies. In: Progress in Hematology (L.M. Tocantins, Ed.) Grune and Stratton, New York, 1, 202.

50. ___, (1957): Fibrination and defibrination. In: Physiologie und Pathologie der Blutgerinnung in der Gestationsperiode. (H. Runge und I. Hartert, Eds.) Friedrich-Karl Schattauer, Stuttgart, p. 15.

51. ___, (1960): Fibrination from abruptio placentae as an accidental cause of eclampsia. Journal of the Japanese Obstetrical and Gynecological Society (English Ed.) 7, 293.

52. ___, (1968): Erythrocyte hemolysis and fibrination-fibrinolysis during retained abruptio placentae with hypovolemia and transient anuria. Obstetrics and Gynecology, 31, 491.

53. ___, (1969): "Obstetric shock" and "shock in obstetrics." Postgraduate Medicine, 45, 185.

54. ___, (1969): Fibrination-fibrinolysis: Toxemia of pregnancy, "obstetric shock" and exsanguinating diathesis. In: Thrombosis. (S. Sherry, K.M. Brinkhous, E. Genton and J.M. Stengle, Eds.) National Academy of Sciences, Washington, p. 71.

55. ___, (1969): Disseminated intravascular coagulation: Thrombosis versus fibrination, in clinical disease states. In: Disseminated Intravascular Coagulation. (E.F. Mammen, G.F. Anderson and M.I. Barnhart, Eds.). Thrombosis et Diathesis Haemorrhagica, Friedrich-Karl Schattauer, Stuttgart, Supplement 36, 1.

56. ___, and Engstrom, R.M. (1954): Experimental pulmonary arterial occlusions: Acute cor pulmonale simulating "obstetrical shock" of late pregnancy. American Journal of Obstetrics and Gynecology, 68, 691.

57. ___, Meyers, N.L., Chaplick, M.J. and Engstrom, R.M. (1967): Transient pulmonary arteriolar constriction, then increased perfusion following serotonin and following fibrination. Bibliotheca Anatatomica, 9, 66.

58. Selye, H. (1966): Thrombohemorrhagic Phenomenon. Charles C Thomas, Springfield, Illinois.

59. Sheehan, H.L. and Davis, J.C. (1959): Renal ischemia with failed reflow. Journal of Pathology and Bacteriology, 78, 105.

60. ___ and Moore, H.C. (1952): Renal Cortical Necrosis of the Kidney of Concealed Accidental Haemorrhage. Charles C Thomas, Springfield, Illinois.

61. Smith, D.D. and Johnstone, J.M. (1958): Staphylocoagulase activity in vivo. British Journal of Experimental Pathology, 39, 165.

62. Spaet, T.H. and Kropatkin, M. (1958): Effects of intravenous blood thromboplastin intermediates on clotting in rats. American Journal of Physiology, 195, 77.

63. Stark, C.R., Abramson, D. and Erkan, V. (1968): Intravascular coagulation and hyaline-membrane disease of the new born. Lancet, 1, 1180.

64. Steiner, P.E. and Lushbaugh, C.C. (1941): Maternal pulmonary embolism by amniotic fluid as a cause of obstetric shock and unexpected deaths in obstetrics. Journal of the American Medical Association, 117, 1245 and 1340.

65. Triantaphyllopoulos, D.C., Muirhead, C.R. and Triantaphyllopoulos, E. (1969): Properities of thrombin and fibrinolysin lysed fibrin. In: Disseminated intravascular Coagulation. (E.F. Mammen, G.F. Anderson and M.I. Barnhart, Eds.) Thrombosis et Diathesis Haemorrhagica, Friedrich-Karl Schattauer, Stuttgart, Supplement 36, 269.

66. Weber, L.L., Meranze, D.R., and Kaplan, F. (1952): Intravascular clotting complications of pregnancy. American Journal of Obstetrics and Gynecology, 64, 1037.

67. Williams, W.J. (1969): The tissue factor system and its possible role in thrombosis. In: Thrombosis. (S. Sherry, K.M. Brinkhous, E. Genton and J.M. Stengle, Eds.) National Academy of Sciences, Washington, p. 345.

68. Winter, P.M., and Lowenstein, E. (1969): Acute respiratory failure. Scientific American, 221, 23.

69. Winternitz, M.C., Mylon, E. and Katzenstein, R. (1941): Studies on relation of the kidney to cardiovascular disease. III. Tissue extract and thrombosis. Yale Journal of Biology and Medicine, 13, 595.

COMPLEMENT AND SHOCK

Desiree Armstrong

Department of Pharmacology, Middlesex Hospital

Medical School, London W. 1, England

Manifestations of shock are lowering of the blood pressure
and pooling of blood in various vascular beds. Since the vascular
system is permeated by the serum, any vasodilator or blood pressure-
lowering agent which serum can make either per se, or because of
foreign surfaces or injured tissues, might be formed in the vascular system. This is particularly true if the intrinsic potential
of the serum for producing such a substance is very great, as it
is for the plasma kinins (1, 2, 3, 4; for review articles, see
5, 6, 7, 8, and 9). "The very high kinin-forming potential of
body fluids and tissues is in sharp contrast with the minute concentrations of kinins required for biological effects. One ml. of
human plasma contains sufficient kininogenase and kininogen to
produce in a few minutes kinin concentrations several thousand
times higher than the levels effective on blood vessels. Full
activation of this system in vivo would probably be lethal. A
small fraction of the total potential is sufficient to produce any
of the pathological changes attributed to kinins." (10). These
changes include vasodilatation and increase in capillary permeability; the large reserve capacity of this system is like those in
various other biological systems such as the blood clotting system.
Another system of the plasma capable of producing vasodilation,
increase in capillary permeability and fall of blood pressure is
the anaphylatoxin system, which seems to operate mainly by means of
the histamine which it releases from the tissues (11, 12, 13, 14,
15, and 16) and by means of certain other blood pressure-lowering,
shock-inducing agents and effects (17, 18, and 19). The kinin
system also may operate through the action of intermediaries subsequent to the liberation of plasma kinin (20). It should not be
forgotten that some of the various enzyme systems activated prior to
the formation of the respective vasodilator, permeability-increasing

end products may themselves also possess these properties.

Research on the anaphylatoxin system preceded that on the kinin-forming system by nearly two decades. Anaphylatoxin was first believed to be an animal system only (in fact, to be found in one species only). Later, it was found in various species, with various relations to anaphylactic shock -- and finally it was found capable of being produced by human serum. The anaphylatoxin system is a complement-requiring system. In 1910, Friedberger (21) showed that guinea-pig serum could be given the properties of inducing reactions resembling anaphylactic shock in guinea pigs by pre-incubating it with immune precipitates. By 1963, it became possible to use purified components of complement; namely, the activated first component, C'l esterase, isolated by Ratnoff and Lepow. They injected it intradermally to guinea pigs and observed the enhanced permeability induced in the post-capillary venules. In the following year these authors, along with Smink and Abernethy (22), created an in vitro system by incubating fresh guinea pig serum with concentrations of C'l esterase below threshold for direct effects in guinea pig skin and thus generated a property capable of enhancing the vascular permeability.

The use of various inhibitors of components of complement applied to the serum pointed to the requirement of certain other components of the complement system in addition to the C'l esterase for the generation of permeability enhancing activity. In this way by analysis, and later by synthesis, Dias da Silva and Lepow (15, 16) were able to show participation of complement system components C1, C4, C2, and C3 in the production of activity characterised as that of anaphylatoxin by the following (see also ref. 21):

1. the ability

    a. to contract the isolated guinea pig ileum with en-
        suing tachyphylaxis,
    b. to cause cross-desensitization of the guinea pig
        ileum to agar-induced anaphylatoxin.

2. failure to cause such contractions if the tissue be
    previously blocked to histamine by specific antihistamine
    drugs.

3. ability to cause degranulation of mast cells (in guinea
    pig mesentery).

4. failure to contract isolated rat uterus.

With this information and with the methods which had become available for preparing highly purified human complement components it was possible to study the human system. Anaphylatoxin was then produced from mixtures of purified human C'1 esterase, C'4, C'2, and C'3 (15, 16). Moreover, introduction of antigen-antibody complexes and insoluble phases to serum could thus be eliminated since the sequence could be entered at the activated C'1 (i.e., C'1 esterase) stage, with the reagents at physiological concentrations. The anaphylatoxin production was associated with major changes in the C'3 component of the serum whilst C'5 appeared to be concerned with the production of a complement-dependent, non-cytotoxic histamine-releasing factor (16). As the anaphylatoxin system is a histamine-liberating system (12, 18), it is reasonable to expect it to produce histamine-type leakage in the vascular tissues. This leakage, examined electronmicroscopically by Cotran and Majno (23), resembles leakage of bradykinin (see below) and was described by them as "an early transient type of response" as follows: "... / there is/ vascular leakage which begins immediately upon local appearance of the mediator, and lasts for a relatively brief period - of the order of 30 minutes...". The essential morphological features are that the leaking vessels are predominantly venules and the cellular mechanism is a partial dissociation of the epithelium. Capillaries have a few leaks only and fluid loss occurs primarily through hydrostatic mechanisms. Arterioles respond with vasomotor changes and no leakage. Whether or not this system accounts for phenomena of anaphylactic shock in a given species is probably related to the extent to which and the ease with which histamine can be liberated in that species and is reflected by the degree to which antihistaminics antagonize the reaction (see also 17, 18, and 19). That the human serum contains the components for anaphylatoxin generation, and that these components are of the complement system, have been shown largely by the work of Dias da Silva, Lepow, and their collaborators. Liberation of anaphylatoxin can also be induced by addition of polysaccharides to the serum, and this particulate material is more effective than when dissolved (12). Moreover, when this happens, there is a sharp decrease in C'1 titre and anti-complementary activity is liberated (24). An anaphylatoxin-like piece from C'3 can be liberated by a non-enzymatic, chemical mechanism (25). The system therefore has properties strongly resembling events taking place when the kinin-forming system is activated. The problem arises of common origins of these two distinct systems (15, 26) existing in normal human serum.

The kinin-forming system of the human serum or plasma also produces vasodilator, hypotensive substances -- polypeptides. It can be activated in several ways, amongst which the foreign surface reaction, the introduction of antigen-antibody aggregates, of Hageman Factor, and the thermo-reversible action induced by exposure of the serum to cold (37° - 0°C) are of great interest (27, 28, 29, 30, 31).

The mechanisms involved appear to implicate complement factors. Also, certain proteolytic enzymes applied to the serum can induce fall in blood pressure and are classical kinin formers, e.g. extract of pancreas, the original kallikrein of Werle and his co-workers (32). These actions on the cardiovascular system may be partly direct enzymatic and partly kinin actions. Solutions of crystalline trypsin, saliva (including human) and certain snake venoms (e.g. that of the rattlesnake, Crotalus atrox) have this property. When the plasma's intrinsic kinin-forming system has been activated by cooling and allowed to manufacture kinin spontaneously, the snake venom is no longer capable of producing kinin from such plasma. This fact suggests that the intrinsic kinin-forming system and the foreign toxic system, which supplies active enzyme, utilize a common substrate (kininogen).

The mechanism of kinin formation induced by cold has been attributed to the unfolding of the Hageman Facor molecule in the cold and the removal of the activity of an inhibitor of the C'1 esterase inhibitor (C'1 EI) type (33, 3, 31, 4). Introduction of Hageman Factor to human plasma containing low concentrations of C'1 EI leads not only to kinin formation (29) but also to activation of C'1 (34). Many of the other mechanisms of formation of human plasma kinin (e.g. exposure of the serum or plasma to glass; precipitation, then resolution of the 33-44% $(NH_4)_nSO_4$ precipitate of the plasma; dilution, heating to $50^\circ C$, acidification to pH 5.5 and below) involve procedures in which the C'1 EI would be inactivated (35, 3, 31), and it has been found that the C'1 EI can inhibit Hageman Factor (36).

It is necessary that Hageman Factor be activated in order that it should form kinins; such activation occurs with foreign surfaces such as glass (29), with crystals of sodium urate (37, 38) and with cold. Such activation, however, is obviously not necessary for the disappearance of hemolytic complement and the marked depletion of C'3 that results when urate crystals are added to serum lacking Hageman Factor. These changes occur without kinin formation. Moreover, human serum stored at $37^\circ C$ rapidly becomes depleted of hemolytic complement activity, but its kinin-forming potential is maintained almost unimpaired for 12 to 24 hours (39). Thus, there is no direct relation between depletion of hemolytic complement and kinin formation.

Heating of the human plasma or serum to $56^\circ C$ for 1 hour inhibits the formation of kinin in the cold and prevents cold-induced loss of kininogen (31). This is the temperature normally used to inactivate the hemolytic complement system, one-half hour at this temperature being usually employed as this destroys the second component, C'2, (also C'3 and C'4) without which the sequence of enzymatic reactions could not progress. When I made detailed examination of the action of pre-heating at 56°C on the residual kininogen present after exposure of the serum to cold (residual kininogen measured by kinin generation on exposure of the serum to equal volume of ten-fold diluted human saliva), I found that 15 minutes or 30 minutes of pre-heating failed to stabilize the cold-induced kinin-forming system. This finding means that C'2, C'3, and C'4 are not participants of the cold-induced kinin-forming system. The system was, however, stabilized by 45 minutes or 60 minutes at 56°C to the extent that no diminution in the saliva-sensitive substrate was detected. It is interesting to note that Heidelberger (40) and Heidelberger, Rocha e Silva and Mayer (41) give 50 minutes at this temperature as being the duration necessary for complete inactivation of C'1. It is, therefore, not unlikely that the first component of human complement could be involved in the intrinsic kinin formation. However, since kinin formation induced by cold (and by certain other means) is promoted by heparin it seems questionable that the kinin formation should proceed through C'1 esterase (i.e., activated C'1; ref. 34). Thus, if C'1 is involved in the kinin formation, it would appear to be at some stage prior to C'1 esterase. Certainly C'1 is a macromolecular complex (42) comprising several enzymes, and Dias da Silva and Armstrong (39) have shown that at least one of these has kinin-forming properties. Moreover, the partially purified C'1 esterase inhibitor made by Pensky is associated with a potent kinin-forming activity. The inhibitory property is destroyed during heating for one hour at 63°C and the kinin-forming activity of the complex appears enhanced by this process; one infers the presence in it of a stable kinin-forming substance. It is suggested that this enzyme inhibited by C'1 esterase could be the kinin-forming system.

Hageman Factor (which is inhibited by the C'1 EI), though stable at 56°C, is labile at 63°C. Thus, evidence is accumulating for participation of Hageman Factor, the C'1 esterase inhibitor, and the first component of complement (C'1) in plasma kinin formations. These bradykinin-like substances, according to Cotran and Majno (23), produce the histamine-type capillary damage already described. Whether this damage occurs in vivo in man, leading perhaps to cold-induced vasodilatation (43, 44), or to burn injuries (45, 46), remains to be evaluated especially in relation to the presence and activities of kinin-destroying enzymes. Nevertheless, it appears that the human serum can use complement components in these two types of blood pressure-lowering systems, the anaphylatoxin and the plasma kinin-forming systems, each of which is theoretically capable of inducing shock in man. It is also possible that these are just two examples out of several or many permeability systems (e.g., the plasmin system) capable of interaction with complement system components.

REFERENCES

1. Armstrong, D. and Stewart, J. W. (1960): Spontaneous plasma
    kinin formation in human plasma collected during labour.
    Nature (London), 188, 1193.

2. Armstrong, D., Mills, G. L., and Sicuteri, F. (1966): Physio-
    logical influence on the liberation of human plasma kinin at
    low temperatures. Hypotensive Peptides, p. 139. Springer-
    Verlag, New York.

3. Armstrong, D. (1969a): Hageman Factor and the spontaneous
    human plasma-kinin generation occurring in homogeneous media.
    Activation and inactivation. Inflammation, Biochemistry, and
    Drug Interaction, p. 153. Excerpta Medica Foundation, Amster-
    dam.

4. Armstrong, D. (1970a): Pain. Heffter's Handbuch der Experi-
    mentellen Pharmakologie, Vol. 25. Springer-Verlag, Heidel-
    berg. In press.

5. Lewis, G. P. (1960): Active polypeptides derived from plasma
    proteins. Physiological Reviews, 40, 647.

6. Lewis, G. P. (1962): Bradykinin -- Biochemistry, Pharmacology
    and its physiological role in controlling local blood flow.
    Lectures on the Scientific Basis of Medicine, 14, 242.

7. Schachter, M. (1964): Kinins -- a group of active peptides.
    Annual Reviews of Pharmacology, 4, 281.

8. Erdos, E. G. (1966): Hypotensive peptides; bradykinin;
    kallidin and eledoisin. Advances in Pharmacology, 4, 1.

9. Erdos, E. G. (1970): Bradykinin: kallidin: kallikrein.
    Heffter's Handbuch der Experimentellen Pharmakologie, Vol. 25,
    Springer-Verlag, Heidelberg. In press.

10. Eisen, V. (1969): Kinin formation in human diseases. Lectures
    on the Scientific Basis of Medicine. Annual Review, p. 146.
    The Athlone Press, University of London, London.

11. Hahn, F. and Oberdorf, A. (1950): Antihistaminica und ana-
    phylaktoide reaktionen. Zeitschrift fur Immunologische-
    forschung, 107, 528.

12. Hahn, F., Lange, A., and Giertz, H. (1954): Anaphylaktoide
    reaktionen durch kunstliche blutersatzstoffe. Archiv fur
    Experimentelle Pathologie und Pharmakologie, 222, 603.

13. Rocha e Silva, M., Bier, O., and Aronson, M. (1951): Histamine release by anaphylatoxin. Nature (London), 168, 465.

14. Rocha e Silva, M. (1954): Anaphylatoxin and histamine release. Quarterly Reviews of Allergy, 8, 220.

15. Dias da Silva, W. and Lepow, I. H. (1965): Anaphylatoxin formation by purified human C'1 esterase. Journal of Immunology, 95, 1080.

16. Dias da Silva, W. and Lepow, I. H. (1967): Complement as a mediator of inflammation. II. Biological properties of anaphylatoxin prepared with purified components of human complement. Journal of Experimental Medicine, 125, 921.

17. Friedberg, K. D., Engelhardt, G., and Meineke, F. (1965): Uber die tachyphylaxie der anaphylatoxinreaction und ihre bedeutung fur die anaphylaxie. International Archives of Allergy and Applied Immunology, 25, 154.

18. Hahn, F. (1967): Anaphylatoxin and anaphylaxis. Allergology, p. 145. Montreal.

19. Vogt, W. (1967): The anaphylatoxin-forming system. Reviews of Physiological Biochemistry and Experimental Pharmacology, 59, 160.

20. Piper, P. J. and Vane, J. R. (1969): Release of additional factors in anaphylaxis and its antagonism by antiinflammatory drugs. Nature (London), 223, 29.

21. Friedberger, E. (1910): Weitere untersuchungen uber eiweissanaphylaxie. IV. Mitteilung. Zeitschrift fur Immunologischeforschung, 4, 636.

22. Smink, R. D., Jr., Abernethy, R. W., Ratnoff, O. D., and Lepow, I. H. (1964): Enhancement of vascular permeability by mixtures of C'1 esterase and normal serum. Proceedings of the Society for Experimental Biology and Medicine, 116, 280.

23. Cotran, R. S. and Majno, G. (1964): A light and electron microscopic analysis of vascular injury. Annals of the New York Academy of Science, 116, 750.

24. Hahn, F. (1960): Anaphylatoxin: formation, actions and role in anaphylaxis. Polypeptides Which Affect Smooth Muscles and Blood Vessels. Pergamon Press, Oxford.

25.   Budzko, D. B. and Muller-Eberhard, H. (1969): Anaphylatoxin
      release from the third component of human complement by
      hydroxylamine. Science, 165, 506.

26.   Rocha e Silva, M. and Carvalho, I. F. (1967): Anaphylatoxin
      and the kinin system. Allergology, p. 160. Pergamon Press,
      New York.

27.   Armstrong, D., Jepson, J. B., Keele, C. A., and Stewart, J.
      W. (1957): Pain-producing substance in human inflammatory
      exudates and plasma. Journal of Physiology, 135, 350.

28.   Movat, H. Z. (1967): Activation of the kinin system by
      antigen-antibody complexes. International Symposium on
      Vasoactive Polypeptides: Bradykinin and Related Kinins,
      p. 177, Edart Livraria Editora Ltda, Sao Paulo.

29.   Margolis, J. (1960): The mode of action of Hageman Factor
      in the release of plasma kinin. Journal of Physiology, 151,
      238.

30.   Armstrong, D. and Mills, G. L. (1965): The reversible cold-
      induced activation of the plasma kinin-forming system between
      37° and $0^{\circ}C$. Journal of Physiology, 179, 89.

31.   Armstrong, D. (1969b): Actions of the human cold-activated
      plasma kinin-forming system of preheating at 56° and $60^{\circ}C$.
      Pharmacological Research Communications, 1, 30.

32.   Frey, E. K., Kraut, H., and Werle, E. (1950): Kallikrein
      (Padutin). Enke, Stuttgart.

33.   Armstrong, D. (1968): The effects of temperature on the
      response of human plasma kinin-forming system to promoting and
      inhibiting agents. British Journal of Pharmacology, 34, 670P.

34.   Donaldson, V. H. (1968): Mechanisms of activation of C'1
      esterase in hereditary angioneurotic edema plasma in vitro.
      The role of Hageman Factor, a clot-promoting agent. Journal
      of Experimental Medicine, 127, 411.

35.   Pensky, J., Levy, L. E., and Lepow, I. H. (1961): Partial
      purification of a serum inhibitor of C'1 esterase. Journal
      of Biological Chemistry, 236, 1674.

36.   Pensky, J. (1969): Personal communication.

37. Kellermeyer, R. W. and Breckenridge, R. T. (1965): The in-
    flammatory process in acute gouty arthritis. I. Activation
    of Hageman Factor by sodium urate crystals. Journal of
    Laboratory and Clinical Medicine, 65, 307.

38. Eisen, V. (1966): Urates and kinin formation in synovial
    fluid. Proceedings of the Royal Society of Medicine, 59, 302.

39. Dias da Silva, W. and Armstrong, D. (1968): Unpublished
    observations.

40. Heidelberger, M. (1941): Quantitative chemical studies on
    complement of alexin. I. A Method. Journal of Experimental
    Medicine, 73, 681.

41. Heidelberger, M., Rocha e Silva, M., and Mayer, M. M. (1941):
    Quantitative chemical studies on complement or alexin. III.
    Uptake of complement nitrogen under varying experimental
    conditions. Journal of Experimental Medicine, 74, 359.

42. Naff, G. B., Pensky, J., and Lepow, I. H. (1964): The macro-
    molecular nature of the first component of human complement.
    Journal of Experimental Medicine, 119, 593.

43. Cuschieri, A., Onabanjo, A. O., and James, P. B. (1969):
    Kinin release during cold vasodilatation. Pharmacological
    Research Communications, 1, 147.

44. Kulka, J. P. (1964): Microcirculatory impairment as a factor
    in inflammatory tissue damage. Annals of the New York Academy
    of Science, 116, 1018.

45. Armstrong, D., Mills, G. L., and Stewart, J. W. (1967):
    Thermally-induced effects on the kinin-forming system of
    native human plasma, $37^{\circ}-0^{\circ}C$ and $37^{\circ}-50^{\circ}C$. International
    Symposium on Vasoactive Polypeptides: Bradykinin and Re-
    lated Kinins, p. 167. Edart Livraria Editora Ltda, Sao
    Paulo.

46. Goodwin, L. G., Jones, C. R., Richards, W. H. G., and Kohn,
    J. (1963): Pharmacologically active substances in the urine
    of burned patients. British Journal of Experimental Pathology,
    44, 551.

THE ROLE OF SPLANCNIC ADRENERGIC VASOCONSTRICTION IN THE

DEVELOPMENT OF IRREVERSIBILITY OF HEMORRHAGIC SHOCK

GIAN PAOLO NOVELLI, CAMILLO CORTESINI, ELIO PAGNI

DEPTS OF SURGICAL PATHOLOGY AND OF ANESTHESIOLOGY OF

THE UNIVERSITY OF FLORENCE, ITALY

In the indefinite picture of the hypoteses related to the pathogenetic events of experimental shock and its irreversibility, some Authors give particular importance to the effects of bacterial endotoxins and to their deficient detoxification from reticulo-endothelial system (RES).

According to this pathogenetic theory, the shock provoking stimuli (namely hemorrhage, trauma, scalding etc.) initiate a condition of sympato-adrenergic overactivity followed by many effects and, particularly, by a state of diffuse and intense vasoconstriction.

This last phenomenon can be sufficient to cause ischemic tissular hypoxia of the intestinal wall with increased passage into general circulation of endotoxins produced by gram-negative bacteria. At the same time the ischemic hypoxia also acts on the RES which lose their capacity to detoxify endotoxin, which so pass into systemic circulation.

1) These studies were supported by grants from the Consiglio Nazionale delle Ricerche.

If this hypothesis is exact, an increase in the total mass of
RES or the abolition of the vasoconstrictive damage both to the
gut, and to the liver and spleen (organs very rich in RES) should
prevent the irreversibility of shock.

In view of the first idea we subjected some dogs to hemorrhagic
shock after eterotopic transplantation of a supplementary omologous
spleen, selectively treated with an alpha-blocking agent to prevent
the precocious vasoconstriction (Novelli et al., 1969). The results
were not such as to confirm the working hypothesis.

In the present paper, on the contrary, are reported the results
of experiments aimed at preventing, by a selective alpha-adrenergic
blockade, the vasoconstriction and subsequent ischemic hypoxia of
the whole splancnic vascular bed, namely of the mesenteric, hepatic
and splenic vascular beds.

MATERIAL AND METHODS

All the experiments were carried out on healthly, apparently
young mongrel dogs, the rate of erythrosedimentation being used to
exclude the existence of infective pathology.

The surgical procedures were performed under general anesthesia,
using intravenous short acting barbiturates (Pentothal Abbott),
orotracheal intubation, nitrous oxide plus oxygen and controlled
respiration (Harvard mod.606).

The alpha-receptor blockade was realized treating the three
main arteries of the splancnic bed directly (namely the superior
mesenteric artery, the hepatic artery and the splenic artery) and
using phentolamine (Regitin Ciba).

Each vessel was first closed , then 20-30 ml of cooled heparinized Ringer solution containing the adrenergic blocking drug were
injected distally to the occlusion ; after this the occlusion was
maintained for a further ten minutes.

Phentolamine (0,4 mg/Kg) was injected into the superior mesenteric artery while in the hepatic and in the splenic artery phentolamine was injected in doses of only 0,1 mg/ kg.

Phentolamine reflowing from the mesenteric and splenic circulation was considered sufficient to block the portal circulation.

In each experiment a certain fall in arterial pressure was observed, caused by the massive splancnic vasodilatation.

Arterial pressure was brought back to normal values by transfusions of citrated blood.

The completeness and selectivity of the alpha-receptor blockade was confirmed by the absence of increase in the vascular resistances of each bed after injection of 5 gamma/kg of noraadrenaline (Noradrec Recordati). Such values in vascular resistances were calculated from values of blood flow (Nycotron) and from mean values of aortic pressure (Statham).

The same injection of noradrenaline was used to establish the absence of an alphablockade of the systemic circulation. Dogs with insufficient increase of systemic blood pressure after selective blockade were discarded from the experiments.

To test of the decrease in vascular resistances could be attributed to opening of peripheral artero-venous shunts, modifications of differences in artero-venous pO2 (Radiometer) in the mesenteric and splenic bed, before and after blockade were controlled.

A flowmetric probe was kept around the superior mesenteric artery during the whole experiment, while a catheter was placed on the aorta to measure the arterial pressure by means of an electromanometer.

After these procedures, the abdominal wall was sutured and anesthetic drugs or oxygen removed so that dogs breathed only air during the following phases of the experiments.

As controls, other animals were subjected, before the start of bleeding, to surgical procedures identical to those carried out on treated animals but the intra-arterial injections were done with Ringer solution without pentolamine.

Hemorrhagic shock was provoked by bleeding at constant pressure of 40 mm/Hg after massive doses of heparin (5 mg/Kg).

The period of hypovolemic hypotension before retransfusion was
5 hours in 12 experiments, 3 and a half hours in 5 experiments and
2 and a half hours in another 5 experiments.

At the end of each period of bleeding all the blood collected
in reservoir was retransfused ; 30 ml/Kg of a plasma-expander
(Hemagel Hoechst) were infused after additional 150 minutes.

During each experiment the hemodynamics of the mesenteric
vascular bed and the modifications of the arterial pressure were
controlled; after death the pathology of the gastro-intestinal apparatus was observed.

RESULTS

Generally speaking, the results were not such to confirm the
working hypothesis reported in the foregoing pages.

Observing Table 1 it appears evident that in the table 1
group of dogs subjected to the longest period of hypovolemic hypotension, the difference in survival between treated and controls
were not significant.

With regard to this group of experiments, it must be noted
that in the control dogs hemorrhagic phenomena were always present
in the intestinal mucosa ; in the selectively blocked dogs, on the
other hand, these phenomena of hemorrhagic necrosis were absent in
the gut, but were very evident in the stomach and duodenum.

In the group of dogs subjected to hemorrhagic hypotension lasting
two and a half hours 4 out of 5 of the controls survived while among
the treated animals 1 out of 5 survived. Therefore control animals
endure a shock better than treated.

Figure 1 shows the selectivity of adrenergic blockade.

In the upper half are recorded the variations in mesenteric
blood flow and arterial pressure after injection of 5 gamma/Kg of
noradrenaline as observed in an animal before treatment.

TABLE 1

RESULTS OBTAINED IN DOGS SUBJECTED TO HEMORRHAGIC SHOCK AFTER SPLANCNIC

SELECTIVE ALPHA-BLOCKADE

	N° experim.	Intestinal hemorrhage	Gastric hemorrhage	Surviving after hours		
				6	12	24
A- 5hours of bleeding						
- controls	12	12/12	0/12	5/12	1/12	0/12
- treated	12	2/12	10/12	4/12	1/12	1/12
B- 3½ hours of bleeding						
-controls	3	2/3	0/3	3/3	2/3	1/3
-treated	5	0/5	5/5	2/5	1/5	0/5
C- 2½ hours of bleeding						
-controls	5	1/5	0/5	5/5	4/5	4/5
-treated	5	0/5	0/5	3/5	1/5	1/5

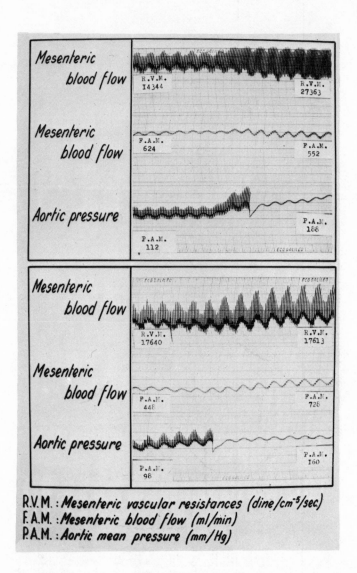

Fig. 1 - Effect of injection of noradrenaline (5gamma/Kg) on the
mesenteric hemodynamics.

Above : before regional alpha-adrenergic blocade
Below : after regional alpha-adrenergic blockade.

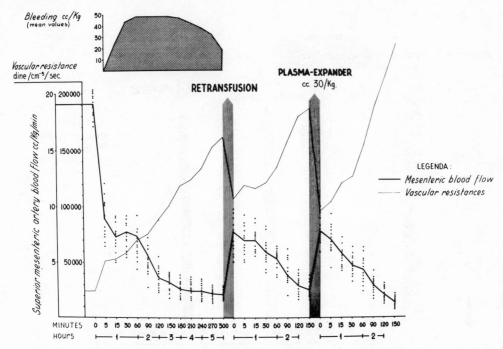

Fig. 2- Variations of regional mesenteric haemodynamics in
control dogs. Points indicate individual values and continuous line the mean values.

TABLE   2

EFFECTS OF SELECTIVE ALPHA-BLOCKADE ON REGIONAL

ARTERO-VENOUS DIFFERENCES IN pO_2

	before	after
Superior mesenteric bed	116	160
	112	143
	101	153
	100	126
	121	137
Splenic bed	90	137
	87	114
	80	121
	74	112
	93	117

Dogs breathing oxygen and nitrous oxide.

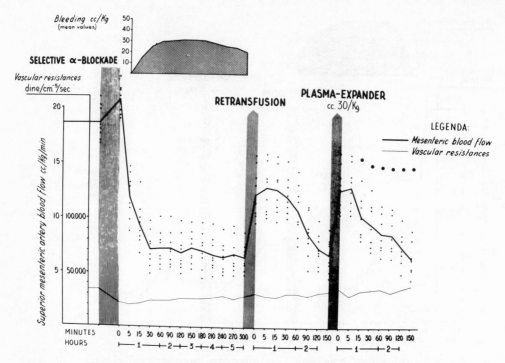

Fig. 3 - Variations of regional mesenteric haemodynamics in dogs
subjected to hemorrhagic shock after selective alpha-adrenergic blockade. Points indicate individual values and continuous line the
mean values. Larger points are values not included.

In the lower half of the same slide, can be seen what happens
in the same animal after selective adrenergic blockade : the increase of aortic pressure is almost unvaried and there is no increase
of vascular mesenteric resistances ; while on the contrary , the
mesenteric flow increases in direct proportion to the increase of
perfusion pressure.

Table II shows the variations in artero-venous difference in
pO2 of the mesenteric and of the splenic bed. After alpha-blockade
such difference increases, showing the improvement of tissular perfusion and the absence of opening of artero-venous shunts.

Additional data can be obtained observing the hemodynamics of
the mesenteric vascular bed during hemorrhagic shock, as referred
in the two following graphs.

Figure 2 gives the data for control experiments and it is noticeable that bleeding is accompanied by a progressive and marked increase of vascular resistances. This condition is not reversed by retransfusion, showing so that intestinal perfusion is always low.

Figure 3 shows the hemodynamics of the mesenteric circulation in dogs subjected to selective splancnic adrenergic blockade. In this condition there is no sign of vasoconstriction.

In figures 2 and 3 it must be noted that the total mean volume of bleeding was lower in the control dogs than in those treated.

DISCUSSION

The presence of an adrenergic factor in the pathogenesis of shock is supported by many facts, that are beyond question. Here it will be sufficient to recall the existence of very high levels of catecholamines in the blood of shocked animals (Rosemberg,1961-64; Richardson, 1965) and the protection offered against shock by phenoxybenzamine (Nickerson,1962-64; Bloch et al., 1966 ; Dietzman and Lillehei, 1968-69).

On the contrary , attempts to solve the enigma of the pathogenesis of shock and its irreversibility on the sole basis of adrenergic hyperactivity, seems to be an excessive simplification of certainly more complex events.

For these reasons the hypothesis of an endotoxic mediator was accepted with a certain degree of enthusiasm and endotoxemia has been widely found (Schweinburg, et al., 1954; Ravin et al., 1958-60) in all the main forms of experimental shock (Schweinburg and Fine, 1960), and probably also in clinical shock (Palmerio C. : personal communication).

The role of RES as detoxifing system of bacterial endotoxins in shock is documented by various papers, starting with that of Rutenburg et al. (1960) and arriving at the recent work of Fine et al., (1968).

Some of such experimental data suggest that the detoxificating properties of RES are active only on bacterial endotoxins but do not

affect catecholamines or vasoactive polypeptides (Palmerio et al.,
1964 ; Rutenburg et al., 1967).

Experiments on RES in shock also underline another important
fact : namely, that detoxification is active only when the implicated organs (i.e. liver and spleen) are well perfused. This has been
demonstrated by Palmerio et al. (1963-1967) investigating the protection afforded by the coeliac blockade against irreversibility of
experimental shock.

Noxious vasoconstrictive ischemia of the RES (i.e. liver and
spleen) and of the gut was prevented during the experiments reported
here, and the perfusion of such tissue was good even when arterial
pressure was at low levels.
In fact the absence of the constrictive vasal tone is able to ensure
a good tissutal perfusion even with low pressure according to the
data of Hochberger and Zweifach (1968) on the isolated ear of rabbit.
In fact our data regarding the variations of artero-venous difference in pO2 demonstrate the high level of perfusion in the tissues
studied.

Furthermore those vasoconstrictive phenomena that should determine the beginning of endotoxemia (Shapiro et al., 1958) were not
observed during shock and their absence in the selectively alpha-
receptor blocked animals shows the high degree of sympatho-adrenal
activity that affects tissues in the shocked animal.

Another proof of the efficiency of the perfusion of the
splancnic tissues lies in the absence of hemorrhagic necrosis
affecting the intestinal mucosa, the absence of hepatic congestion
or of any reduction of the splenic volume.

In spite of such an efficient perfusion of the gut and RES,
control animals endured shock better than those treated.

One could criticize the selectivity of the splancnic alpha-
receptor blockade in this experimental model. Admittedly free phentolamine may escape into the systemic circulation, but in such case
survival should increase and not decrease.

Another aspect of these experiments that might be opened to
criticism is the difference in the mean values of bleeding between

treated and control dogs; but this is also irrelevant as the lowest
levels of bleeding were observed in the treated animals.

It is also feasible that phentolamine directly injures the RES
but this has never been proved.

To explain the data given above one should take into account
the hemorrhagic necrosis of the stomach and duodenum. Such phenomena should probably be accepted as lesions provoked by adrenergic
overactivity , whose appearance was not observed in untreated animals, owing to the prevalence of intestinal damage.

So, in the experimental conditions here described no increase
of endotoxemia was possible as there was no intestinal ischemia.
Furthermore, the absence of ischemia of RES excludes an insufficiency
of detoxification.

Nevertheless, shock evolved regularly towards irreversibility.
Therefore one must search for some lethal circulating factor other
than endotoxin.

In this case, it is probable that the letality of hemorrhagic
shock in the dog is dependent on the action of catecholamines in
the whole organism (thus explaining the gastric hemorrhage observed)
or on the action of vasoactive agents such as kinins or histamine.

CONCLUSION

From the foregoing data it has been confirmed :
a) that the splancnic vasoconstriction of hemorrhagic shock in dogs
   is dependent on adrenergic factors,
b) that such splancnic vasoconstriction is not fundamental in the
   genesis of shock.

Moreover it is suggested that in the pathogenesis of experimental hemorrhagic shock endotoxin is of limited importance, while
catecholamines, histamine or kinins are probably the main factors.

SUMMARY

According to the hypothesis of a role of ischemia of the gut
and RES in the pathogenesis of irreversibility of shock, hemorrhagic

shock was carried out on dogs subjected to selective alpha-adrenergic
blockade of mesenteric, hepatic and splenic vascular beds.

    Animals so treated endured shock worse than controls.
    Considering the good level of perfusion of the splancnic tissues
it may be possible that the importance of endotoxins in pathogenesis
of shock has been overstressed and that a significant role may be
played by other vasoactive agents.

BIBLIOGRAPHY

1) Bloch, J.H., Pierce, C.H. and Lillehei, R.C. (1966) : Adrenergic
   blockings agents in the treatment of shock. Annual Review of
   Medicine, 17 : 483.

2) Dietzman, R.H. and Lillehei,R.C. (1968) : The treatment of cardiogenic shock. IV : The use of phenoxybenzamine and chlorpromazine.
American Heart Journal, 75,136.

3) Dietzman, R.H., Bloch , J.H., Lyons , G.W. and Lillehei, R.C.
(1969) : Prevention of lethal cardiogenic shock in epinephrine tolerant dogs.
Surgery,65,623.

4) Fine, J., Palmerio, C. and Rutemburg,S. (1968) : New developments
in therapy.
Archives of Surgery, 96, 163.

5) Hochberger, A.I. and Zweifach , B.W. (1968) : Analysis of critical closing pressure in the perfused rabbit ear.
American Journal of Physiology, 214, 962.

6) Nickerson,M. : Drug therapy of shock. in : "Shock, pathogenesis
and therapy" Springer, Berlin 1962.

7) Nickerson,M. (1964): Vasoconstriction and vasodilatation in shock.
International Anesthesiology Clinics, 2,385.

8) Novelli, G.P., Pagni, E., Patumi,F., Cortesini, C. and
Ristori,M. (1969): Il sistema reticolo-istiocitario nella patogenesi

e nella evoluzione dello shock sperimentale. Policlinico, Sezione Chirurgica,76,2.

9) Palmerio,C., Zetterstrom, B., Shammash, J., Euchbaum,E., Frank , E. and Fine , J. (1963) : Denervation of the abdominal viscera for the treatment of traumatic shock. The New England Journal of Medicine, 269, 709.

10) Palmerio , C., Zetterstrom, B., Tudor,J., Rutenburg,S.H. and Fine,J.(1964). Further studies on the nature of the circulating toxin in traumatic shock. Journal of reticuloendothelial Society, 1,243.

11) Palmerio, C., Nahor,A., Minton,R. and Fine, J. (1967) : Limitation of antiadrenergic therapy for refractory traumatic shock. Proceedings of the Society for Experimental Biology and Medicine, 124,623.

12) Ravin,H.A., Schweinburg , F.B. and Fine,J. (1958) : Isolation of toxic factor from hemorrhagic shock plasma. Proceedings of the Society for Experimental Biology and Medicine, 99,426.

13) Ravin, H.A., Rowley,D., Jenkins,C. and Fine , J. (1960) : On the absorption of bacterial endotoxin from the gastro-intestinal tract of the normal and shocked animal. Journal of Experimental Medicine, 112,783.

14) Richardson,J.A.(1965) : Catecholamines in shock.in :Mills & Moyer : "Shock and hypotension" Grune & Stratton.

15) Rosemberg,J.C. (1961) : Studies on hemorrhagic and endotoxin shock in relation to vasomotor changes and endogenous circulating epinephrine, nor-epinephrine and serotonin. Annals of Surgery, 154, 611.

16) Rosemberg,J.C. (1964) : Circulating serotonin and catecholamines following occlusion of the superior mesenteric artery. Annals of Surgery, 160, 1062.

17) Rutenburg,S.H., Schweinburg,F.B. and Fine , J. (1960) : "In vitro" detoxification of bacterial endotoxin by macrophages. Journal of Experimental Medicine, 112, 801.

18) Rutenburg, S.H., Skarnes, R., Palmerio,C. and Fine, J. (1967) :
Detoxification of endotoxin by perfusion of liver and spleen.
Proceedings of the Society for Experimental Biology and Medicine,
125,455.

19) Schweinburg,F.B.,Frank,H.A. and Fine,J. (1954) : Bacterial factor
in experimental hemorrhagic shock : evidence for development of,
bacterial factor which accounts for irreversibility to transfusion
and for loss of normal capacity to destroy bacteria.
American Journal of Physiology, 179,532.

20) Schweinburg,F.B. and Fine, J. (1960) : Evidence for a lethal
endotoxemia as the fundamental feature of irreversibility in three
types of traumatic shock. Journal of Experimental Medicine,112,793.

21) Shapiro, P., Rutenburg,S.H., Rutenburg,A.M. and Fine,J.(1958) :
Host resistance to hemorrhagic shock. Role of deficient flow through
intestine in the development of irreversibility.
Proceedings of the Society for Experimental Biology and Medicine,
97,372.

CIRCULATORY FUNCTION IN THE EARLY POSTOPERATIVE PERIOD AFTER PULMONARY SURGERY

Bengt Wranne

Departments of Clinical Physiology, Anesthesiology

and Thoracic Surgery, University Hospital, Uppsala, Sweden

The circulatory adaptation after major surgical trauma was studied with the objective to elucidate patophysiological mechanisms in postoperative complications. Such changes may also have importance for understanding the early development of clinical shock.

Fortyfour patients were operated on because of suspected or diagnosed pulmonary malignancy. They had no history, signs or symptoms of cardiovascular disease. They were fully informed about the investigation and gave their free consent. Pneumonectomy was performed in 12 cases, lobectomy in 19, explorative thoracotomy in 5 and exstirpation of benign tumors or cysts in 8 cases. There were 31 male and 13 female patients. The average age was 51.7 years.

Preoperative circulatory data were obtained through a conventional right heart catheterization. After operation pressures were recorded by means of indwelling catheters in a systemic artery, in the pulmonary artery and in the left and right atria. The cardiac output was determined according to the FICK principle.

The patients were breathing air spontaneously during the investigations. After operation a subathmospheric pressure of 15 cm H_2O was used in the thorax drainage tubes (after pneumonectomy 5 cm H_2O). Clamping the tubes did not affect the recorded intravascular pressures.

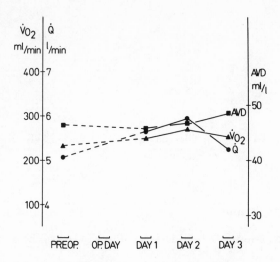

Fig 1. Cardiac output (●),oxygen uptake (▲) and arteriovenous oxygen difference (■) before and on 3 consecutive days after operation.

Cardiac output: The cardiac output $(\dot{Q})$ increased slightly during the postoperative period (Fig. 1), mostly parallel with
an increased oxygen uptake $(\dot{V}_{O_2})$. The rectal temperature during the same time was elevated by about 1 ^{o}C, as an average.
The arteriovenous oxygen difference (AVD_{O_2}) did not change
consistently, although a slight increase was seen on the
average.

Stroke volume: The stroke volume (SV) decreased consistently
(Fig. 2) and the heart rate (HR) increased by about 20 beats/
min as an average during the postoperative period. The mechanisms concerning the SV decrease were considered. A myocardial failure seemed less probable as the left atrial pressure (LA_M) decreased after operation and also for other reasons.
An inadequate venous return instead seemed a probable cause,
and may have been provoked by a decrease in or unfavourable
distribution of the total blood volume.

Blood volume: The possibility of a decrease in total blood
volume (TBV) was investigated by simultaneous blood and stroke
volume determinations. For TBV determinations the double indicator technique was used (Bratteby, 1967). There was a positive correlation between TBV decrease and SV decrease (Fig. 3).

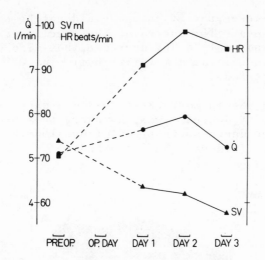

Fig. 2. Cardiac output (●), heart rate (■) and stroke volume (▲) before and on 3 consecutive days after operation.

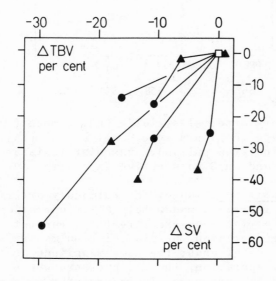

Fig. 3. Percentage change in blood (TBV) and stroke volume (SV) one (●) and three (▲) days after operation in relation to preoperative value (□) in 5 patients.

In all cases, however, the SV change could not be explained simply by a simultaneous TBV decrease. The conclusion was therefore drawn that not only a TBV decrease, but also other factors, possibly an unfavourable distribution of TBV contributed to the SV decrease.

The TBV decrease was in most cases due to a decrease in plasma
volume (PV). The PV decrease was, however, less pronounced than
expected from the decrease in circulating albumin. An inflow
of extravascular fluid had thus occurred.

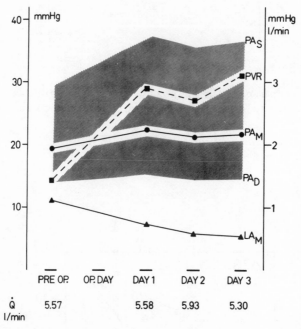

Fig. 4. Pulmonary arterial systolic (PA_S), mean (PA_M) and
diastolic (PA_D) pressure, left atrial (LA) pressure
and calculated pulmonary vascular resistance (PVR)
before and on 3 consecutive days after operation.

Pulmonary vascular resistance: The pulmonary arterial mean
pressure (PA_M) increased moderately after operation (Fig.4),
while the left atrial mean pressure (LA_M) consistently decreased. Before operation the diastolic pulmonary arterial
(PA_D) pressure was of about the same magnitude as the LA_M
pressure. After operation, the PA_D pressure was considerably
higher than the LA_M pressure. Therefore, the diastolic pulmonary arterial pressure should not under such conditions
be used as an index of the filling pressure of the left ventricle.

The pulmonary vascular resistance (PVR), when calculated as $(PA_M - LA_M)$: $\dot{Q}$, was found to be about double after operation compared to before. The mechanisms responsible for the increase in calculated PVR were considered

A moderate arterial hypoxaemia was present during the postoperative period. One factor of interest was therefore the possibility of a hypoxaemic pulmonary vasoconstriction. The presence of such a vasoconstriction was tested by oxygen administration. It was found that the pulmonary arterial pressure decreased consistently on oxygen administration. Cardiac output decreased simultaenously in some of the patients. The calculated PVR decreased in all cases but one. The effect of oxygen breathing speaks in favour of this possibility although its quantitative role cannot be ascertained.

The left atrial pressure was found to decrease consistently after operation. Therefore in the uppermost parts of the lungs the alveolar pressure may exceed the left atrial pressure, giving a passive increase in resistance (cf. West,1966).

Another possible cause of postoperative increase in the PVR would be some mechanical obstruction or else other vasoconstrictive factors than hypoxia. An interesting observation in this connexion is the consistent decrease in thrombocyte concentration seen after operation in our patients. There might be a relationship between these observations, either because thrombocytes may have formed aggregates in the lungs, causing mechanical obstruction or because vasoactive substances may have been liberated from the trombocytes.

Sympathetic activity. After operation there were signs of increased sympathetic activity, as indicated by an increased urinary excretion of free catecholamines (Fig. 5.). A myocardial 'tachyphylaxis' to repeated doses of adrenaline in dog was reported by Bendixen, Laver & Flacks (1963). The possible occurrence of such a mechanism in man under the present conditions was tested in 15 patients by short periods (5 min) of intravenous infusion of adrenaline (0.06 µg/kg · min) before and on 3 consecutive days after operation.

Before operation the circulatory reactivity was similar to that reported earlier in the literature (cf. v. Euler, 1958). After operation the stroke volume increase during infusion of adrenaline was less pronounced than before operation (Fig. 6). The heart rate increase was unaltered as was also the metabolic and respiratory response.

Changes in arterial pH and P_{CO_2} are known to alter the reacti-

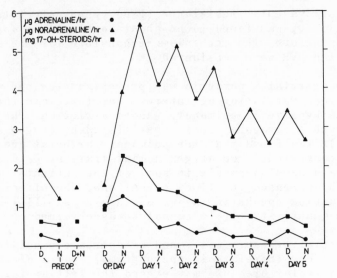

Fig. 5. Urinary excretion of adrenaline (●), noradrenaline
(▲) and 17-hydroxycorticosteroids (■) before and
on 5 days afteroperation. D = day value, N = night
value.

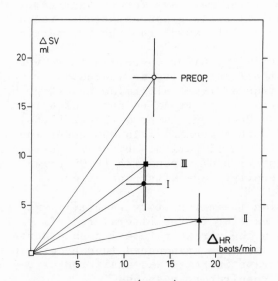

Fig. 6. Changes in heart rate (Δ HR) and stroke volume (Δ SV),
during adrenaline infusion compared with the control
value (□) of the same day before and on 3 consecutive
days after operation.

vity to adrenaline (Campbell, Houle, Crisp, Weil & Brown,1958) as is also severe arterial hypoxaemia (Surtshin, 1948). In the present study such changes did not occur, however.

Under normal conditions the stroke volume increase during the adrenaline infusion is partly due to a 'peripheral' factor, i.e. venoconstriction which enhances the venous return to the heart, and partly due to a 'central' factor, i.e. a positive inotropic effect. After operation an increased venous tone is probably present even before the adrenaline infusion, as concluded indirectly from our observations. The volume displacement of a one unit change in the radius of an already constricted vessel is less than that of a dilated vessel. Therefore the decrease in effect of the adrenaline infusion on the stroke volume response after operation may perhaps be even fully explained by the peripheral geometrical change. Our observations therefore neither demonstrate nor exclude the occurrence of a myocardial tachyphylaxis to adrenaline.

Acknowledgements

Financially supported by grants from the Swedish National Association against heart and chest diseases, the Medical Faculty of the University of Uppsala, Viktor and Albertina Molinder's and Gunnar Forsner's foundations.

References

Bendixen, H.H., Laver, M.B. & Flacks, W.E. (1963): Influence of respiratory acidosis on circulatory effect of epinephrine in dogs. Circulation Research, 13, 64.

Bratteby, L.E. (1967): Studies on erytro-kinetics in infancy. VIII Mixing disappearance rates and distribution volume of labelled erythrocytes and, plasma proteins in early infancy. Acta Societas Medicorum Upsaliensis, 72, 243.

Campbell, G.S., Houle, D.B., Crisp, N.W., Weil, M.H. & Brown, Jr. E.B. (1958): Depressed response to intravenous sympathicomimetic agents in humans during acidosis. Diseases of the Chest, 33, 18.

Euler, U.S. v. (1958): Some aspects of the role of noradrenaline and adrenaline in circulation, American Heart Journal, 56, 469.

Surtshin, A., Rodbard, S. & Katz, L.N. (1948): Inhibition of
epinephrine action in severe hypoxaemia. American Journal of
Physiology, 152, 623.

West, J.B. (1966): Regional differences in blood flow and ventilation in the lung. IN: Caro C.G. Advances in Respiratory
Physiology. Edward Arnold (Publishers) Ltd, London.

The results presented here will be published in more extensive
form:

Circulatory effects of moderate alterations in body position
before and in the postoperative period after pulmonary surgery. Acta Societas Medicorum Upsaliensis (1969) in press.

Central circulatory function in the early postoperative period
after pulmomary surgery. To be published in Scandinavian Journal of Thoracic and Cardiovascular Surgery. Together with
L. Johansson, C.J. Westerholm.

Circulatory reactivity to adrenaline and urinary excretion of
noradrenaline and adrenaline in the early postoperative period after pulmonary surgery. To be published in Scandinavian
Journal of Clinical and Laboratory Investigation.

Circulatory effects of Digoxin and Propranolol in the early
postoperative period after pulmonary surgery. To be published
in Scandinavian Journal of Thoracic and cardiovascular surgery.

Changes in total blood volume early after pulmonary surgery
and its relation to changes in stroke volume. To be published
in Acta anaesthesiologica scandinavica. Together with L.E.
Bratteby.

Effects of oxygen on the circulation and the pulmonary vascular resistance in the early postoperative period after pulmonary surgery. To be published in Acta anaesthesiologica scandinavica.

PROPOSED MECHANISMS FOR THE AMELIORATIVE EFFECTS OF

CORTICOSTEROIDS IN SHOCK*

J. C. Houck and J. A. Gladner,

Children's Hospital of the D. C., Washington, D. C.

20009 and N.I.A.M.D., N.I.H., Bethesda, Md. 20014

The authors of this paper make the assumption that corticosteroid administration is helpful to the patient in shock. Experts
in the clinical management of shock debate this proposition elsewhere in this volume; we simply assume it! If this assumption is
true, and at least some clinicians will maintain this proposition,
then why and how can corticosteroids influence the clinical course
of shock? We would propose that corticosteroids can influence
shock both during the initial and the latter phases of this condi-
tion--namely, by inducing bradykininase and stimulating collagen
catabolizing enzymes to provide free amino acids for energy production to the patient.

Previosuly, we have shown that cortisol administration to the
rat results in the induction of both proteolytic and collagenolytic
activities in the extracellular space of their skin (1,2). This
induction has also been shown for collagenase in diploid human
fibroblasts (3) and thus is not unique to the rat. The postulated
significance of these induced enzymes to shock will be developed
below.

The dialyzed and lyophilized 0.15M NaCl extract of normal
rat skin prepared in the cold as described previously contains no
proteolytic activity upon denatured hemoglobin at pH 7.5 or upon
native insoluble collagen at pH 5.5 (1,2). If a similar cutaneous
extract is made from groups of 12 rats each which have received
3mg/kg of cortisol or prednisolone 16 hours prior to sacrifice,
then both of these enzymatic activities can be determined in these
extracts.

---

* Supported in part by NIH grant AM-08168 and ONR grant NR 105-325.

Table I demonstrates the amounts of trichloracetic acid (TCA) soluble tyrosine equivalents released by 5mg/ml of these extracts from denatured hemoglobin after 16 hours incubation (1,2). The amount of soluble hydroxyproline released from insoluble rat skin collagen (10mg/ml) are also reported in this table.

TABLE I

The proteolytic and collagenolytic activities of 5mg/ml of dialyzed and lyophilized 0.15M NaCl extracts of the skin of groups of 12 rats each which had received various steroids and inhibitors of protein biosynthesis.

	Protease (pH 7.5) (µg tyrosine/ml TCA)	Collagenase (pH 5.5) (µg hypro/ml)
Control (solvent)	0	0
Cortisol	280	60
Cortisol+cycloheximide	0	0
Cortisol+actinomycin D	0	0
Prednisolone	270	70
Prednisolone+cycloheximide	0	0
Prednisolone+actinomycin D	0	0
Cortisone	0	0
Prednisone	0	0
Deoxycorticosterone	0	0

These results demonstrate firstly that cortisol and predni-solone, but not cortisone, prednisone or deoxycorticosterone, will effect the release of proteolytic and collagenolytic activity into the extracellular compartment of rat skin and secondly that the prior treatment of these animals with an inhibitor of peptide bound synthesis (cycloheximide) or of RNA synthesis (actinomycin D) completely eliminated the appearance of these enzymes in the skin of these rats. Since the appearance of these enzymes was not associated with increased quantities of acid phosphatase, β-glucu-ronidase, β-galactosidase or aryl sulfatase (1,2) all enzymes of lyosomal origin (4), we conclude that those corticosteroids that the rat can respond to (i.e. these with β-11 OH groups) induce the synthesis of the proteolytic and collagenolytic enzymes, rather than their being released from the lyosomes of skin cells.

The properties of the induced proteolytic activity was studied by incubating crude cortisol released protease preparation (CRPP) with various natural and synthetic substrates. The results are described in Table II, and show that both hemoglobin and fibrin clots could be partially digested by CRPP. The difference in fibrinolytic activity found between heated and unheated fibrin plates suggests that thermolabile plasminogen had been activated by CRPP as well as demonstrating a direct fibrinolytic activity. If fibrin thrombus formation is important to the circulatory prob-

lems of shock patients then perhaps these two fibrinolytic activities of this cortisol induced proteolytic preparation might be
helpful!

TABLE II

Substrate specificity of the induced proteolytic activity of the
0.15M NaCl extracts for the skin of cortisol treated rats.

	Control Extract	Induced Extract
Hemoglobin[1]	0	280μg tyrosine/ml TCA
Fibrin clots[2]		
normal	0	205 sq. mm.
heated	0	145 sq. mm.
TAME[3]	0	0
ATEE[4]	0	5%
APEE[5]	0	+
CBZ pro-phe-[6]	0	+
CBZ pro-phe-o-me[7]	0	+

1) Tyrosine equivalents released into 1 ml of TCA by 5 mg of
extract. 2) Clot lysis in Astrup fibrin plates units per mg extract.
3) Tosyl arginine methyl ester (quantitative pH stat). 4) Acetyl
tyrosine ethyl ester (qualitative). 5) Acetyl phenylalanine ethyl
ester (qualitative). 6) Carbobenzoxy proline-phenylalanine (qualitative). 7) Carbobenzoxy proline-phenylalanine methyl ester.

Table II further indicates that while CRPP was not active
against a trypsin substrate (TAME) it was active against both
chymotrypsin substrates (ATEE and APEE). Associated with this
chymotrypsin-like activity were unique activities against proline-
phenylalanine and pro-phenyl-methyl ester bonds. The significance
of the last point will be discussed later on in this paper.

The demonstration of chymotrypsin-like activity by CRPP
suggested that this enzyme, like chymotrypsin, might attack bradykinin, the pain producing polypeptide which is believed to be
involved importantly in the changes in the permeability of the
microcirculation with injury and shock(5). Male Sprague-Dawley
rats (usually from a germ-free colony) weighing 250 grams were
injected with cortisol, the enzyme preparations were extracted from
the skin and partially purified as described above. Bradykinin
activity was assayed by measuring the smooth muscle contractibility
of either rat uterus or guinea pig ileum employing a transducer-
balance apparatus as described by Erdos (5). Bradykinin breakdown
products were isolated by column chromatography employing suitable
solvent systems. The analysis and amino acid sequences of the
bradykinin peptide fragments were determined by conventional
methods. The detailed biochemistry of these latter investigations
will be reported in a subsequent publication elsewhere.

Incubation of either natural or synthetic bradykinin with
various quantities of cortisol released protease preparation at
pH 7.5, 25°C, produced a rapid and irreversible destruction of the
smooth muscle contraction activity of this compound. Within the
limits of the quantities of enzyme preparations, the loss of bradykinin activity was proportional to the quantities of enzyme preparation employed. When isotonic extracts of rat skins from animals
untreated by cortisol were employed as controls, there was no
bradykinin destruction.

Previously, we have shown that the action of CRPP on denatured
hemoglobin, ATEE and APEE could be completely inhibited by di-
isopropylphosphorofluoridate, (DFP), and that this activity was
maximal at pH 7.5. Prior incubation of CRPP with DFP at pH 7.5
also rapidly inhibited its bradykinin-destroying activity.

In an effort of discern the exact molecular mode of CRPP
activity towards bradykinin, the following investigations were
performed:

Bradykinin was inactivated by a quantity of CRPP sufficient to
give complete inactivation in one hour. The time course release
of products was followed by high voltage paper electrophoresis,
thin layer chromatography, and column chromatography. The hydrolysis products so obtained are compared to bradykinin in Table III.

TABLE III

Products of cortisol induced proteolytic activity acting upon
purified bradykinin.

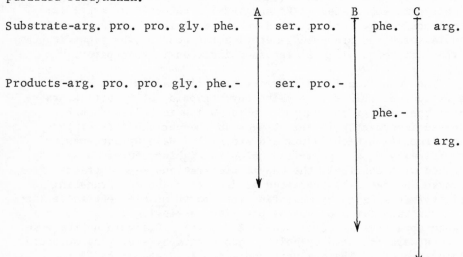

Examination of the final products following the action of CRPP on bradykinin disclosed that the protease preparation must contain at least three individual enzymes which act either independently or in concert upon bradykinin. These results lend themselves the following conclusion and could be verified by further experimentation. As shown in Tables II and III, endopeptidase A hydrolyzes the phe-ser bond very rapidly and is the primary induced enzyme insofar as bradykinin inactivation, hemoglobin hydrolysis, and ATEE and APEE hydrolysis is concerned. Judgin by its slow rate against hemogloblin and synthetic substrates versus its rapid inactivation of bradykinin, it is most interesting to consider that it is a specific bradykininase and a "limited protease" of a rather high order of specificity.

Peptidase B is a very unique carboxypeptidase in that it liberates free phenylalanine from a penultimate proline. No such enzyme has been reported to date. Rats which were not cortisol treated do not contain the enzyme. This exo-peptidase could be examined against the specific substrate cbz-pro-phe. The reaction of CRPP towards this substrate yeilded free phenylalanine. From the examination of the bardykinin degradation products, it is obvious that the free phenylalanine comes from position 8 since one can identify the peptides ser-pro and the peptide arg-pro-gly-phe. At no time was there any arg-pro-pro-gly-present. Thus, the enzyme appears to be a very unusual carboxypeptidase which requires a penultimate proline residue. Whether or not it is specific for only the prolylphenylalanine bond is still under investigation. The activity of this enzyme toward release of free phenylalanine from cbz-pro-phe was also inhibited by DFP, a most unusual finding for a carboxypeptidase. A further testing of validity for the existence of peptidase A and B activities in the CRPP is the ability of the preparation to yield free phenylalanine from cbz-pro-phe-0-Met. Peptidase A hydrolyzes the substrate to cbz-pro-phe and methanol, followed by the reaction of peptidase B to yield free phenylalanine.

Finally, peptidase C appears to be similar, but not necessarily the same as classical carboxypeptidase B. Close examination indicates that following incubation with DFP, CRPP shows a very slow reaction leaving to the release of free arginine coupled with the loss of activity when reacted with bradykinin. However, this reaction is very slow. It is more probable that peptidase A must first hydrolyze the bradykinin into the two peptides before peptidase C acts upon it. The action of peptidase C is, of course, the rate determining step for the subsequent release of free phenylalanine during the bradykinin breakdown mediated by CRPP.

The induced collagenolytic activity was found to be soluble in 65% saturated ammonimum sulfate and was excluded from Sephadex-100 columns. This partially purified collagenase was concentrated

by electric focusing at pH 5.2 into one double band in subsequent
acrylamide gel electrophoresis. This collagenase was thus purified
over 400 fold from its concentration is the initial saline extract.

A comparison of the properties of CRPP [at pH 5.5, the
optimal pH for collagenolysis (1,2)] and the purified induced
collagenase and CRPP attacked only collagen at pH 5.5.

The products from insoluble collagen-collagenase or CRPP
incubation mixtures (16 hours) were then subjected to molecular
sieving using Amicon graded molecular sieves in series under
pressure. The relative amounts of these products were determined
from the 220mμ absorptive capacity of the various solutions and
free hydroxyproline was determined according to Prockup and Udenfreund (6). These results are presented in Table IV and indicate
that while no free hydroxyproline was found using pure collagenase,
the induced skin preparation (CRPP) did release free imino acid
and in general more hydrolysis products of a smaller molecular
size than did the pure collagenase itself.

TABLE IV

Substrates and products hydrolyzed and released by crude and purified collagenase from cortisol induced rat skins.

Substrate	Crude Skin Extract (pH 5.5)	Purified Collagenase
Hemoglobin	0	0
Soluble Collagen	+	+
Insoluble Collagen	+	+
ATEE	0	0
TAME	0	0
Products (<100,000)		
>50,000	±	+
>30,000	+	++
>10,000	+	+++
>1,000	+++	+
<1,000	++	±
Free hydroxyproline	+	0

These results suggest that a number of enzymes participated in the
further degradation of the products of the cortisol induced
collagenase resulting in the release of free amino acids! This
is turn suggests that since as much as 30% of the insoluble collagen
of rat skin can be mobilized by cortisol administration (1,2,7),
these amino acids might be valuable to the energy metabolism of
the animal via liver glyconeogenesis.

Therefore, a larger number 'of 200 gm rats were fasted for 24 hours and then received <u>via</u> stomach tube some 40μ moles of one of four amino acids found in large amounts in collagen while other rats received similar amounts of amino acids <u>not</u> commonly found in collagen. After four hours, these animals were sacrificed and their liver glycogen determined (8). The results are summarized in Table V and indicate that the amino and imino acids of collagen

TABLE V

The effects of various amino acids upon liver glyconeogenesis when administered by stomach tube to fasted rats.

Strongly glyconeogenic	Weakly glyconeogenic
1) glycine	5) tyrosine
2) hydroxyproline	6) tryptophane
3) proline	7) phenylalanine
4) alanine	8) methionine

(these four consititute over 70% of the amino acids in collagen) were all extremely potent in producing liver glyconeogenesis while the four amino acids uncommon to collagen were barely glyconeogenic at all!

Thus, it appears possible that one of the consequences of corti-sol administration is the mobilization of skin collagen amino acids (via collagenase induction) which produce increased amounts of liver glycogen and hence energy to the host. Approximately one-third of the body protein of the rat is collagen (9) and almost one-half of the body collagen is found in the skin! Thus, the catabolism of cutaneous collagen by cortisol induction of a colla-genase could represent a very significant metabolic reserve pool!

The demonstration of C^{14} labeled liver glycogen after cortisol administration to animals whose collagen was prelabled C^{14} proline, would not be helpful since a number of non-collagen proteins in-corporate proline and cortisol is known to produce protein catabo-lism. We therefore tried another approach--namely, we administered 100 μ curies of C^{14} proline to BN rats and then after making sure that their skin collagen contained C^{14} hydroxyproline (converted from C^{14} proline), large numbers of small pieces of radioactive skin from these rats were grafted onto other BN rats (these animals are immunotolerant to each others skin grafts). After two or three weeks, these animal grafts had taken and were grossly healed. Serum samples from the tail vein were taken, precipitated with 4-5 volumes of ethanol and the free hydroxyproline isolated from the ethanol supernatant chemically (6). The specific activity of this free circulating hydroxyproline was approximately 40cpm per μ mole. By six hours after administration of cortisol this

specific activity had increased to about 600 cpm per μ mole!
Thus, significant amounts of free amino acids can be demonstrated
to be released from cutaneous collagen into the circulation with
cortisol administration!

Summary and Conclusions

1) Cortisol induces the synthesis of at least three proteolytic
and one collagenolytic enzyme which appears in the extracellular
compartment of rat skin.

2) The proteases digest fibrin and can activate plasminogen.

3) The proteases destroy bradykinin very rapidly.

4) The collagenase released products of collagenolysis which
can be degraded to free amino acids which in turn are powerful
inducers of liver glyconeogenesis and hence can provide reserve
energy to the host.

5) Therefore, steroid induced enzymes might be important in
restoring the microcirculatory blood flow (via fibrinolysis and
the destruction of bradykinin)and for providing extra energy (via
collagenolysis and consequent liver glyconeogenesis) to the patient
in shock!

REFERENCES

1) Houck, J. C., Patel, Y. M. and Gladner, J. A.: Biochemistry
   Pharmacol. 16: 1099 (1967).

2) Houck, J. C., Sharma, V. K., Patel, Y. M. and Gladner, J. A.,
   Ibid, 17: 2081 (1968).

3) Houck, J. C. and Sharma, V. K.: Science 161: 1361 (1968).

4) Weissmann, G. New Eng. J. Med.273: 1084 (1965).

5) Erdos, E. G., Advan. Pharmacol. 4: 1 (1966).

6) Prockup, D. A. and Udenfreund, J.: Anal. Biochem. 1:228 (1960).

7) Houck, J. C. Amer. J. Pathol. 41: 365 (1962).

8) Stetten, D. and Boxer, G. J. Biol. Chem., 115: 131 (1944).

9) Neuberger, A. Symp. Soc. Exp. Biol., 9: 72 (1955).

SECTION 2

BIOCHEMICAL PATHOLOGY OF SHOCK

PARTICIPATION OF THE KININ-SYSTEM IN DIFFERENT KINDS OF SHOCK[(+)]

M. Rocha e Silva

Department of Pharmacology, Faculty of Medicine

U.S.P., Ribeirão, Prêto, São Paulo, Brazil

The evidences of the participation of the Kinin-system in the etiology of different manifestations of shock derive from the following lines of considerations: a) Activation of proteolytic or estero-lytic enzymes in many kinds of shock: anaphylactic, peptone, bacterial toxins, hemorrhagic, scalding (thermic) etc; b) Variations of the bradykininogen (Bkg) content of plasma following the injection of proteases, animal venoms or in different kinds of shock; c) Detection of free kinins in the blood under shock-like conditions; d) Activation of the Kinin-system in in vitro conditions produced by tissue trauma or by the action of shock-producing agents (Ag-Ab, trypsin, animal venoms, cellulose sulfate, and so forth); e) By the use of inhibitors of the kininogenin-kininogen system or by antagonists of the kinin itself.

We are going to analyse briefly each one of the classes of evidences indicated, with recourse to our own experience and to data that can be found in the literature.

a) ACTIVATION OF PROTEASES IN SHOCK-LIKE CONDITIONS

By far the most important evidence in favor of the release of vaso-active peptides in shock has been the unambiguous demonstration that the fibrinolytic system in plasma is activated under conditions of anaphylactic, peptone and other kinds of shock. As early as in

(+)Aided in part by Research Grant HE 10074-03 from the NIH(USPHS).

1946, with Andrade and Teixeira we could demonstrate that fibrinoly--
sis takes place when the incoagulable blood from animals submitted
to peptone shock is made to clot by addition of the proper amount of
protamine to counterbalance the released heparin. This protamine-fi-
brinolytic test indicated that as soon as the blood of peptone shock
animals is made to clot, a process of redissolution of the coagulum
starts and can be complete in one to three hours as indicated in Table I. By using a different technique Ungar (1947) has shown that
even in vitro, peptone can activate the fibrinolytic system and later on Beraldo (1950) showed that a bradykinin-like material can be
released in anaphylactic and peptone shock. With Holzhacker we have
reported that peptone releases a bradykinin-like activity when normal rats plasma is put in vitro in contact with peptone (Rocha e Silva and Holzhacker, 1959). As far as other kinds of shock (or stress)
are concerned we have to refer to the work by MacFarlane and Biggs
(1946) who observed increased fibrinolysis associated with trauma

Table 1

PROTAMINE - FIBRINOLYTIC TEST IN DOGS SUBMITTED
TO   PEPTONE   SHOCK (Rocha e Silva et al. 1946)

PROTAMINE ADDED (μg/0.5 ml)	OBSERVATION	BEFORE	BLOOD SAMPLES AFTER SEVERAL INTERVALS FOLLOWING THE INJECTION OF 300 mg OF PEPTONE PER KILO OF BODY-WEIGHT:							
			1st injection					2nd injection		3rd injection
		I	II	III	IV	VI	VII	VIII	IX
100	Clotting time (min)	10	12	13	10	8	20	15	10
	fibrinolysis	0	++++	++++	++++	0	++++	0	0
50	Clotting time (min)	8	11	12	8	7	14	9	10
	fibrinolysis	0	+++	++++	+++	0	++	0	0
25	Clotting time (min)	5	8	10	7	9	17	7	8
	fibrinolysis	0	+	+++	+++	0	0	0	0
10	Clotting time (min)	5	6	11	9	10	12	5	5
	fibrinolysis	0	++	+++	0	0	0	0	0
0	Clotting time (min)	4	∞	∞	∞	∞	∞	∞	∞
	fibrinolysis	0	−	−	−	−	−	−	−

++++. Total fibrinolysis in less than 1 hr.; +++. total fibrinolysis in less than 2 hr.; ++. total fibrinolysis in less
than 3 hr.; +. partial fibrinolysis; 0, no fibrinolysis for at least ˙24 hours. The minimum clotting time indicates
the optimum amount of protamine and therefore the amount of heparin present in the blood samples.

and surgical operations and of Tagnon et al.(1946) on fibrinolysis
and fall of fibrinogen during hemorrhagic shock. It would be difficult to review the pertinent literature ever since these basic data
have been obtained. Reviews and additional data can be found in Ungar and Hayashi (1958), Gans et al. (1963), Rocha e Silva (1968),
Back et al.(1968) and many others.

The scheme presented in Fig. 1, shows the complexity of the phenomena and the variety of mediators that might take a part in the
three kinds of shock mentioned: anaphylaxis, traumatic and scalding.

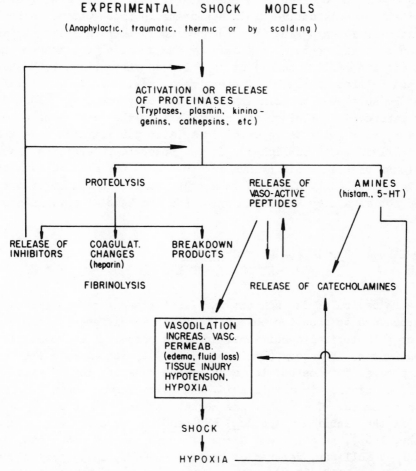

Fig. 1 – Operational scheme on the participation of proteases in
the etiology of shock. Modified from Back et al.(1968).

However, the main lines of evidences on activation of proteases in shock refer to activation of fibrinolysin or of plasmin, because it is easier to show activation of a fibrinolytic activity. But, on the other hand, doubts have been cast on the efficacy of plasmin to release active kinins from their precursor (bradykininogen) in plasma. Another enzyme in plasma that has been called plasma-kallikrein, that we can call plasma-kininogenin (or ase) might also be activated under certain circumstances, and Vogt (1964) assumed that plasmin would act through activation of the above mentioned enzyme. In a series of papers, however, Henriques et al.(1966,69) have shown that plasmin acting upon pure bradykininogen would release active kinin, that apparently is methionyl-lysyl-bradykinin. In fresh plasma this material could be changed into bradykinin, since there are indications that the only active kinin appearing in fresh plasma is bradykinin itself. To this line of evidence should be paralleled the activation of a kininogenin in plasma by the drastic treatment of heating it (to the boiling point) at pH = 2.0 as shown first by Rocha e Silva and Holzhacker (1959). The enzyme so activated is completely blocked by soya bean trypsin inhibitor and only partially blocked by Kunitz pancreatic inhibitor and not at all by the Kazal pancreatic inhibitor, as it will be reported in a later publication (Reis and Rocha e Silva, to be published). It is, however, interesting that the release of bradykinin by heating the rat's paw at 46ºC is also completely blocked by SBTI and less so by Kunitz inhibitor or trasylol and not at all by Kazal inhibitor (Garcia Leme et al., in the press).

b) FALL IN Bkg IN PLASMA FROM ANIMALS SUBMITTED TO SEVERAL
KINDS OF SHOCK

The reduction of Bkg content was first thought to constitute a safe procedure to show the release of kinin in different kinds of shock or pathological conditions. For this purpose a micromethod was devised in our laboratory (Diniz et al., 1961) to estimate the total Bkg in plasma. This method is based on the denaturation of plasma proteins by heating in acetic acid, and releasing the total activity with an excess of trypsin. The method was applied to anaphylactic shock (in the rabbit and the dog) and hemorrhagic shock (Diniz and Carvalho, 1963), in different kinds of anaphylactoid reactions, such as shock by Kollidon, dextran or heating (Greeff, 1965), cellulose sulfate (Rothschild, 1968) and in shocks produced by proteolytic enzymes (Corrado et al., 1966). In all cases, a significant fall in

Bkg occurred.

The method, however, has two main pitfalls:
1) the occurrence of a Bk potentiating factor generated in
plasma, by the action of trypsin (Aarsen, 1968; Hamberg, 1968); and
2) the possibility that a decrease of total Bkg might occur as a consequence of a destruction of the precurssor without the release of
active kinin.

There is a third possibility stressed recently by Urbanitz and
Habermann (1969), that the fall in Bkg can simply reflect the decrease in total protein in plasma. This last inconvenience, however, can
be simply overcome by a simultaneous estimation of the total protein
in parallel with the Bkg estimations. Since we dont know the fate of
the Bkg leaving the circulation, this situation may introduce a serious incertitude in the method.

The first objection can also be overcome by using as standard,
natural bradykinin prepared by making the venom of B. jararaca to
act upon fresh plasma, or trypsin to act upon denatured plasma. If
the standard is made with the plasma of the same animal, the differences arising from potentiating factors could be overcome.

But, the second objection, namely that of the shocking agent to
produce a destruction of the kininogen without the release of active
kinins is of course a serious pitfall to the method and has been the
object of a fresh investigation in our laboratory. The diagrams presented in Fig. 2A,B, show that drastic reductions of Bkg in vitro
can be observed under conditions which are not parallel to the release of active kinins. Nagarse and pronase, which are very poor re-
leasers of kinins in vitro, produced the most drastic falls in Bkg
content, especially in the dog, though trypsin that can easily be
shown to release kinin in vitro and in vivo, did affect very slightly the Bkg content of fresh plasma (Reis, 1969).

The failure to show active kinins when such enzymes as pronase,
nagarse and even kallikrein (Padutin) are put in vitro in contact
with fresh plasma might derive from the rapid destruction of the active material formed by a different component of the enzyme preparation. This was actually shown as regards pronase, where two fractions
were separated by electrophoresis, one which releases and the other
that destroys the active kinin (Reis, 1969). It is possible, however,
that in vivo a situation can arise in which the releasing activity

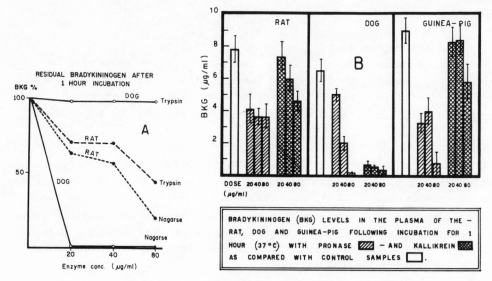

Fig. 2 – Residual Bkg after 1 hour incubation with: A) Trypsin
and Nagarse in the rat and dog plasma; and B) Pronase
and Kallikrein, at the doses indicated in the abscis-
sae. According to Reis (1969).

is more powerful than the destroying one, as it appears to be obvious with the common commercial preparation of kallikrein (Padutin).
In fact with large doses of nagarse injected _in vivo_ producing a fatal shock in the dog, the Bkg vanished and active kinins could be detected in the circulation, as shown in Fig. 3.

c) DETECTION OF FREE KININS IN THE BLOOD IN SHOCK-LIKE CONDITIONS

As mentioned in the last paragraph, the great difficulty of detecting kinin activity when proteases are injected into the intact
animal, comes from the rapid inactivation of the kinin by natural kininases present in blood and tissues, and possibly also by the action
of the enzyme itself. In the case of trypsin, slight variations in
Bkg content of fresh plasma can be detected, when the shock is produced by moderate doses of the enzyme. However, if a profound shock
is produced by injection of large amounts of the enzyme, a deep fall
in the Bkg levels could be detected with appearance of active kinin
in the circulating blood (Corrado et al., 1966).

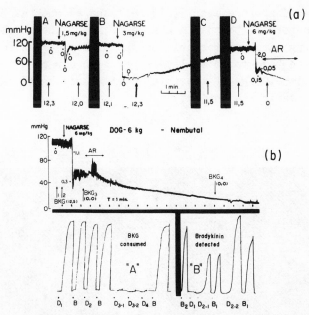

Fig. 3 - (a) Injections of increasing doses of Nagarse showing
the effect upon blood pressure, free kinins (see figures under tracings) and Bkg (figures under arrows).
(b) A single injection of 6 mg/kg of Nagarse in a dog
of 6 kg body weight. Note that the Bkg falls rapidly
to 0, with appearance of active kinin, in B, in the
circulating blood. According to Corrado et al.(1966).

The experiments mentioned above were done in the conventional
way, by collecting samples of blood before and after the injection
of the enzyme. In a more recent contribution of our laboratory (Ferreira and Rocha e Silva, 1969) the sophisticated technique of super-
fusion described by Vane (1964) using the cat jejunum strip (very
sensitive to bradykinin) and the rat colon (sensitive to angiotensin)
cascaded with the blood of the dog to which minute amounts of chymotrypsin, trypsin and nagarse were given intravenously was employed.
A definite release of kinin with doses of nagarse or trypsin that
hardly affected the total Bkg content could be observed, as shown in
Figs. 4 and 5. The activity released was potentiated by BPF (bradykinin potentiating factor). These experiments would further stress
the fact that release of kinin can occur without any detectable fall
in blood Bkg. This can be well understood if we consider that a dog
with 2.5 liters of plasma can have as much as 2.50 mg of bradykinin
as Bkg, and that a few µg of bradykinin can produce a deep fall in

blood pressure. Therefore even if it releases as much as 50 μg of
bradykinin, there will be only a change of 2% of the total, such a
difference being hardly detectable by the biological estimation of
Bkg. Actually we have to go to levels of the order of 5 to 10% (equivalent to 125 to 250 μg) of the total content of Bkg to have a significant decrease in its content.

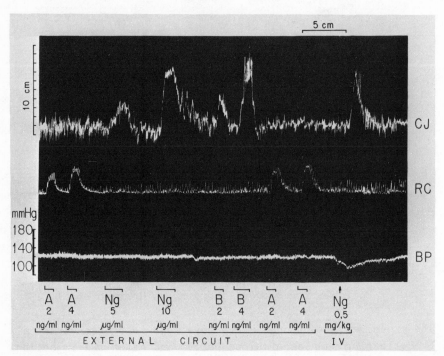

Fig. 4 - Vane's cascade to detect release of kinin in the in-
        tact dog. CJ, cat jejunum preparation; RC, rat colon;
        BP, blood pressure in mm Hg. The injection of nagarse
        (Ng) in the external circuit produced contraction of
        CJ, but not of RC indicating release of bradykinin but
        not of angiotensin. Much larger doses of nagarse by in-
        travenous route (IV) produced similar effect and defi-
        nite fall in BP. Angiotensin (A) produced a contraction
        of the rat colon, but not of the cat jejunum; and Bra-
        dykinin (B) did the same as nagarse. According to Fer-
        reira and Rocha e Silva (1969).

    A last remark about the attempts to detect free kinin in the
circulating blood. In experiments, of heating of the rat's paw to

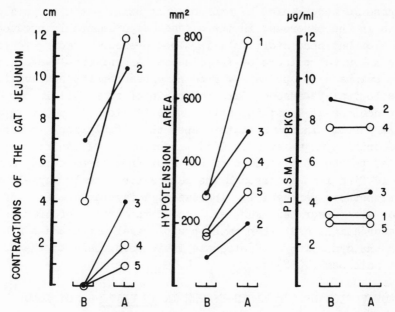

Fig. 5 — Vane's cascade with record of BP (hypotension area).
The points represent 5 experimental animals receiving
trypsin (o——o) or nagarse (●——●) intravenously,
in the doses of 0.4 mg/kg and 1 mg/kg respectively.
Left and middle panel, B and A represent the effects
before and after injection of BPF (bradykinin potentiating factor). Right panel, indicates plasma Bkg,be-
fore (B) and after (A) the injection of the enzymes.
According to Ferreira and Rocha e Silva (1969).

46ºC (thermic edema), in which a conspicuous bradykinin-like activity can be detected we had to perfuse the subcutaneous tissue in order to show such kinin-like activity, as mentioned in other papers
(Rocha e Silva and Antonio, 1960; Rocha e Silva, Garcia Leme and Souza, 1969). We might therefore wonder whether we are not looking at
the wrong place, namely the circulating blood, to detect active kinins under conditions in which a prolonged fall of blood pressure,
producing deep hypoxia of the tissues, might establish the conditions
for activation of the kinin system outside the blood vessels.   The
same remark could be done about attempts to detect active kinin in
the blood of ischemic limbs after temporary ligature of the main artery.

The interest of these facts is great to understand the etiology
of shock and pain in acute pancreatic necrosis. The first stage of

the disease is accompanied by excruciating pain, edema and small hemorrhages in the pancreas. In the disease experimentally produced in
dogs, a slow but persistent fall in blood pressure leading to fatal
shock is the usual outcome of the disease (experimental pancreatitis
in dogs, guinea pigs and rats). From numerous reports now available
it seems logical to assume that the origin of such fall in blood
pressure derives at least in part from activation of the kinin system arising from kininogen that escaped the circulation. In experiments reported by Ryan et al.(1965) the severity of shock was well
correlated to the total amount of Bkg lost from circulation, and
that would find its way through the pancreatic vessels largely dilated and with their permeability increased. A favorable effect of trasylol was also described. Further data on the effect of trasylol in
acute pancreatitis and other pathophysiological phenomena can be
found in the Symposium on Proteinase Inhibitors, held at the N.Y.
Acad. of Sciences (1968).

d) ACTIVATION OF THE KININ-SYSTEM IN IN VITRO CONDITIONS

In spite of the large body of evidence showing the participation
of the kinin system in inflammatory reactions, and here I can refer
to the several Symposia on the subject (New York Academy of Sciences
1964,66; Florence Symposium, 1965; Ribeirão Prêto Symposium, 1966;
Como Symposium, 1968; Fiesole Symposium, 1969), we have relatively
few data upon the release of kinin in trauma produced upon the tissues (see mainly data in Keele and Armstrong, 1964). On scalding of
the skin, at 96ºC for 15 seconds (Rocha e Silva and Rosenthal, 1961)
or heating the rat's paw at 43-46ºC, the data are more abundant. By
using the double coaxial perfusion we have now (Garcia Leme, Hamamura and Rocha e Silva, in the press) a large wealth of data showing
the direct release of kinins when the temperature reaches 46ºC and
the experimental conditions varied at large limits of pH and under
the action of inhibitors, such as SBTI, pancreatic inhibitors, trasylol, hexadimethrine and so forth. The interesting point already
mentioned is the indication that the enzyme so activated under mild
temperatures (43-46ºC) and around the normal pH of the tissues, is
possibly the same that is activated by drastic treatment of boiling
at pH = 2.0 and adjusted to pH 7.4. At least the behavior of such an
enzyme toward the pancreatic inhibitors and the soya bean trypsin
inhibitor is surprisingly parallel. The contention by others (Urbanitz and Habermann, 1969) that activation of the kinin system by heating the paw to 46ºC depends upon collection of the perfusates upon
ice, could not be confirmed. The material can pass directly from the

paw to the bath containing the rat uterus, without any difference in detectable activity.

As far as the in vitro activation of kininogenins in guinea pig plasma by the complex Ag-Ag is concerned definite evidences have been presented by Movat and colleagues (1969) and at least two diffe- rent enzymes appear to be activated under such conditions.

Along these lines we have to consider activation of the kinino- genin-kininogen system in vitro and probably also in vivo by sulfat- ed polysaccharides or polymers (Rocha e Silva et al., 1969). Since Dr. Rothschild is going to present the results of his group, I leave that point open.

d) EVIDENCES DERIVED FROM THE USE OF ANTAGONISTS OF THE KININOGENIN-
   -KININOGEN SYSTEM AND OF BRADYKININ ITSELF

It would be impossible to review the innumerable papers in which trasylol has been utilized in a critical or uncritical way to show amelioration of shock symptoms, as an indirect evidence of the par- ticipation of kinin in such pathophysiological phenomena. We can re- fer to several symposia in which trasylol and other protease inhibi- tors have been studied as agents to counteract shock symptoms (Gross and Kroneberg, 1965; New York Academy of Sciences, 1968 and others).

Both trasylol and its simile Kunitz inhibitor are not very pow- erful inhibitors of the release of kinin by plasma enzymes. This was shown to be particularly true in the activation of kinin by heating the rat's paw at 46ºC and collecting the active material by the dou- ble coaxial perfusion. Not only huge doses are needed, but there is always an "escape" phenomenon, namely reactivation of the kinin sys- tem in spite of the trasylol being kept in the perfusion fluid. The same "escape" phenomenon was observed in the in vitro activation of the kininogenin in plasma boiled at pH = 2.0. Kazal pancreatic inhi- bitor had no effect at all in either system.

The most powerful inhibitor of the plasma system has been the SBTI, that can stop activation in both cases mentioned and the inhi- bition persists while the inhibitor is kept in the system. An inter- mediary antagonist of the release has been the polybrene, or hexadi- methrine bromide, which can be applied intraperitoneally and had a reducing action upon thermic edema in the rat's paw.

In the case of trasylol we can make the remark that under certain conditions it can prevent destruction of the active kinin and therefore it might even potentiate the kinin in the case it has been released (Greenbaum et al., 1969). It might be possible to explain in that way the "escape" phenomenon described above, but we have so far no evidences in favor of such an interpretation.

Finally we can think of the possibility of using antagonists of bradykinin to evidence its participation in shock. As far as specific antagonists of bradykinin are concerned we still are in the preliminary phase to try several classes of compounds looking for a specific anti-bradykinin agent. The ones we have found are either weak or unspecific, blocking also the actions of histamine, 5-HT or acetylcholine (Rocha e Silva and Garcia Leme, 1964; Garcia Leme and Rocha e Silva, 1965). Some inhibition of thermic edema was found with tricyclic compounds (imipramine, cyproheptadine, phenothiazines such as chlorpromazine) and the α-adrenolytic compounds, dibenzyline and dibenamine. These compounds were found to antagonize the effects of bradykinin upon the smooth muscle of the guinea pig ileum but to potentiate the duration of the hypotensive effect of bradykinin in the dog. This apparent paradox might be explained by recent experiments of Al-Katib and Baba (1969) showing that phenoxybenzamine (dibenzyline) blocks the venoconstricting action of bradykinin in the rabbit and reduces the vasopressor action of bradykinin in animals submitted to hemorrhagic shock. Whether this finding might contribute to explain the therapeutic effect of dibenzyline in shock can be a matter for speculation, at the present moment.

CONCLUSIONS

With the rapid review of the main points concerning the participation of the kinin system in different kinds of shock, we have to be satisfied mainly with indirect evidences in most cases. We have to deal separately with each kind of shock: anaphylactic, peptone, traumatic, hemorrhagic or by scalding or heating, to ponder over the evidences so far collected. We have to consider also other mediators, such as histamine, 5-HT, and now the classes of compounds, the prostaglandins and the so-called slow-reacting substances (SRS-A). In anaphylactic shock, histamine plays probably a major role, though anti-histamines are rather ineffective in preventing the fall in blood pressure in many species or the protracted shock in guinea pigs. The evidences for the participation of the kinin system in ana-

phylaxis derive indirectly from the observation that the Ag x Ab complex is able to activate the kinin system in vitro in guinea   pig
plasma and that the bradykininogen (Bkg) content is reduced in vivo
in anaphylactic shock in the dog and the rabbit. In peptone shock,
a direct activation of the kinin system has long been observed in
the dog and later confirmed in the rat, for instance. The basis to
consider participation of the kinin system in any kind of traumatic
shock derives from the known fact that lesions inflicted on tissues
bring about activation of the kinin system. As far as thermic shock
is concerned, we have considerable evidence that a release of bradykinin takes place in the rat treated by heat as soon as the temperature reaches a level of 43-46ºC. No histamine is released under such
mild heating conditions. On the other hand, it has been shown by the
air-pouch technique that large amounts of histamine and kinins are
released from the rat's skin when scalded at 96ºC for 15 seconds.
In the case of shock by bacterial endotoxins the evidences of an activation of the kinin system are scanty, the drop in circulating bradykininogen being the only indication . A direct activation of the
kinin system could not be obtained by direct contact of endotoxins
with plasma. Concerning shocks produced by enzymes, such as trypsin,
nagarse, pronase, snake venoms containing proteases, work from our
laboratory has shown that: a) a small drop in blood pressure is
usually connected with slight reduction in circulatory Bkg; b) in
order to reduce conspicuously the content of Bkg in dog plasma, large amounts of such enzymes have to be injected leading to an irreversible fall in blood pressure; c) in such severe cases, active kinins
could be detected in the circulating blood.

On the basis of such results a general discussion of the available evidences of the participation of the kinin system in several
kinds of shock will be presented.

REFERENCES

Aarsen, R.N. (1968): Sensitization of guinea pig ileum to the action
   of bradykinin by trypsin hydrolysate of ox and rabbit plasma.
   Brit. J. Pharmacol., 32, 453.

Al-Katib, H.A. and Baba, W.J. (1969): The action of certain haloal-
   kylamines on some biological activities of bradykinin. Brit. J.
   Pharmacol., 36, 635.

Back, N., Wilkens, H. and Steger, R. (1968): Proteinases and pro-

teinase inhibitors in experimental shock states. Ann. N.Y.Acad.
Sci., 146, 491.

Beraldo, W.T. (1950): Formation of bradykinin in anaphylactic and
peptone shock. Am. J. Physiol., 163, 283.

Corrado, A.P., Reis, M.L., Carvalho, I.F. and Diniz, C.R. (1966) :
Bradykininogen and bradykinin in the cardiovascular shock produced by proteolytic enzymes. Biochem. Pharmacol., 15, 959.

Diniz, C.R. and Carvalho, I.F. (1963): A micro–method for determination of bradykininogen under several conditions. Ann. N.Y.Acad.
Sci., 104, 77.

Diniz, C.R., Carvalho, I.F., Ryan, J. and Rocha e Silva, M. (1961):
A micro–method for the determination of bradykininogen in blood
plasma. Nature (London) 192, 1194.

Ferreira, S.H. and Rocha e Silva, M. (1969): Liberation of a bradykinin–like substance in the circulating blood of dogs by trypsin, chymotrypsin and nagarse. Brit. J. Pharmacol., 36, 611.

Gans, H., Hanson, M. and Krivit, W. (1963): Effect of endotoxin on
clotting mechanism. III. On the relationship between hypercoagulability, plasminogen activator activity and antithrombin activity. Surgery 53, 792.

Garcia Leme, J., Hamamura, L. and Rocha e Silva, M. (1969): Effect
of anti–protease agents and hexadimethrine bromide upon the
release of a bradykinin–like substance during heating (46ºC) of
rat's paw. In the Press.

Greeff, K. (1965): Die Kininogengehalte des Plasmas beim experimen-
tellen Schock. In: Gross, R. und Kroneberg, G., Edit., Neue
Aspekte der Trasylol Therapie. F.K. Schattauer–Verlag, Stuttgart, pg. 135.

Hamberg, U. (1968): Plasma protease and kinin release with special
reference to plasmin. Ann. N.Y. Acad. Sci., 146, 517.

Henriques, O.B., Lavras, A.A.C., Fichman, M. and Picarelli, Z. P.
(1966): Plasma enzymes that release kinins. Biochem. Pharmacol.
15, 31.

Henriques, O.B., Gapanhuk, E., Kauritcheva, N. and Budnitskaya, P.
(1969): Methionyl–lysyl–bradykinin release from plasma kininogen by plasmin. Biochem. Pharmacol., 18, 1788.

Keele, C.A. and Armstrong, D. (1964): Substances producing pain and itch. E. Arnold (Publishers), Ltd., London.

MacFarlane, R.G. and Biggs, R. (1946): Observations on fibrinolysis spontaneous activity associated with surgical operations, trauma, etc. Lancet 2, 862.

Movat, H.Z., Treloar, M.P., Burrowes, C.E. and Takeuchi, Y. (1969): Isolation and partial purification of two kininogenases and of permeability factors from plasma. Fiesole Symposium. Pharmacol. Res. Commun., 1, 176.

Reis, M.L. (1969): Liberação de cininas por enzimas proteolíticas. Tese: Fac. Farm. e Odontol., Ribeirão Prêto, São Paulo.

Reis, M.L. and Rocha e Silva, M.: To be published.

Rocha e Silva, M. (1968): Pharmacological actions of proteolytic enzymes (proteases). Ann. N.Y. Acad. Sci., 146, 448.

Rocha e Silva, M., Andrade, S.O. and Teixeira, R.M. (1946): Fibrinolysis in peptone and anaphylactic shock in dog. Nature 157, 801.

Rocha e Silva, M. and Antonio, A. (1960): Release of bradykinin and the mechanism of production of a thermic edema (45ºC) in the rat's paw. Med. Exper., 3, 371.

Rocha e Silva, M., Cavalcanti, R.Q. and Reis, M.L. (1969): Anti-inflammatory action of sulfated polysaccharides. Biochem. Pharmacol., 18, 1285.

Rocha e Silva, M. and Garcia Leme, J. (1963): Antagonists of bradykinin. Med. Exper. (Basel) 8, 287.

Rocha e Silva, M., Garcia Leme, J. and Souza, J.M. de (1969): The significance of the kinin-system in inflammatory reactions. In: Intern. Symp. on Inflammation, Biochemistry and Drug Interaction (Como, 1968). In the Press.

Rocha e Silva, M. and Holzhacker, E. (1959): Liberation of bradykinin from plasma by treatment with peptone or by boiling with HCl. Arch. Intern. Pharmacodyn., 122, 168.

Rocha e Silva, M. and Rosenthal, S.R. (1961): Release of pharmacologically active substances from the rat skin in vivo following thermal injury. J. Pharmacol. Exptl. Therap., 132, 110.

Rothschild, A.M. (1968): Some pharmacodynamic properties of cellulose sulphate, a kininogen–depleting agent in the rat. Brit. J. Pharmacol., 33, 501.

Ryan, J.W., Moffat, J.C. and Thompson, A.G. (1965): Role of bradykinin in the development of acute pancreatitis. Nature 204, 1212.

Symposia:

Acute Inflammatory Response (1964). Ann. N.Y. Acad. Sci., 116, 747.

Fross, R. und Kroneberg, G. Edit. (1965). Internationales Symposion, Grosse Ledder, on Neue Aspekte der Trasylol Therapie. F.K. Schattauer–Verlag, Stuttgart.

International Symposium on Hypotensive Peptides (1966): Florence (1965); Erdös, E.G., Back, N., Sicuteri, F. and Wilde, A.F. Editors, Springer–Verlag, New York, Heidelberg.

International Symposium on Vaso–Active Polypeptides: Bradykinin and Related Kinins (1966). Rib. Prêto, M. Rocha e Silva and Hanna A. Rothschild, Editors, Edart Edit. São Paulo (1967).

International Symposium on Inflammation Biochemistry and Drug Interaction (1968). A. Bertelli and J.C. Houck, Editors, Como, Italy. Excerpta Med. I.C.S. 188,

Chemistry, Pharmacology, and Clinical Applications of Proteinase Inhibitors (1968). N. Back, Edit., Ann. N.Y. Acad. Sci., 146, 361–787.

International Symposium on Cardiovascular and Neuro–Actions of Bradykinin and Related Kinins (1969). M. Rocha e Silva and F. Sicuteri, Editors, Fiesole, Pharmacol. Res. Commun. Vol. 1, 127–209.

Tagnon, H.J., Levenson, S.M., Davidson, C.S. and Taylor, F.H.L.(1946): The occurrence of fibrinolysis in shock with observation on the prothrombin time and the plasma fibrinogen during hemorrhagic shock. Am. J. Med. Sci., 211, 88.

Ungar, G. (1947): Release of proteolytic enzyme in anaphylactic and peptone shock "in vitro". Lancet 1, 708.

Ungar, G. and Hayashi, H. (1958): Enzymatic mechanisms in allergy. Ann. Allergy 16, 542.

Urbanitz, D. and Habermann, E. (1969): In vivo investigations on the role of the kinin system in tissue injury and shock syndrome. In: Intern. Symp. on Cardiovascular and Neuro-Actions of Bradykinin and Related Kinins, Fiesole Symposium. Pharmacol. Res. Commun., 1, 201.

Vane, J.R. (1964): The use of isolated organs for detecting active substances in the circulating blood. Brit. J. Pharmacol., 23, 360.

Vogt, W. (1964): Kinin formation by plasmin, an indirect process mediated by activation of kallikrein. J. Physiol. (London) 170, 153.

THE GENERATION OF KININS IN THE CIRCULATION OF THE

DOG DURING HYPOTENSION DUE TO BLOOD LOSS

H. Berry, J.G. Collier and J.R. Vane

Department of Pharmacology, Institute of Basic Medical
Sciences, Royal College of Surgeons of England,
Lincoln's Inn Fields, London W. C. 2

Many authors have suggested that kinins circulate in the
blood of shocked animals (Erdös, 1966) . The methods used for
measuring kinins have been either indirect , in which kininogen
levels have been serially estimated and any reduction taken to
infer kinin release (Webster & Clark, 1959) or direct in which
lengthy and difficult extraction is required (Brocklehurst & Zeitlin,
1967). Both approaches have disadvantages; they share the
limitation inherent in estimating concentrations from intermittently
sampled blood, and furthermore neither method necessarily
reflects the intrinsic activity of kinins in the animal during shock.
The recent observation of Habermann (Symposium on kinins,
Fiesole, 1969) that the fall in kininogen level in shock parallels
the fall in other plasma proteins, makes the 'kininogen depletion'
method for kinin estimation especially difficult to interpret.

We have used the blood-bathed organ technique (Vane, 1964)
which overcomes the problems outlined above, to investigate
kinin release during hypotension induced by blood loss in the dog.
This technique provides immediate, continuous, and direct
estimation of changes in concentration of selected circulating
vaso-active hormones.

Methods

The experiments were carried out on dogs of both sexes
weighing 12-30 kg. Anaesthesia was induced using halothane, and

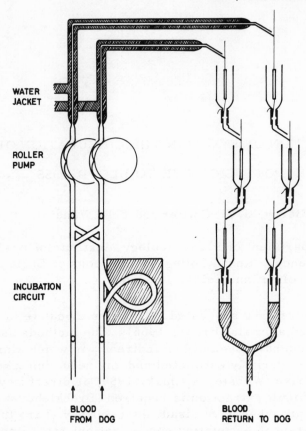

Fig. 1. Diagram of the extracorporeal circuit of the blood-
bathed organ technique.

and maintained by chloralose (100 mg/kg I.V.) and injections of
pentobarbitone sodium. The dogs were respired with air by inter-
mittent positive pressure ventilation. Blood for assay was withdrawn
through polyethylene cannulae in the femoral artery, right atrium,
portal vein, or superior mesenteric vein depending on the nature
of the experiment. The intra-abdominal vessels were approached
through a mid-line incision. After cannulation the dogs were
anticoagulated with heparin (1000 i.u./kg I.V. 4 hourly).

Portal, arterial or venous blood was delivered at a constant
rate (10ml/min) by a roller pump (see Fig. 1) to two separate
banks of assay tissues, thus enabling simultaneous assay of kinins
in each stream. After passing over these tissues the blood was
collected in the resevoir from whence it drained back to the dog

via a femoral vein cannula. Strips of cat jejunum, kept at 4°C
for 2-6 days, were used to assay the kinins. These respond
selectively to kinins by contracting or increasing their rhythmic
activity (Ferreira & Vane, a). Changes in tissue length were
detected by auxotonic levers attached to Harvard transducers,
and recorded on a Beckman dynograph.

The sensitivity of the tissues was assayed by infusions of
known concentrations of synthetic bradykinin (0.5-8ng/ml) into
the blood after it had left the dog. The strips of cat jejunum were
usually sensitive to bradykinin in concentrations of 1-2 ng/ml.

The transit time of the blood between dog and tissues was
sometimes prolonged by including a length of tubing which would
cause the blood to be incubated for a further 1 or 2 min before
reaching the tissues.

Hypotension was produced by bleeding the dogs into a raised
resevoir, through a cannula in the femoral artery. The blood loss
was measured as an increase in resevoir weight , by attaching
the resevoir to an isometric transducer. Initially the resevoir was
held 150 cm above the table, but in order to maintain a hypotension
at 35-50 mmHg the resevoir was intermittently lowered to a height
of 55-90 cm above the table. During bleeding there was free flow
between dog and resevoir. Blood was returned to the dog either by
elevating the resevoir or by using a syringe to pump the blood
back in 20 ml. aliquots.

Mean arterial blood pressure was recorded from a side arm
of an arterial cannula connected to a pressure transducer. Central
venous pressure was similarly recorded through a cannula
inserted into the vena cava.

Results and interpretation

When dogs were bled to produce hypotension, kinins were
consistently detected in the arterial stream. In some dogs they
appeared within 12 min of blood loss while the blood pressure was
still falling, but in others they were found only after 190 min of
maintained hypotension. The kinin concentration gradually increased
to amounts equivalent to 2-3 ng/ml bradykinin. When blood was
returned and hypotension reversed the kinin concentration waned
until it became undetectable (i.e., the strips of cat jejunum
returned to their original base line).

In order to discover the source of these kinins, two streams, chosen from arterial or venous blood were simultaneously assayed throughout a period of hypotension. When comparing arterial with mixed venous (right atrial) blood, no difference in time of appearance or final concentration of kinins was detected. However, when portal and arterial blood were compared differences were observed: kinins appeared in portal blood before arterial blood, with delays of up to 160 min. The kinin concentration in portal blood was usually 1-2 ng/ml greater than that in the other stream.

In one experiment where portal and superior mesenteric vein blood were compared, kinins appeared in the blood draining the the small intestine at the same time as it did in the portal venous blood and in a concentration similar, if not higher than that in the portal venous blood. Although this does not exclude the pancreas as the source of kinins, it does suggest that the small gut is the probable site of generation.

Were these kinins being released into the blood stream from a single organ, such as the small intestine, or were they being generated throughout the body by circulating activated kininogenase, such as kallikrein? It is possible to differentiate between these two alternatives by taking advantage of their different half-lives in dog's blood, that of bradykinin being 15 sec (Ferreira & Vane, 1967a) and that of kallikrein 2-4 min (Ferreira & Vane, 1967b). In several experiments the blood transit time from dog to tissues was increased by up to 2 min by including a 20 ml incubation circuit in the delivery tubing. This manoeuvre had no effect on the kinin concentration detected by the strips of cat jejunum; from this it is inferred that the kinins were produced by a circulating kallikrein. This conclusion is reinforced by our observation that the concentration of kinins in mixed venous and arterial blood during hypotension were similar. This could only occur if kinins were being produced by a circulating kininogenase, as 90% of kinins are removed in one circulation through the pulmonary bed (Ferreira & Vane, 1967a).

The mechanism by which kallikrein enters the circulation is a matter of speculation. Our experiments show that kallikrein originates initially in the portal circulation probably through the release of intracellular kallikrein from the cells of the gut wall, where in carnivores it is particularly abundant (Werle, 1963). In man adrenaline has been shown to release kallikrein from carcinoid tumours (Oates, 1964), which are derived from cells normally found in the intestinal wall. The appearance of kinins sometimes within 10 min of bleeding certainly suggests that physiological stimuli are the most likely cause of kallikrein release, rather than cell death, although the latter may contribute to the release at a later stage.

The effect on the dog of circulating kinins in concentrations of 1-4 ng/ml was investigated by infusing kallikrein (Glumorin, 0.5 units/min I.V.) for an hour into anaesthetised dogs. During the length of the infusions the strips of cat jejunum maintained a constant contraction inferring that the kinin concentration remained the same and therefore there was no depletion of either kininogen or kininase. The effect of this circulating kinin on the blood pressure was not maintained. Initially the arterial blood pressure fell by 60 mm Hg, but this was followed by a gradual increase in pressure until by the end of the infusion it was only 10 mm Hg below the pre-infusion level. Central venous pressure was increased by 3-4 cm H_2O at the start of the infusion, and this too waned to be only just greater than normal by the end of the infusion. Blood kinin levels of 1-4 ng/ml are therefore sufficient to produce a profound drop in arterial blood pressure.

Conclusion

When anaesthetised dogs were bled to produce hypotension kinins appeared in the circulation in amounts equivalent 1-4 ng/ml bradykinin. When the blood pressure was restored this output was reversed. These kinins appeared in the portal blood before they appeared in the arterial blood and in higher concentrations. They were produced by a circulating active kallikrein. The concentration of kinins detected in the arterial blood would be sufficient to lower the blood pressure of an otherwise healthy dog.

References

Erdös, E.G.,Advances in Pharmacology, 1966,4,1.
Webster, M.E.& Clark, W.R., Amer. J. Physiol., 1959,197,406.
Brocklehurst, W.E.& Zeitlin, I.J., J. Physiol., 1967,191,417.
Habermann, E., et al., Kinin Symposium, 1969, Fiesole, Italy.
Vane, J.R., Br. J. Pharmac. Chemother., 1964,23,360.
Ferreira,S.H.&Vane,J.R. (a), ibid. 1967,29,367.
Ferreira,S.H.&Vane,J.R. (b), Nature,1967,215,1237.
Werle, E.&Trautschold,I., Ann. N. Y. Acad. Sci., 1963,104,117.
Oates, J.A., et al., Lancet,1964,1,514.

Pathophysiologic Mechanisms in Endotoxin Shock and
its Therapeutic Approaches

H. Neuhof, E. Glaser, D. Hey, and H.G. Lasch
Department of Internal Medicine,
Justus Liebig-University, Giessen, Germany

In comparative shock studies, one of the main problems
is to find a parameter suitable for measuring the
extent of organ damage during shock. Measuring the
arterial, central venous and right ventricular
pressure only yields very unreliable parameters, as
f.i. even with an extremely diminished cardiac output,
the arterial blood pressure may, as a compensatory
mechanism, be raised above normal. The characteristic
common to all forms of shock, regardless of their
causative factor, is the acute insufficient blood flow
in the circulation periphery. The limiting factor in
shock is the insufficient oxygen supply of organs,
which results in anaerobic metabolism with all its
well-known metabolic consequences (1, 2). The continuous registration of the cardiac output, however, is
rather intricate, and up to know has been mainly used
in animal experiments. Besides, measuring the cardiac
output without simultaneously measuring arterial and
central venous blood gases, would not permit a quanti-

tative conclusion as to the oxygen supply of the
circulation periphery.

In animal experiments, direct continuous measuring of
the body's total oxygen uptake is relatively easy.
Figure 1 shows the measuring procedures applied by us.

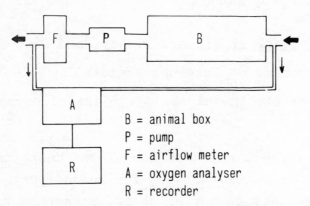

B = animal box
P = pump
F = airflow meter
A = oxygen analyser
R = recorder

Fig. 1: Block diagram showing the various subunits of
        the continuous oxygen uptake measuring
        arrangement.

Shock patients are supervised according to the same
principle with only minor changes. The deviation of
the actual oxygen uptake from the oxygen requirement
during steady state or from an empirically obtained
value permits continuous calculation of the oxygen
debt. The oxygen debt developed by the body must be
understood as the total balance of all aerobic metabolic processes that did not take place and does not
give any indication of its distribution in the various
organ systems.This disadvantage, however, is inherent
in all other studies on metabolic alterations.

GUYTON, CROWELL and SMITH were the first to describe a
direct connection between the oxygen debt developed by
the body and the severity of the body's damage in
shock (3, 4). In our experience, especially in comparative shock studies, continuous registration of the
oxygen uptake constitutes the most valuable parameter.

Experimental investigations reported here were performed in unanesthetized rabbits of both sexes. We wanted
to clarify whether the alterations observed in the
coagulation system during endotoxin shock are of
causalpathogenic importance for the course of shock.

Endotoxin shock in the rabbit is characterized by a
typical biphasic course caused by two different pathophysiologic mechanisms in the initial and final stages.
15 to 20 minutes after a single intravenous injection
of endotoxin (Escherichia coli, 100 μg/kg) as a rule a
sudden increase in the pressure of the right ventricle
and the right atrium is observed, whereas the arterial
pressure in the systemic circulation drops. The oxygen
uptake of experimental animals decreases rapidly and
pronouncedly to a mean value of 64,4% of the initial
value. This decreased oxygen uptake in the initial
stage is caused by an acutely reduced cardiac output,
as a consequence of an acutely increased resistance
in the pulmonary circulation. The diminished oxygen
uptake runs parallel to the alterations of the cardiac
output, as our studies with implanted flow-transducers
indicate (Fig. 2). The oxygen debt measured thus
permits direct conclusions to the perfusion debt of
the circulation periphery. The arterial blood pressure
can, as a compensatory mechanism, still be raised above

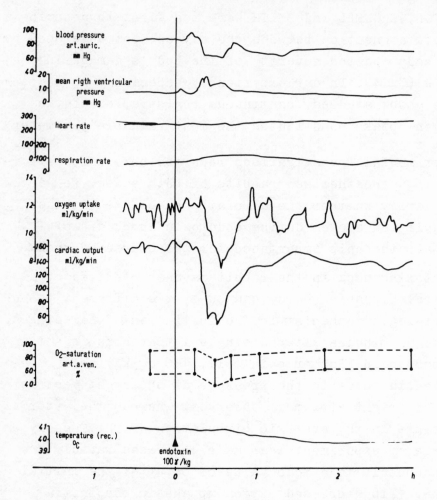

Fig. 2: Endotoxin shock in the rabbit: the early stage
of endotoxin shock is characterized by a
sudden increase of the resistance in the pulmonary circulation, whereas the arterial
pressure drops. The diminished oxygen uptake
runs parallel to the decrease of the cardiac
output.

normal, when oxygen uptake and cardiac output have
already dropped to 30 to 40% of their initial values,
thus proving itself an unreliable parameter for
assessing microcirculatory conditions (Fig. 3).
21,4% of our experimental animals already died in the

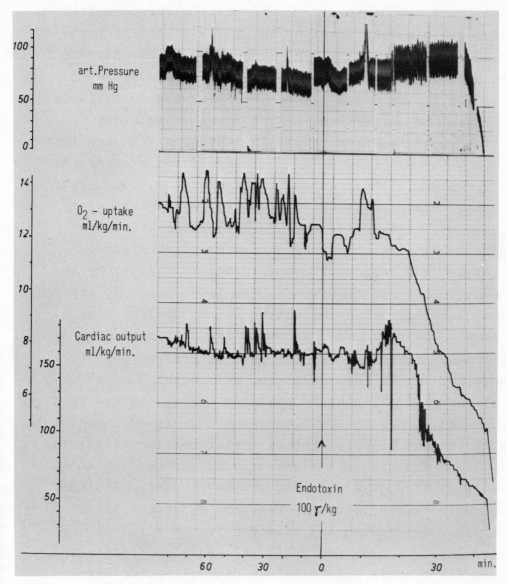

Fig. 3: In the early stage of endotoxin shock in the
         rabbit arterial blood pressure can still be
         elevated above normal, when oxygen uptake and
         cardiac output have already critically dropped.

initial stage of endotoxin shock, displaying symptoms
of acute cor pulmonale. In 53,6%, alterations of the

initial stage had partly or completely receded after
15 to 30 minutes. After an interval of varying duration, in 39,9% a slow continuous drop in the oxygen
uptake and later also in arterial blood pressure
results in the final stage, however, with no symptoms
of pulmonary hypertension, and these animals die
within 6 hours after endotoxin injection. The question,
in how far alterations of the coagulation system are
of pathogenic importance for the processes described
during endotoxin shock, therefore, is of particular
interest, as this form of shock is accompanied by
pronounced alterations of the coagulation system.
Platelet and leukocyte counts drop; initially, hypercoagulability is observed, which later leads to hypo-
coagulability, thus indicating a consumption coagulopathy (5, 6) (Fig. 4). As causative factor of the
increased resistance in the pulmonary circulation
occuring in the initial stage, an occlusion of the
pulmonary circulation by platelet aggregates has been
proposed, since following endotoxin application several
authors were able to demonstrate aggregated platelets
by light and electron microscopy in the small lung
vessels (7, 8, 9). In order to clarify this question,
we measured circulation parameters in anesthetized
rabbits, which with the aid of an extra corporal
circulation system had been rendered almost platelet-
free (10). After endotoxin administration, no significant difference in the increase in the pulmonary
circulation was observed between control animals and
"platelet-free" animals (Fig. 5). Therefore, platelet
aggregates cannot be responsible for the increased
resistance in the pulmonary circulation as a causative
factor or essentially contribute to it. Reversely,

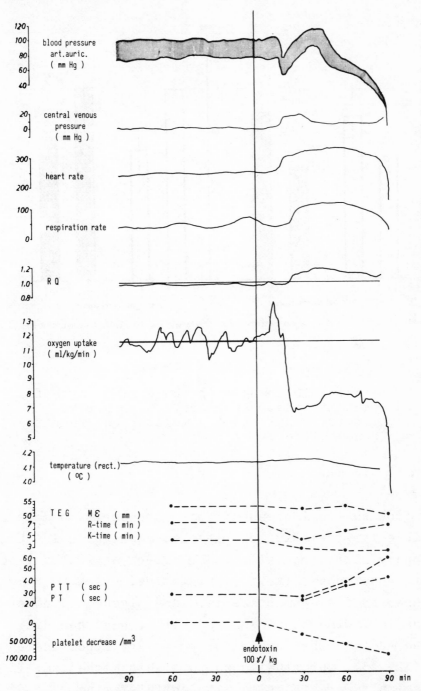

Fig. 4: In the endotoxin shock in the rabbit hemodynamic changes and the decrease in oxygen uptake are accompanied with alterations in the blood coagulation system.

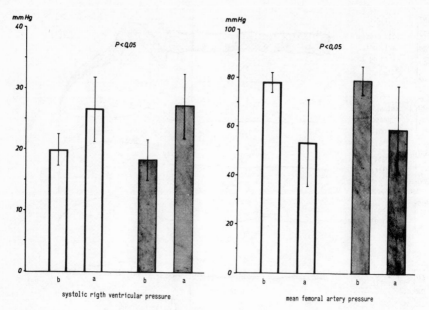

Hemodynamic changes in the early phase of endotoxin shock in the rabbit : b = before , a = after injection of endotoxin (3000 γ/kg)

☐ normal rabbits
■ "platelet-free" rabbits

Fig. 5: Hemodynamic changes in the early stage of
endotoxin shock in rabbits with normal
platelet count and "platelet-free" rabbits
do not differ.

slow flow due to increased resistance seems to make
possible the formation of platelet aggregates in the
pulmonary microcirculation. The direct action of vasoactive substances like f.i. histamine, which is
released by tissue mast cells, lung tissue and other
organs following endotoxin injection, has been discussed as a further cause for pulmonary hypertension
(11, 12, 13). Our studies support this mechanism. If
the animals were injected with antihistamine

(Neo-Bridal = N-dimethylaminoaethyl-N-p-methoxybenzyl-
-aminopyridin: 100 µg/kg), only one out of 6 animals
displayed a drop in the oxygen uptake in the initial
stage; in the control group 21 out of 28, this are 75%,
behaved likewise. Oxygen uptake following endotoxin
injection remained stable in the remaining 5 animals,
and they survived the next 6 hours. If in another
group of 6 rabbits the animals were heparinized
(1500 IU/kg/h) before endotoxin injection and heparin
infusions were continued, half of the animals displayed typical alterations of the initial stage; the
mean oxygen debt incurred corresponded to that of
untreated animals. None of the animals developed the
final stage, all the animals survived the 6-hour
limit with normal behaviour of metabolic parameters
and oxygen uptake.

These studies suggest the following: the initial stage
of endotoxin shock is determined by primarily hemodynamic alterations. Platelet aggregates are not responsible for the increased resistance in the pulmonary
circulation. Alterations in the coagulation system in
this stage are not of causal pathogenic importance,
although they do occur. Inhibition of the coagulation
system by heparin cannot influence the initial stage,
but antihistamines can. In contrast to the initial
stage, alterations in the blood coagulation system
seem to assume increasingly causal pathogenic
importance in the final stage. In this stage, intravascular fibrin deposits may be detected (14, 15).
By prophylactic inhibition of blood coagulation the
final stage could be prevented in all animals despite
unchanged reaction in the initial stage.

The **successful** heparin prophylaxis of septic shock in patients with septic abortion, as it has been applied for some time now by KUHN and GRAEFF of the Heidelberg Womens Hospital, is based on this assumption (16). The favorable effect of inhibition of the coagulation system can also be observed in other forms of shock (17,

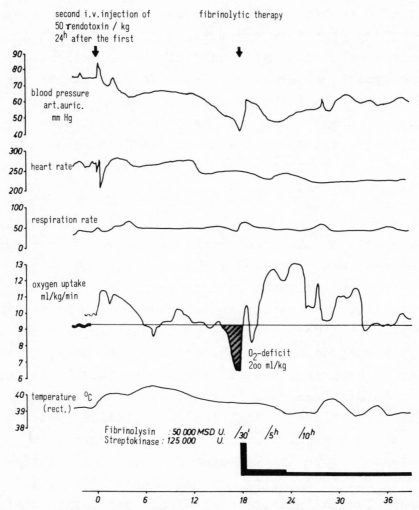

Fig. 6: In the generalized Sanarelli Shwartzman reaction in the rabbit an increasing oxygen debt becomes reversible and circulatory conditions normalize under fibrinolytic therapy.

18). In the hemorrhagic shock of the rabbit, which was not treated by volume substitution, we were able to demonstrate that all experimental animals receiving heparin infusions could develop an oxygen debt 30% higher than control animals.

If in the course of shock states intravascular coagulation has already manifested itself, heparin therapy will not be very successful. On the basis of present pathophysiologic knowledge, only an active fibrinolytic therapy will be effective (19). The last figure is to represent such a case. The lethality of the Generalized Shwartzman Reaction in the rabbit, which is dominated by intravascular coagulation, can be prevented by active fibrinolytic therapy. An already developed and increasing oxygen debt becomes reversible under therapy, and circulatory conditions normalize, although it has been proven that intravascular processes with beginning renal cortical necrosis have already taken place. It is for the therapy of final stages of shock that fibrinolytic therapy offers a possibility which has to be further investigated and used.

References

1 Isselhard, W.:   DMW 8: 349 (1965)

2 Bing, R.J.:   Fed. Proc. 19(9): 72 (1961)

3 Guyton, A.C. and J.W. Crowell:
                      Fed Proc. 20(9): 51 (1961)·

4 Crowell, J.W. and E.E. Smith:
                      Am.J.Physiol. 206(2): 313 (1964)

5 Lasch, H.G.:   Med.Welt 31: 1780 (1967)

6   Müller-Berghaus, G. und H.G. Lasch:
                        Thrombos.Diathes.haemorrh. 9:
                        335 (1963)

7   McKay, D.G.:   Disseminated Intravascular
                        Coagulation (New York 1965)

8   Hardaway, R.M., E.A. Husni, E.F. Geever,
    H.E. Noyes and J.W. Burns:
                        Ann.Surg. 154: 791 (1961)

9   Robb, H.J.:   Angiology 16: 405 (1965)

10 Neuhof, H. und G. Kaufmann:
                        Verh.Deutsch.Ges.Kreislaufforsch.
                        34: 218 (1968)

11 Hinshaw, L.B., J.A. Vick, C.H. Carlson and Y.L.Fan:
                        Proc.Soc.exp.Biol. 104: 379 (1960)

12 Hinshaw, L.B., M.M. Jordan and J.A. Vick:
                        J.Clin.Invest. 40: 1631 (1961)

13 Hinshaw, L.B., R.E. Emerson, P.F. Iampietro and
    C.M. Brake: Am.J.Physiol. 203: 600 (1962)

14 Lee, L.:   Z.exp.Med. 115: 1065 (1962)

15 Sandritter, W. und H.G. Lasch:
                        Meth.Achievm.exp.Path. 3: 86
                        (1967)

16 Kuhn, W. und H. Graeff:
                        Septischer Abort und bakterieller
                        Schock. Springer-Verlag, Berlin
                        (1968)

17 Crowell, J.W. and W.L. Read:
                        Am.J.Physiol. 183: 565 (1955)

18 Lasch, H.G. und H. Neuhof:
                        Therapeutische und experimentelle
                        Fibrinolyse. F.K.Schattauer-Verlag.
                        Stuttgart (1969)

SEVERAL PHARMACOLOGIC AND BIOCHEMICAL ASPECTS

OF CYSTEAMINE- AND CYSTAMINE-INDUCED SHOCK

P. van Caneghem, J. Lecomte, Z. M. Bacq
and M. L. Beaumariage

Laboratory of Radiobiology, Léon Fredericq
Institute and Laboratory of Physiopathology,
University of Liège

INTRODUCTION

Cysteamine $[HSCH_2CH_2NH_2]$ and cystamine $[(H_2NCH_2CH_2)_2S_2]$ provide remarkable protection against the action of ionizing radiation (1, 2). Numerous attempts to explain the mode of action of these substances followed the initial discovery of their radioprotective effects by Bacq and coworkers in 1951(3). The present study was undertaken in order to elucidate the cardiovascular properties of these radioprotectors. A clearer understanding of their effect on oxygen distribution at the cellular level seemed desirable, since anoxia is known to provoke marked biochemical changes which enhance cellular radioresistance.

Cysteamine and cystamine, particularly the latter, produce a state of shock when injected at radioprotective dose levels. Both compounds possess pharmacologic properties which contribute to the animal's collapse; for example, they are generally hypotensive and vasodilative (4, 5, 6, 7, 8, 9, 10). They also enhance vascular permeability (5, 9, 11, 10). Cysteamine- and cystamine-induced shock is accompanied by a number of metabolic disturbances resulting from decreased exchanges between the vascular and extravascular compartments and from changes in vascular permeability. These nonspecific disturbances, whose intensity varies with the degree of shock, produce alterations in the concentrations of various plasma constituents (12, 13, 14, 15). The present study attempted to ascertain whether these

171

properties underlie the radioprotective effects of the
two compounds.

MATERIALS AND METHODS

Adult cats, rabbits and rats, and 20-35 day old
chickens were used in this study. The experimental
techniques utilized have been described elsewhere (9,
10, 12, 14, 15).

RESULTS

Vasomotor Properties in Different Species.
Cysteamine. When injected intravenously at low
dose levels (2.5-5 mg/kg) in the cat, rabbit, rat and
chicken, cysteamine induces a drop in blood pressure
after a short period of latency (Fig.1).The rat and
chicken are more sensitive, but in all four animals the
decrease in arterial tension is proportional to initial
blood pressure and to dose provided that the dose administered is lower than 20 mg/kg. Blood pressure then
rises to normal or above-normal levels. Tachyphylaxis
does not occur.

Repeated intravenous injections of cysteamine (2.5-
5 mg/kg/30 sec.) bring about immediately after the
first injection a moderate decrease in arterial pressure followed by a rise of variable magnitude and duration. Finally, the blood pressure falls slowly until
the animal's death in circulatory collapse, with irre-
gular bradypnea convulsions and cyanosis. The rat sometimes dies in acute pulmonary oedema.

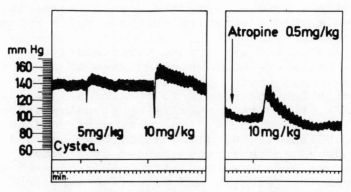

Fig. 1. Cat (2 kg) anesthetized with Dial; carotid
        pressure. Cysteamine was injected into the
        femoral vein; atropine was administered sub-
        cutaneously (10).

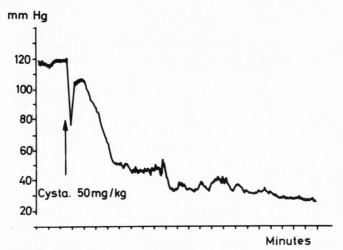

Fig. 2. Rat (200 g) anesthetized with nembutal; carotid
        pressure. Cystamine was injected intraperito-
        neally (9).

  Cystamine. We found, as Robbers had (1937), that
at equimolecular doses cystamine is between two and
three times as hypotensive as cysteamine. Certain
cats (5) and chickens (10) which are particularly
sensitive to cystamine respond to doses smaller than
1 mg/kg. In the cat, there is no secondary increase in
blood pressure following cystamine; in the chicken, this
rise is inconstant.
  When injected continuously, the compound produces
a fall in blood pressure followed by a rise and stabilization under the normal level; the pressure drops
abruptly shortly before the animal's death.
  The effects of intraperitoneally injected cystamine (Fig. 2) or cysteamine are analogous to those obtained when the compound is infused intravenously.
  Action of various pharmacologic agents on the tension effects of cysteamine and cystamine. If the cat
(Fig. 1) or chicken is atropinized prior to the injection of small doses of cysteamine, the primary hypotensive response is reversed. Atropine nevertheless
does not antagonize the hypotensive effects of cystamine. Bilateral vagotomy seems to be without effect in
the cat, an animal which tolerates vagus resection very
well.
  In the four species studied, antihistamines and
histamine liberators do not increase tolerance to high
doses of cystamine. These pharmacologic agents fail to
diminish the hypotensive response to small doses of

TABLE I.

Epinephrine Level of Suprarenals in Rats
Injected with Cysteamine or Cystamine $(16^{(1)}$,
$9^{(2)})$.

Treatment (i.p.)	Dose (mg/Kg)	% Decrease in Blood Pressure	Average Epinephrine Level* (μg/10 mg)
1st Series[1]			
NaCl 0.9%	-	-	4.07
Cysteamine	50	8 - 13	4.29
Cysteamine	100	17 - 25	4.11
Cysteamine	200	collapse	2.21**
Cysteamine	400	collapse	1.24**
2nd Series[2]			
NaCl 0.9%	-	-	7.20
Cystamine	50	25	6.70
Cystamine	100	50	5.00**
Cystamine	200	collapse	3.10**
Cystamine	400	collapse	3.40**

  * Suprarenals were removed 30 min. after i.p.
    injection of cysteamine or cystamine.

 ** $P < 0.01$ (Student t test).

cystamine in the rabbit and rat; in the cat and chicken,
however, a decrease in cystamine's cardiovascular effects
can be observed.
    The secondary rise in blood pressure produced by
these compounds may be due, at least in part, to the
release of catecholamines from the suprarenals (17, 18).
However, it is interesting to note that while this secondary rise is more pronounced following cysteamine administration, the decrease in the epinephrine content of
rat suprarenals is greater after cystamine (Table I).
    Cysteamine and cystamine, in addition, have a sym-
pathicomimetic action in various species, but phentolamine at adrenolytic dose levels fails to modify this
property in the rat. The hypertensive and tachycardiac
effects of exogenous catecholamines are reduced in animals pretreated with cysteamine or cystamine, whereas
the vasomotor properties of histamine, 5-hydroxytryp-
tamine and bradykinin are little if at all modified.

Action on Vascular Permeability

The inflammatory properties of cysteamine and cystamine have been investigated in man (5, 19,), the dog (11), the rabbit (5), the rat (9) and the mouse (10). These phenomena have been studied especially thoroughly in the rat. Subcutaneous administration of cystamine (500 μg) in the plantar region of the animal's paw provokes marked edema of the distal end of the paw. The area becomes distended and warm. Edema, which begins to appear toward the end of the injection period, progresses for an hour and finally is slowly resorbed. Macroscopically, the lesions resemble those produced by dextran administration (9). The magnitude and duration of edema are reduced by promethazine, an antihistamine, and by methysergide, a serotonin antagonist. In animals pretreated with chlorazol blue (i.p. injection), the increase in vascular permeability is reflected by the movement of dye into the interstitial spaces. Van Cauwenberge and Lecomte showed in 1955 (20) that the speed with which dye flowed into the interstitial spaces in the irritated area was unmodified by adrenocorticoids but that it was slowed by large doses of promethazine. The two types of treatment were not tried in combination.

Similar modifications of cystamine's permeability effects have been observed in the rabbit injected with trypan blue.

Studies in the mouse have shown that cysteamine is as effective in this respect as cystamine. In this species, moreover, the two compounds produce a greater increase in permeability than histamine, 5-hydroxytryptamine or compound 48/80 (a histamine liberator). The increase is inhibited by methysergide, Trasylol® and mepyramine, but in order to produce the same degree of inhibition this last compound must be administered at a dose level capable of producing shock.

Assays of cutaneous histamine in the plantar region of the rat hind paw following intracutaneous cystamine injection indicate that marked changes occur in the course of the edema's development (Table II). During the first 5 minutes, histamine decreases and rapidly disappears from the tissue; when edema is maximal (45 minutes after the injection), histamine has reached normal or above-normal levels. This rise is probably due to the increase in histamine-rich formed elements of the blood which accumulate in situ and which tend to compensate for the loss of histamine from the damaged region.

In the mouse, cystamine seems to lack a histamine-liberating action despite the fact that the cutaneous

TABLE II.

Average Cutaneous Histamine Levels in the Plantar
Region of the Rat Hindpaw Following Intracutaneous
Injection of Cystamine (500 μg) (9).

Treatment	Min. after Injection	n	Weight Fresh Tissue (mg)	Average Histamine Levels (μg/g)
Hindpaw injected with NaCl 0.9%	5-90	100	67	29.0
Hindpaw injected with cystamine	5	25	94	5.9**
	15	25	175	13.7**
	45	25	205	30.5
	90	25	218	32.7*

* P⩽0.05   ** P⩽0.01 (Student t test).

histamine reserves of this species are as abundant as
those of the rat. However, the compound does reduce by
half the cutaneous levels of 5-hydroxytryptamine (10).

Modifications in Composition of the Blood.
Hemoconcentration. In the rat, the intraperitoneal
injection of cystamine rapidly produces a marked degree
of hemoconcentration (Table III). This effect is less
pronounced after cysteamine administration (21). The
conditions under which the compound is administered
affect the animal's response. Hemoconcentration is less
intense when the intravenous route is used. Anesthesia
also diminishes the effect of intraperitoneal cystamine.
An increase in the cell: plasma volume ratio can likewise be elicited in the rabbit and chicken.
Plasma Proteins. The administration of cystamine
in the rat (Table III) induces hypoproteinemia, a decrease in -SS- and -SH groups bound to proteins (including
the albumins) and a drop in sialic acid, a glycoprotein
constituent. A correlation has been found between the
hypoproteinemia and the decrease in sialic acid and
protein-bound -SS- and -SH groups. These changes are
also observed in the rabbit and chicken. In the latter
animal, sialic acid normally exists at low levels and
becomes unassayable by our techniques after cystamine
administration. The great increase in free -SS- and
-SH groups in the plasma after cystamine is due in part
to the influx of -SS- groups provided by this compound

TABLE III.

Average Changes in Plasma Constituents Following Intraperitoneal Cystamine-2HCl Administration (150 mg/kg) in Rats (12).

Time after Injection	n	Cell:Plasma Ratio (v:v)	Proteins (gr %)	Sialic Acid (mg %)	SS+SH Groups (μg Cysteine/ml) Bound	Free
0	10	0.99 ± 0.05	6.01 ±0.07	93 ± 3.4	720 ± 34	12.4 ± 1.0
10 min.	10	1.52**± 0.08	5.78* ±0.05	83* ± 3.5	787 ± 39	54.6**± 2.7
1 h	10	2.07**± 0.12	5.47**±0.10	74**±2.6	720 ± 62	65.2**± 2.1
2 h	10	1.99**± 0.13	5.30**±0.06	72**± 2.7	658 ± 62	75.6**± 6.2
3 h	10	1.45**± 0.11	5.31**±0.08	68**± 1.9	584**± 24	45.0**± 5.1
4 h	10	1.54**± 0.13	5.23**±0.10	74**± 2.7	633 ± 58	56.1**±10.6
5 h	10	1.44**± 0.12	5.11**±0.06	71**± 1.0	600 ± 75	43.4**± 6.9

* Indicates statistically significant difference (P≤0.05).

** Indicates highly significant difference (P≤0.01).

TABLE IV.

Comparison of Plasma Disturbances Observed in Different Types of shock (12, 14).

Treatment	Time* before Sacrifice	Cell:Plasma Ratio (v:v)	Proteins	Alb:Glob. Ratio	Sialic Acid	SS+SH Groups	
						Bound	Free
NaCl 0.85%**	3-4 h	100.0	100.0	100.0	100.0	100.0	100.0
Cystamine (iv)	3h	101.0	82.2	100.4	79.3	84.7	161.9
Cystamine (ip)	3h	141.0	77.7	98.6	70.2	82.2	332.4
Epinephrine (ip)	3h	177.2	87.3	84.6	80.3	97.5	125.0
Burns	4h	158.8	81.9	78.8	87.9	77.8	146.0
Ag*** (iv)	4h	86.7	88.3	99.4	88.5	83.7	144.6
Tourniquet	3h	91.3	92.9	-	90.8	-	-

 * Animals were sacrificed when shock appeared clinically most severe.

 ** The experimental values are expressed as a percentage of the control values.

*** Colloidal preparation (Collargol).

and in part to the liberation of -SS- and -SH groups
which ordinarily occurs in other types of shock (Table
IV). Another possible factor is that the cysteamine
which is formed by the reduction of cystamine in the
body may destroy disulfide bridges in proteins and thus
give rise to smaller soluble fractions, as Lorber and
coworkers have shown (22) using other compounds with
-SH or -SS- groups. Among the proteins, the albumins
show a smaller decrease than the α-globulins. In contrast to the situation in other types of shock, with
cystamine there is no tendency for the albumin:globulin
ratio to become inverted. Table IV makes it possible
to compare the changes observed in various types of
shock (produced by burns, collargol, the application of
a tourniquet, epinephrine administration) to those observed in cystamine-induced shock. In each case, the
blood samples were drawn at the moment at which shock
seemed to have reached its maximum clinical intensity.
The absence of hemoconcentration after collargol and
after loosening of the tourniquet is most likely due to
the poor choice of the time at which blood was drawn.
　　Twelve hours after the injection of cystamine sialic acid has once again returned to normal; after this,
it rises above the pre-injection value and remains at
abnormally high levels for approximately one week (van
Caneghem and Stein, unpublished observations). This response corresponds to a hyperglycoproteinemia, a response

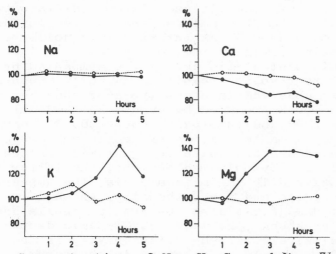

Fig. 3. Concentration of Na, K, Ca and Mg after i.p.
　injection of cystamine- 2 HCl (150 mg/kg) in the rab-
　bit. Ordinate:cation concentrations expressed as a
　percentage of the pre-injection value. Abcissa:time
　in hours---Animals injected with 0.9% NaCl.___Animals
　injected with cystamine (13).

which has been observed in various types of shock (23)
and in the course of inflammatory reactions. These alterations are potentiated by epinephrine and are diminished in intensity if cystamine is injected by the
intravenous route.

Following cysteamine administration, the decrease
in plasma sialic acid is less pronounced. This is explained by the fact that cysteamine induces a less marked state of shock than cystamine.

Plasma Cations. In the rabbit injected with cystamine, there is an increase in plasma potassium and
magnesium (Fig.3) just as in other types of shock (24).
The intracellular localization of these cations suggests
that there is a disturbance of permeability at the cellular and subcellular level. In contrast, plasma sodium
remains unchanged and there is a slight drop in plasma
calcium.

Increase in Enzyme Activities. The electron microscopy studies of Firket and Lelièvre (25) have shown
that cystamine damages certain subcellular structures,
including the mitochondria, in the hematopoietic organs.
These lesions occur rapidly and are reversible. As the
result of the increase in cell membrane permeability
and the destruction or increased fragility of subcellular structures (mitochondria, lysosomes), various
enzymes which were linked to these structures now appear
in the blood. Figure 4 shows the increase in the plasma
activities of lactic, malic and glutamic dehydrogenase,
glutamic oxalacetic transaminase and β-glucuronidase
after cysteamine as well as the rise in aldolase and the
serum cathepsins after cystamine. There is an increase
in the serum's proteolytic activity accompanied by a
decrease in its trypsin-inhibiting capacity. Such modifications are observed in other types of shock as well.
Anoxia (26), shock produced by burns (27, 28), hemorrhagic shock (29) and endotoxin shock (30, 31) can
increase the plasma activities of lactic dehydrogenase,
aldolase, malic dehydrogenase and glutamic oxalacetic
transaminase, all cytoplasmic enzymes; the latter two
are also localized in the mitochondria. The appearance
of β-glucuronidase and the cathepsins, which is a sign
of lysosomal damage, is also observed in anoxia and
other types of shock (32, 14, 26). Glutamic dehydrogenase, an exclusively mitochondrial enzyme, is increased
in anoxia (26). Lastly, a decrease in the serum's trypsin-inhibiting capacity is characteristic of traumatic
shock (33), epinephrine-induced shock and shock produced by burns (14).

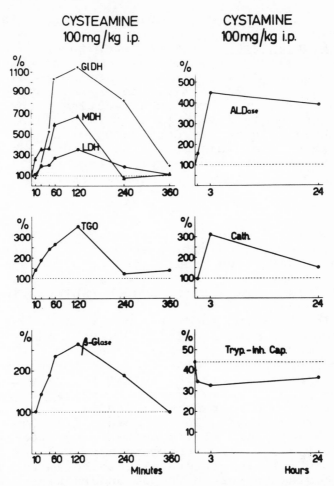

Fig. 4. Activities of plasma lactic, malic and glutamic
        dehydrogenase (LDH, MDH, GlDH), glutamic oxa-
        lacetic transaminase (GOT) and β-glucuronidase
        (β- Glase) after cysteamine. The activity of
        plasma aldolase (Aldase) and the serum cathep-
        sins (Cath.) and the trypsin-inhibiting capacity
        (Tryp-Inh Cap) of the serum after cystamine.
        Ordinate: specific plasma activities of the
        various enzymes expressed as a percentage of
        control values. Abscissa: time in minutes or
        hours (15).

Lipemia. After cystamine administration, esterified fatty acid levels rise in the plasma, reaching
0.803 mval/100 ml after 24 hours as compared with control values of 0.662 mval/100 ml. The serum can remain

milky for several days. This also occurs in other forms
of shock (34).

    Pyruvic Acid. The intraperitoneal administration
of cysteamine or cystamine in the rat causes a pronounced drop in hepatic glycogen, a rise in blood glucose
induced by the liberated epinephrine (35), and considerable urinary excretion of lactic and pyruvic acid (36).
Plasma pyruvate levels (12.9 μM/100 ml in the control
rat) have practically doubled 25 minutes after cystamine injection. This metabolic disturbance, which is
also observed in other types of shock (37), reflects
an increase in anaerobic glycolysis.

DISCUSSION

    When injected intravenously or intraperitoneally
into the cat, rabbit, rat and chicken, cystamine and to
a lesser degree cysteamine induce a non-specific state
of shock marked by cardiovascular symptoms, alterations
of cellular permeability and characteristic metabolic
disturbances.

    The fall in blood pressure triggers a number of
compensatory homeostatic reflexes. Among these reflexes
is the release of catecholamines from the adrenal medulla, a phenomenon observed in both the rat and dog (7)
and which can ensure the animal's survival. Adrenal-
ectomy greatly increases the toxicity of the radio-
protector, and this in turn can be corrected by an intraperitoneal injection of epinephrine (38) despite
the possible adrenolytic action of cysteamine and cystamine (39). Various pharmacologic studies have shown
that the release of adrenal catecholamines is not the
determining factor in the secondary hypertensive response observed after cysteamine and cystamine in the
cat and rat. The radioprotectors themselves have a sym-
-pathicomimetic action (18) which can be abolished by
an adrenergic blocking agent in the cat and chicken.
However, the liberated catecholamines may be involved
in producing the biochemical manifestations described
earlier in this paper since epinephrine is known to be
able to reproduce or reinforce certain effects exerted
by cystamine.

    The histamine liberated from certain tissues (9)
plays only a small role in the hypotension and shock
generated by cysteamine or cystamine. Repeated injections of these radioprotectors fail to cause tachyphylaxis. In the rabbit, rat and chicken, no preventive
effect is obtained with either antihistamines or histamine liberators. However, in the cat the magnitude of
the blood pressure drop can be reduced by pretreatment

with an antihistamine. The same effect has been reported in the dog (6). Nevertheless, histamine can play
a role notably in areas which are directly exposed to
high concentrations of the radioprotectors. This is
suggested by the considerable degree of peritoneal
exudation observed in the dog (11) and also in the rat
(van Caneghem, unpublished observations) when cysteamine or cystamine is injected intraperitoneally at
radioprotective dose levels. Further evidence is provided by the finding that the intracutaneous injection
of the radioprotectors is followed by irritation and
edema in both these animals as well as in the mouse.
Such inflammatory reactions are diminished by the administration of antihistamines and, in the rat, also
by methysergide, a serotonin antagonist. Serotonin's
role in the production of this phenomenon has been
confirmed in the mouse (10). It should also be recal-
led that cysteamine administration in the rabbit,
guinea pig and rat prolongs certain effects of histamine, most likely via a temporary block of diamine oxi-
dase (40).

The plasma changes observed after cystamine and,
to a lesser extent, after cysteamine (Van Caneghem and
Stein, unpublished observations) reflect an increase
in permeability between the vascular and extravascular
compartments (hemoconcentration, changes in plasma
proteins), an alteration of cellular permeability, and
lesions of subcellular structures (increase in potassium and magnesium, rise in plasma enzyme activities).
Damage to cellular structures in turn brings about severe metabolic disturbances, as illustrated by the modifications in carbohydrate metabolism (2), acidosis
(36, 14) and hyperlipemia. The cardiovascular properties
of cysteamine and cystamine are not related to the presence of thiol or disulfide groups since these actions
can be mimicked by substances lacking the groups (e.g.
epinephrine, histamine) and since, inversely, both β-
mercaptoethanol and mercaptoethane sodium sulfonate
which contain an -SH group are unable to produce shock.

Is there a relationship between the shock induced
by cysteamine and cystamine and their ability to confer
radioprotection ? This question must be answered with
caution for the following reasons:

1. Cysteamine, which is as effective a radiopro-
tector as cystamine in the rat, causes a less severe
state of shock. According to Heiffer (8), it does not
bring about hypoxemia.

2. In the mouse, the two compounds are equally
effective in conferring radioprotection despite the

fact that they act differently on arterial tension and
on tissue oxygen pressure. Cysteamine is often hypertensive whereas cystamine produces a moderate reduction
in blood pressure (41, 42).

3. There have been varied and conflicting reports
on the changes in tissue oxygen pressure recorded in
response to cysteamine (43, 44, 45). Depending on the
author, cysteamine can either increase, fail to modify
or decrease oxygen tension in the hematopoietic organs.
However, cystamine is generally believed to cause anoxia (44, 45).

The underlying cause of the radioprotective properties of cysteamine and cystamine appears to be their
inhibition of cellular multiplication by means of severe but reversible metabolic disturbances, a decrease
in available oxygen, or the two effects combined. When
cells are in the resting stage, they are more radio-
resistant. It is known that cysteamine and cystamine,
like other sulphur-containing radioprotectors (46),
are able to inhibit mitosis (47). However, when cellular damage is so severe as to be irreversible, there
is of course no possibility of radioprotection. This
is true in the chicken, an animal in which cysteamine
and cystamine potentiate the severe hypotensive effects invariably seen after irradiation (48).

SUMMARY

The intravenous or intraperitoneal injection of
cysteamine or cystamine is followed in the cat, rabbit
and chicken by complex vasomotor reactions. The predominant response is a fall in blood pressure, followed by mechanisms which tend to normalize the tension.
The decrease in blood pressure triggers a number of
homeostatic reflexes, including stimulation of the
adrenal medulla.

Cystamine and cysteamine produce changes in vascular permeability which are reflected by hemoconcentration and various alterations of the plasma proteins.
When administered via the intracutaneous route, the
two radioprotectors cause local irritation accompanied
by edema; histamine and 5-hydroxytryptamine are involved in these phenomena.

The increase in some plasma cations and in the
plasma activities of several intracellular enzymes
reveals that damage has been sustained by cell membranes and structures. Hyperlipemia and acidosis are
two results of the metabolic disturbances produced by
these lesions.

Most of these non-specific modifications are also encountered in other types of shock.

ACKNOWLEDGEMENTS

The authors wish to thank Bracco Industria Chimica and Bayer-Pharma for kindly providing the cysteamine and the Trasylol®.

REFERENCES

1. Z.M. Bacq and P.Alexander, Fundamentals of Radiobiology, 2nd edition, Pergamon Press, Oxford, p. 459 (1961).

2. Z.M. Bacq, Chemical Protection against Ionizing Radiation, Charles C. Thomas Publ., Springfield, Illinois, p.80 (1965).

3. Z.M. Bacq, A.Herve, J.Lecomte, P.Fischer, J.Blavier, G.Dechamps, H.Le Bihan et P. Rayet, Arch. Intern. Physiol. 59, 442 (1951).

4. H. Robbers, Arch. Exper. Path. Pharmakol. 185, 161 (1937).

5. J. Lecomte, Arch. Intern. Physiol. 60, 179 (1952).

6. R. L. Mundy and M. H. Heiffer, Radiation Res. 13, 381 (1960).

7. R. L. Mundy, M. H. Heiffer and B. Mehlman, Arch. Intern. Pharmacodyn. Ther. 130, 354 (1961).

8. M. H. Heiffer, R. L. Mundy and B. Mehlman, Radiation Res. 16, 165 (1962).

9. J. Lecomte, A. Cession-Fossion, J. Cl. Libon et Z. M. Bacq, Arch. Intern. Pharmacodyn. Ther. 149, 487 (1964).

10. M. L. Beaumariage, P. Van Caneghem et Z. M. Bacq, Strahlentherapie 131, 342 (1966).

11. R. L. Mundy, M. H. Heiffer and B. Mehlman, Amer. J. Physiol. 204, 997 (1963).

12. P. van Caneghem et F.Stein. Arch. Intern. Physiol. Biochim. 75, 769 (1967).

13. P. van Caneghem, J. G. Henrotte et Z.M. Bacq, Arch. Intern. Physiol. Biochim. 75, 469 (1967).

14. P. van Caneghem, C. R. Soc. Biol. 162, 2331 (1968).

15. G. Plomteux, M. L. Beaumariage, Z. M. Bacq et C. Heusghem, Biochem. Pharmacol. 16, 1601 (1967).

16. J. Cl. Libon, J. Lecomte et A. Cession-Fossion, C.R. Soc. Biol. 157, 685 (1963).

17. J. Lecomte, Arch. Intern. Physiol. 62, 431 (1954).

18. M. Goffart, Arch. Intern. Physiol. 63,500 (1955)

19. J. Lecomte et C. Bohrenstayn, C. R. Soc. Biol. 147, 369 (1953).

20. H. van Cauwenberge et J. Lecomte, Bull. Acad. Roy. Med. Belg. IIème série, 3, n° 7, 3 (1955).

21. P. van Caneghem, Strahlentherapie, 137, 231 (1969).

22. A. Lorber, C. M. Pearson, W. L. Meredith and L. E. Gantz-Mandell, Ann. Intern. Med. 61, 423 (1964).

23. J. Owen, In: Advances in Clinical Chemistry, H. Sobotka and C. Stewart Eds., Academic Press, New York, 2, p. 1 (1961).

24. J. G. Henrotte, J. Troquet et D. Collinet-Lagneaux, Arch. Intern. Physiol. Biochim. 75, 77 (1967).

25. H. Firket et P. Lelièvre,Intern. J. Rad. Biol. 10, 403 (1966).

26. G. Plomteux, M.L. Beaumariage, Z. M. Bacq et C. Heusghem, Second International Symposium on Radio-sensitizing and Radioprotective Drugs. In press (1969).

27. G. P. Lewis, J. Physiol. 191, 591 (1967).

28. A. F. Blyuger, M. L. Belen'Kii and Ya. Ya. Shuster, Fed. Proc., 24, T 93 (1965).

29. E. S. Vesell, M. P. Feldman and E. D. Frank, Proc. Soc. Exper. Biol. Med. 101, 644 (1959).

30. E. S. Vesell, C. F. P. Palmerio and E. D. Frank, Proc. Soc. Exper. Biol. Med. 104, 403 (1960).

31. A. Konttinem, M. Rajasalmi and J. Paloheimo, Amer. J. Physiol. 207, 385 (1964).

32. A. Janoff, G. Weissmann, B. Zweifach and L. Thomas, J. Exper. Med. 116, 451 (1962).

33. H. Fürstenberg, Langenbecks Arch. Clin. Chir. 301, 714 (1962).

34. C. Harvengt and M. Jeanjean, Med. Pharmacol. Exper. 15, 233 (1966).

35. J. E. Sokal, E. J. Sarcione and K. E. Gerszi, Amer. J. Physiol. 196, 261 (1959).

36. P. Fischer, Arch. Intern. Physiol. Biochim. 64, 130 (1956).

37. L. Mignone, In: Shock Pathogenese und Therapie, K. Bock Ed., Springer Verlag, Berlin, p. 85 (1962).

38. P. Fisher, J. Lecomte et M. L. Beaumariage, Arch. Intern. Physiol. Biochim. 63, 121 (1955).

39. V. Varajic, R. Debijadji and S. Elčić, Arch. Intern. Pharmacodyn. Ther. 142, 206 (1963).

40. C. De Marco, B. Mondovi and P. Cavallini, Biochem. Pharmacol. 11, 509 (1962).

41. C. van der Meer, P. W. Valkenburg, C. A. ter Kuile and J. A. Neyhoff, Afdrukken van Medish Biologisch Laboratorium RVO-TNO 25, 19 (1960).

42. V. DiStefano, J.J. Klahn and D. E. Leary, Radiation Res. 17, 792 (1962).

43. E. Y. Grayevsky, I. M. Shapiro, M. M. Konstantinova and N. F. Barakina In: The Initial Effects of Ionizing Radiation on Cell, R. J. C. Harris Ed., Academic Press, New York, p. 237 (1961).

44. C. van der Meer, P. W. Valkenburg and M. Remmelts, Nature 189, 588 (1961).

45. P. Lelièvre, V. Smoliar and E. H. Betz, Abstracts of 6th Annual Meeting of the European Society for Radiation Biology, p. 70 (1968).

46. R. Goutier, Irradiation, Radioprotection et Synthèse de l'Acide Désoxyribonucléique, Thèse d'Agrégation de l'Enseignement Supérieur, Editions Arscia, Bruxelles, 238 pages (1967).

47. R. Bassleer et S. Chèvremont-Comhaire, Bull. Acad. Roy. Med. Belg. 25, 709 (1960).

48. S. P. Stearner, A. M. Brues, M. Sanderson and E. J. Christian, Amer. J. Physiol. 182, 407 (1955).

EFFECT OF VARYING BLOOD SUGAR LEVEL IN ANAPHYLACTIC SHOCK

H.L. DHAR

DEPT. OF PHARMACOLOGY, JAWAHARLAL INSTITUTE OF

POSTGRADUATE MED.EDUCATION & RES. PONDICHERRY -INDIA

Rats and mice are known to be resistant to anaphylactic shock (Gallivallerio, 1910; Longcope, 1922). Procedures used to increase the susceptibility of these species to anaphylactic shock include hypophysectomy (Molomut, 1939), suprarenalectomy (Weiser, Golub & Hamre, 1941), the use of <u>Bordetella pertussis</u> vaccine along with the sensitising dose of antigen (Malkiel & Hargis, 1952) and injection of insulin a shortwhile before challenge (Dhar & Sanyal 1963; Adamkiewicz, Sacra & Ventura, 1964). These procedures have a common factor in the production of hypoglycaemia and as such attempts have been made to analyse the mechanism involved by which alterations in the blood sugar level modify the severity of anaphylactic shock.

We have recently reported that severity of anaphylactic shock is much altered by varying the level of glucose in the blood (Dhar, Sanyal & West 1967a; Dutta & Dhar 1968). It has been shown that when hypoglycaemia is induced by injection of insulin before challenge, systemic anaphylactic shock is potentiated in rats, mice, guinea pigs and rabbits. We could not produce fatal anaphylactic shock in the dog, but the degree of fall in blood pressure during anaphylactic shock was increased by pretreatment with insulin.

When animals were made hyperglycaemic either by alloxan pretreatment or by hypertonic glucose infusion the systemic anaphylactic shock was markedly reduced in the rat, the mouse and in the rabbit.

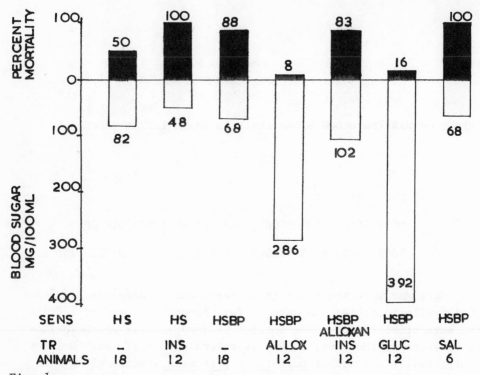

Fig. 1:
Relationship of blood sugar level with severity of anaphylactic
shock in the rat. Sens: sensitized; TR: treatment; HS: horse
serum; B. P.: <u>Bordetella pertussic</u> vaccine; Ins: insulin; Allox:
alloxan; Gluc: glucose; Sal: saline.

We failed to produce alloxan diabetes in the guinea pig and glucose
infusion did not afford significant protection. However glucose
infusion either abolished or reduced the degree of fall in blood
pressure during anaphylactic shock in the dog.

    We have tried to analyse the relationship of blood glucose
level at the time of challenging dose of antigen with the degree
of anaphylactic shock in the rat (fig.1.)
It is evident that when hypoglycaemia is induced by <u>B.Pertussis</u>
vaccine in sensitised animals, per cent mortality increases as in
the case with insulin. When however, blood sugar level is high
either due to alloxan treatment or due to glucose infusion, per
cent mortality is minimal. Injection of insulin in alloxan treated
animals before challenge increases the percentage of mortality along
with a reduction in blood sugar. In those animals where death could

not be prevented it was seen that higher the blood sugar level at the time of challenge, longer the animal survived after anaphylactic shock.

The protective effect of glucose on dextran anaphylactoid reaction has been reported earlier (Adamkiewicz & Adamkiewicz 1960). However, local cutaneous anaphylactic reaction is unchanged with altered blood sugar level (Dhar et al., 1967b).

The mechanism of the protective effect of hyperglycaemic state has been studied as follows :

i) Antibody formation : action on antibody formation was ruled out as hyperglycaemia was induced before challenge when antibody formation was over.

ii) Antibody uptake : Isolated uteri of vergin guinea pigs were incubated with anti horse serum rabbit antibodies at 37°C, for one hour and then one horn was challenged as such with antigen and the other horn was challenged in presence of 0.5 per cent glucose in the bath fluid. However, anaphylactic contraction was similar in presence and in absence of glucose.

iii) Dale Schultz reaction : Presence of glucose on Dale Schultz's reaction of isolated uterus or ileum obtained from sensitized guinea pigs and rats was not significantly different from control. Anaphylactic reaction with uterus from diabetic rats or from rats treated with insulin behaved in similar manner to that noted with uterus from normoglycaemic animals.

iv) Antigen antibody union : precipitation reactions and complement fixation tests were positive in 1 : 10 dilution of antisera. The reactions were unchanged in presence of 0.1, 0.3 or 0.5 per cent glucose.

v) Response of smooth muscle to metabolites ; Response of guinea pig ileum to graded doses of histamine was reduced in presence of 0.3 and 0.5 per cent glucose in the bath fluid. Response of rat uterus to graded doses of 5HT under similar conditions was unaltered. Effect of bradykinin was confusing. Whereas presence of 0.5 per cent glucose increased the sensitivity of rat oestus uterus to bradykinin, the response of guinea pig ileum under similar conditions was either unaltered or reduced.

vi) Glycemic states and sensitivity to histamine and 5HT : Insulin rendered the rats three times more sensitive to histamine (control LD50 : 600 mg. of histamine base i.p.).

TABLE I

Histamine content (r/g/ml $\pm$ S.E) of the lung, intestine and blood in sensitized rats before (Pre) and after (Post) anaphylactic challenge as such and after glucose pretreatment. Sensitized and glucose : blood sugar in sensitized animals before and after glucose treatment without challenge. Glucose (25%/w/v in water) 1 ml/100 g. was given subcutaneously one hour before.

N° of animals	Treatment	Blood histamine r/ml Pre	Post	Lung histamine r/g Pre	Post	Intestine Hist. r/g Pre	Post
6	Sensitized & challenged	0.09+0.01	0.15+0.07	11.8+1.4	7.5+0.38	16.5+1.7	12.0+0.67
6	sensitized, glucose and challenge	0.08+0.02	0.09+0.05	6.2.+0.12	4.8+0.26	10.5+1.2	9.2+0.86
6	Sensitized & Glucose	0.11+0.04	0.16+0.02	9.2.+0.65	5.5+0.25	11.9+0.19	7.6+0.22

5HT sensitivity under similar condition was two times (control
LD 50 :117 mg. of 5HT base s.c.). In hyperglycaemic states
induced by injection of alloxan, rats were two times more resistant to histamine than with untreated animals whereas resistance
to 5HT under similar conditions was not significantly different
from control.

vii) Capillary permeability and glycemic states : Increase
capillary permeability induced by local injection of antigen
to sensitized rats was unaltered either by insulin pretreatment
or by alloxan induced diabetic state or glucose infusion.

viii) Effect of glucose on the blood and tissue histamine has
been studied in sensitized rats as such and during anaphylactic
shock (table 1). It will be seen that there is considerable
release of histamine from lung and intestine and consequent rise
in the blood level during anaphylactic reaction. Pretreatment
with glucose one hour before challenge has the similar effect and
subsequent challenge in these animals does not produce additional
histamine release.
Chakravarty (1962) has shown that glucose does not inhibit anaphylactic release of histamine from minced guinea pig lung. However,
hyperglycaemia induced by continued administration of cortisone
produces rise in blood histamine (Kovacs & Suffiad, 1968). It is
possible that hyperglycaemia induced either by alloxan or slow
infusion of hypertonic glucose, produces slow release of tissue
histamine and prevent the animals from deleterious effects of sudden
release of histamine during anaphylactic shock.

Thus it seems that hyperglycaemia reduces the sensitivity of
histamine and to a less extent to 5HT and that there is slow and
sustained release of histamine during hyperglycaemic state. But
the role of histamine in anaphylactic shock in the rat is doubtful,
in as much as systemic anaphylactic shock can be produced in these
species by almost complete depletion of tissue histamine (Sanyal &
West 1968.).

Mechanism of anaphylactic sensitization has been next studied.
Since B. Pertussis vaccine has been known to produce hypoglycaemia
in mice (Parfentjev & Schleyer, 1949) and rats (Dhar,1963) and
increases the susceptibility to anaphylactic shock, it is possible
that antigenic sensitisation also produces hypoglycaemia. As such
effect of horse serum and egg-white, two commonly used antigens have been studied on blood sugar level in rats.(Fig.2).

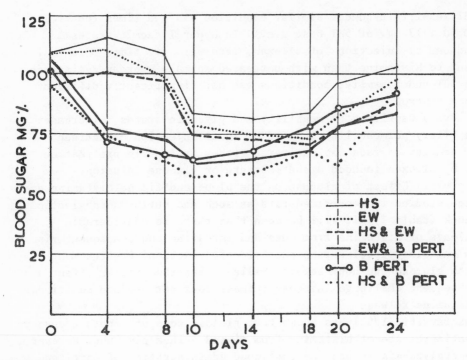

Fig. 2:
Graph showing the blood sugar level in rats before and at different days after sensitization with antigen as such in combination with B. Pertussis vaccine and two antigens together.

It will be seen that both egg-white and horse serum produce fall in the blood sugar level 10 days after sensitization which persists up to 18th day. The degree of fall in the blood sugar is higher with egg white than with horse serum. Addition of B.pertussis vaccine with either antigen produces further fall in the blood sugar level. However ,the result is not significantly different from B. Pertussis when used alone. Use of both antigens together does not make any difference.

It is interesting to note that maximum period of sensitization to anaphylactic shock in the rat occurs between 12th to 18th day after sensitisation and that anaphylactic shock induced by egg white is comparatively more severe than produced with horse serum (Sanyal & West 1958).

B. Pertussis vaccine has been known to produce β adrenergic
blockade in mice (Fishel & Szentivanyi, 1963) and rats (Dhar,1969).
Recently horse serum and egg white has also been shown to possess
week β - adrenergic blockade in rats (Dhar,1969) which may contribute in the formation of hypoglycaemia.
Similar studies have been done in other species as well.

In some preliminary experiments it has been found that in the
guinea pig, the rabbit and the dog horse serum produces hypoglycaemia
only after 20th day of injection and that the addition of B. Pertussis
vaccine on the 16th day of injection does not produce any significant
change in the blood sugar in the guinea pig and in the rabbit. In
the dog however the use of B.Pertussis vaccine produces futher fall
in the blood sugar level. The results in mice are similar to rats.
It is known that successful anaphylactic shock can be produced in
the dog, the guinea pig or the rabbit only after 3 weeks of sensitization and that these animals are very much suceptible to anaphylactic shock. In our laboratory we could not produce severe anaphylactic shock in the dog and use of B. Pertussis vaccine has been
found to be useful in producing systemic anaphylactic shock in this
species.

SUMMARY

1) Anaphylactic shock is potentiated by hypoglycaemia and
prevented by hyperglycaemia. However, here is a species variation.

2) The mechanism of protective effect is still obscure though
reduced resistance to histamine might be a contributing factor.

3) Hypoglycaemia is associated with antigenic sensitization .
B. adrenergic blockade which also produces hypoglycaemia may be an
associated factor.

4) Antigenic sensitization produces hypoglycaemia after 10
days in rats and mice. In the guinea pig, the rabbit and in the
dog under similar conditions hypoglycaemia occurs 20 days after
injection of antigen

5) While B. pertussis vaccine produces additional fall in
blood sugar in rats, mice and dogs, it does not do so in the other
species.

BIBLIOGRAPHY

Adamkiewicz & Adamkiewicz (1960) Glucose and dextran anaphylactoid Inflammation. Am.J. Physiol. 198; 51

Adamkiewicz V.W., Sacra P.J. and Ventura J. (1964) Glycemic state and the horse serum and egg-white anaphylactic shock in rats. J. Immunol. 92; 3.

Chakravarty , N. (1962) Aerobic metabolism in anaphylactic reactions in vitro. Am. J. Physiol.203; 1193.

Dhar, H.L. (1963) Investigations on the mechanism of anaphylaxis Ph.D.Thesis. Calcutta University.

Dhar, H.L. (1969) Comparison of hypoglycaemia induced by horse serum and egg white with B. Pertussis vaccine in rats. Aspt. Allerg. Appl. Immunol.(Press).

Dhar, H.L. and Sanyal, R.K. (1963) Carbohydrate metabolism and anaphylaxis. J. Pharm. Pharmacol. 15; 628.

Dhar, H.L., Sanyal , R.K. and West, G.B. (1967a) . The relationship of the blood sugar level to the severity of anaphylactic shock Brit. J. Pharmacol. 31; 351.

Dhar, et al (1967b) . Anaphylactic shock and the blood sugar level 19; 699.

Dutta, S.N. and Dhar,H.L. (1958). Carbohydrate metabolism and anaphylaxis. Aspt. Allerg. Appl. Immun. 1; 15.

Fishel, C.W. and Szentivanyi A. (1963). The absence of adrenaline induced hyperglycaemia in pertussis -sensitized mice and its relation to histamine and serotonin hypersensitivity. J. Allergy.34; 439.

Galli-Vallerio,B. (1910). Peut-on utiliser Mus rattus et decumann pour le diagnostic taches de sang par le procédé 1 anaphylaxi. Z. Immun. Forsch. 5; 659.

Kovacs, E.M. and Suffiad , K. (1968). Histamine release by cortisone induced hyperglycaemia. Brit. J. Pharmacol. 32 ; 362.

Malkiel, S. and Hargis, B.J. (1952) Anaphylactic shock in pertussis vaccinated mouse. Proc. Soc. Exp. Biol. Med. 80;122.

Molomut, N. (1939). The effect of hypophysectomy on immunity and hypersensitivity in rats with a brief description of the operative technique. J. Immun. 37; 113.

Parfentjev, I.A. and Schleyer, W.L. (1949) . Influence of histamine on blood sugar level of normal and sensitized mice.
Arch. Biochem. 20; 341.

Sanyal , R.K. and West G.B. (1968) Anaphylactic shock in the albino rat . J. Physiol. 142; 571.

Weiser, R.S., Golub O.J. and Hamre, D.M. (1941). Studies on anaphylaxis in the mouse. J. infect. Dis. 68; 97.

SECTION 3

PHARMACOLOGY OF SHOCK

THE INFLUENCE OF BLOOD pH ON PERIPHERAL VASCULAR TONE: POSSIBLE ROLE OF PROTEASES AND VASO-ACTIVE POLYPEPTIDES

H. Wilkens, N. Back, R. Steger, and J. Karn

Department of Biochemical Pharmacology, School of
Pharmacy, State University of New York at Buffalo,
New York

The ability of the microvasculature to respond to the ever
changing metabolic needs of the various tissues is a fundamental
requirement for maintaining homeostasis. The underlying
mechanism is probably a complex one, involving a multiplicity
of mediators, the release of which may be initiated by a primary
metabolic stimulus.

Vasodilatation following a lowering of blood pH was demonstrated nearly a century ago by Gaskell (1), and has been confirmed
since by numerous investigators (2-7). Conversely, it has been
found that muscular activity is accompanied by a decreased pH of
the effluent venous blood (8-11). Although the physiologic importance of this phenomenon has been emphasized repeatedly
by past and recent investigators, (1, 12, 13) the mechanism of
pH-mediated vasodilatation has remained elusive until this day
(13).

In the light of our continuing investigations into the biochemistry of peripheral vascular regulation and failure, a
clarification of the underlying mechanism may be of fundamental
importance not only in physiology, but also in pathologic states,
particularly shock. A body of evidence suggests that decreases
in the pH of the blood and tissue fluids, such as occur during increased metabolic activity or during under-perfusion, (11, 14-17)

may represent a stimulus capable of activating the three major
biological systems concerned with blood coagulation, fibrinolysis,
and kinin formation (Fig. 1).   Activation of these functionally

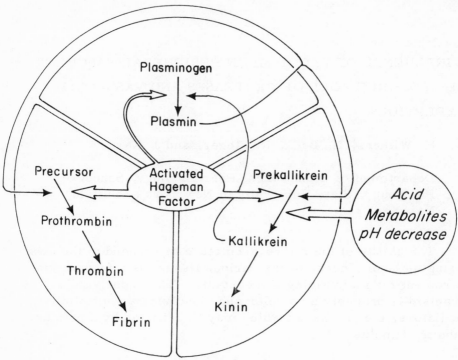

Fig. 1   Triad of blood coagulation-, fibrinolysin-, and
           kallikrein kinin system.

closely interrelated systems may occur either simultaneously
through activated Hageman Factor (18), or sequentially with
either one of the systems activating the other two (19).   Of particular importance is the fact that the kallikrein-kinin system
can be activated, inter alia, by a lowering of pH and by way of
dilution (Fig. 2).   Thus, a slight decrease of pH either effects
the release of kallikrein from the inactive Kallikrein-Inhibitor
Complex prevailing at "normal" physiologic pH (20), or causes
the conversion of inactive pre-kallikrein to kallikrein (21).

        The potential significance of such pH mediated release of
kinins must be viewed in light of the potent pharmacologic properties of kinins.   Nanogram quantities of these potent polypeptides suffice to effect a pronounced degree of vasodilatation and a

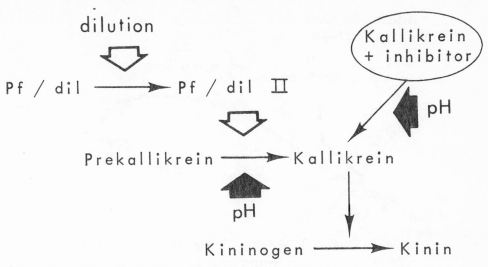

Fig. 2   Effect of pH and dilution on kallikrein-kinin system.

proportionate increase of blood flow in a variety of vascular beds
(22-25).   All these considerations and the important fact that
kinins are very rapidly destroyed by kininases (26), present in
both plasma and tissue fluids, have suggested the possibility that
a pH-mediated release of kinin might very well represent a
decisive link within a metabollically controlled biochemical
mechanism or peripheral vascular autoregulation.   In order to
test this hypothesis, isolated perfusions of canine hind limbs were
carried out in which pH mediated changes in peripheral vascular
resistance were induced by means of injections of buffered solutions.   Changes in the kinin-forming, fibrinolysin and blood
coagulation systems were studied to determine whether and to
what extent a correlation could be established between them and
any observed hemodynamic changes.

Methods and Materials

In situ perfusions of canine hind limbs.   Perfusions of
canine hind limbs in situ were established.   Heparinized arterial
blood obtained from the right carotid artery of the dog was mecha-
nically pumped at a constant flow rate into the left femoral artery
(Fig. 3).   Pressure changes in the perfused limb, representing
changes in peripheral vascular resistance, were measured and
recorded on a polygraph.   A flexible tubing interconnecting the
left femoral vein with the right jugular vein facilitated the with-

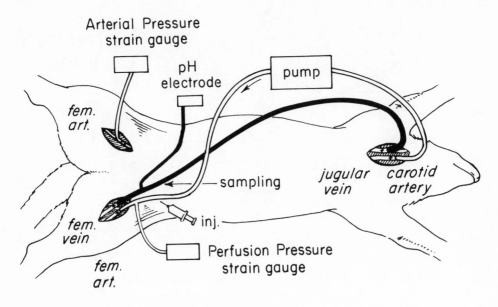

Fig. 3.   In situ perfusion of canine hind limb.

drawal of blood samples. Changes in the pH of the effluent
venous blood were measured and recorded with the aid of a
small gauge catheter inserted deeply into the left femoral vein.
The systemic arterial pressure was obtained and recorded by
means of a catheter introduced via the right femoral artery up to
the aortic bifurcation. The buffer solutions were injected intra-
arterially in close proximity to the perfused limb. Monosodium-
disodium phosphate buffers were selected because the phosphate
ion is not vaso-active (27). Two different buffers, adjusted to
pH 7.4 and 5.8 respectively, were used. The difference in osmo-
ality between these two buffers is only 50 millimols/liter and of
insufficient magnitude to produce a change in vascular resistance
(7). Femoral venous blood samples were obtained immediately
before and at frequent intervals following the injection of buffer.

Perfusions of the severed hind limb.   Perfusion of the
severed hind limb was conducted in essentially the same manner,
except that the venous outflow from the perfused limb drained
into a specially designed bubble type oxygenator, which was aer-
ated by a mixture of 97% O_2 and 3% CO_2, (29) (Fig. 4).

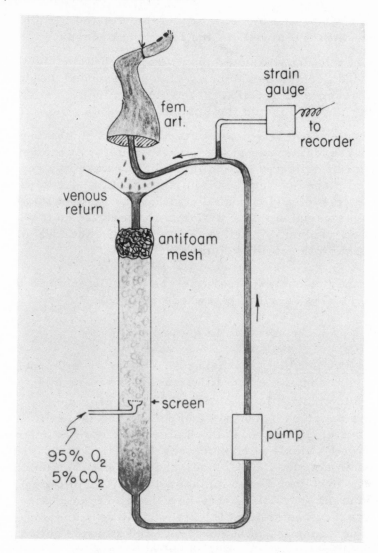

Fig. 4   Perfusion of severed dog hind limb.

In addition to the recording of changes in arterial pressures, blood hydrogen concentrations, and hematocrits of the effluent venous blood, the blood samples were subjected to analysis for the following biochemical parameters: kinin, kininogen, kininase, pre-kallikrein, fibrinogen, prothrombin time, circulating anticoagulants, plasminogen and euglobulin clot lysis times.

Kinin activity was bio-assayed on the isolated rat uterus in accordance with one or both of the following methods:

1. Freshly drawn whole blood was placed immediately into the emptied perfusion chamber with the suspended uterine tissue in the absence of aeration, (to avoid foaming). Thus, direct activity of the blood on the smooth muscle was measured.

2. Whole blood was drawn into a test tube containing crystalline o-phenanthroline as a kininase inhibitor at the ratio of 1 mg per ml of collected blood, immediately mixed by repeated inversion, and placed on ice. This method permitted assays to be carried out at leisure and repeatedly without loss of activity. Frozen samples remained fully active for at least 24 hours. The assays were carried out by adding 0. 5 to 1 ml of either whole blood or plasma to the 10 ml-volume tissue bath.

The other biochemical parameters were determined by methods previously described elsewhere (19, 28).

Results and Discussion

a. In situ perfusions.   In a preliminary experiment (Fig. 5) five ml each of the two different buffers were injected in order to study their effects on the hind limb perfusion pressure and on some principal components of the kalli-krein-kinin system.   Control data obtained prior to the injection of buffer showed a stable perfusion pressure of 115 mm Hg, no detectable kinin activity in the blood, and what may be considered normal levels of kininogen and kininase activity.   Following injection of the pH 7. 4 buffer, a 20 mm Hg drop in perfusion pressure occurred and kinin in the blood appeared, accompanied by a sizable decrease in kininogen levels and kininase activity. Following the injection of the pH 5. 8 buffer, there occurred not only a much greater fall in perfusion pressure, but at the same time a greatly increased kinin activity in the blood, accompanied by correspondingly greater decreases in both kininogen and kininase activity.

A comparison of both sets of data clearly suggests that injection of fluid per se is capable of forming kinin, most probably due to dilution factor Pf/dil. II, which converts pre-kallikrein into active kallikrein (Fig. 2).   In view of the fact that an identical degree of dilution was introduced with the injection of 5 ml of the pH 5. 8 buffer, it may be concluded that the marked

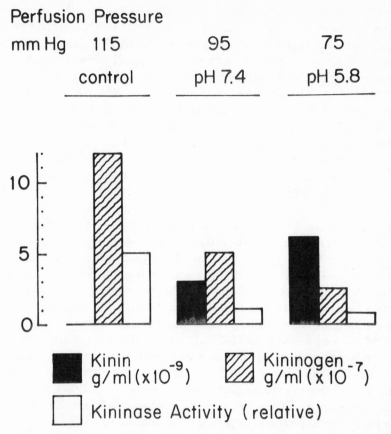

Fig. 5   Comparison of the effects of 5 ml phosphate buffer
          pH 7.4 and pH 5.8 on perfusion pressure and plasma
          kinin system in the in situ perfused canine hind limb.

increase in effect upon the perfusion pressure and the kinin
formation produced by the latter buffer must be due to its
greater hydrogen ion concentration.   Identical conclusions have
been drawn by other investigators who did not study the kinin
system and thus explained the hypotensive effect of dilution on
the basis of lowered blood viscosity (5, 12).

        In view of these preliminary findings, and in order to
reduce the number of complex variables to a minimum, the
intra-arterial injection of 5 ml of phosphate buffer pH 5.8 was
adopted as a uniform procedure for all subsequent experiments.
This procedure caused a . 006 unit decrease of pH in the effluent
venous blood.

Figure 6 summarizes the results of a typical experiment using the perfused canine hind limb in situ. In this experiment the systemic arterial pressure was stable at the outset, but later on declined somewhat, caused perhaps by the frequent blood sampling. The limb perfusion pressure, likewise stable in the beginning, shows a short peak immediately upon injection of the buffer. This peak is without doubt due to a temporary fluid overload. After this peak there occurred a 35 mm Hg fall in perfusion pressure, followed by a slow recovery. A similar injection of buffer given 90 minutes later produced quite similar effects. The kinin level at the outset was below the threshold detectable by bio-assay technique. Fifty seconds following the first buffer injection, however, kinin activity sharply rose to a pronounced peak. Following this peak, kinin activity quickly declined. Interestingly, there occurred a second smaller rise 5 minutes after the injection. This biphasic response, though less pronounced in this particular experiment than in most others, was seen in all our experiments. Whether these secondary increases in kinin activity are caused simply by a recirculation of small amounts of undestroyed kinin (which appears unlikely in view of its very short half-life), or whether they are reflective of a de novo release of kinin, has not been determined. A blood sample taken 10 minutes after the first buffer injection showed no detectable kinin activity. At the 35 minute mark a seemingly spontaneous rise in kinin activity was observed, which was not accompanied by a change in perfusion pressure. Also, no increase in kinin activity was detected following the second buffer injection. The blood kininogen level, as might be expected, showed a decline coinciding with the first kinin peak. Likewise, in keeping with expectations, there was a decrease in kininogen in parallel with the spontaneous rise of kinin activity near the 35 minute mark, and again following the second buffer injection. The incongruous rise in kininogen seen near the 5 minute mark is not easily explained, but may perhaps be assumed to reflect an out pouring of additional substrate from systemic or tissue storage sites in response to unidentified stimuli. Release of kininogen from storage sites possibly may account for the absence of a direct relationship between kinin release and blood kininogen levels reported previously (28, 30-32). A marked decline in blood kininogen whenever observed argues much more positively for a simultaneous release of kinin.

A very good correlation was obtained between kinin release and the consumption of prekallikrein. Both these parameters pre-

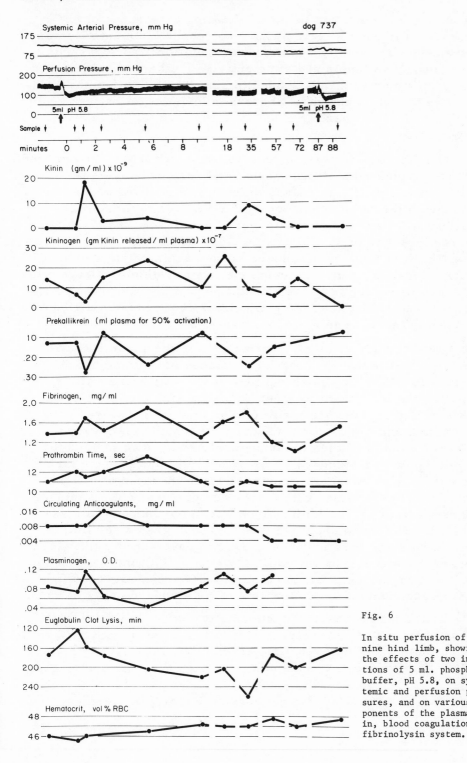

Fig. 6

In situ perfusion of canine hind limb, showing the effects of two injections of 5 ml. phosphate buffer, pH 5.8, on systemic and perfusion pressures, and on various components of the plasma-kinin, blood coagulation, and fibrinolysin system.

sent a near perfect mirror image, indicating a decrease of pre-
enzyme levels in each instance where increased kinin activity was
measured. An apparently significant correlation also was seen
between fibrinogen levels and kinin activity. Likewise, changes in
prothrombin times generally tended to run parallel with both fibrinogen levels and kinin activity, whereas no meaningful pattern could
be established with regard to changes in the level of circulating
anticoagulants.

        The fibrinolysin system was obviously affected, as evidenced
by changes in both plasminogen levels and euglobulin lysis times.
The latter significantly increased following each of the two buffer injections, with fluctuations occurring during the interim. These
alterations in fibrinolytic activity were by and large matched by
concurrent changes in plasminogen levels. Apparent imperfections
in agreement must in our opinion be viewed again relative to a
possible release of additional substrate from systemic storage sites.
Finally, the hematocrits of the effluent venous blood showed no abrupt changes following the buffer injections, but revealed a steady
and moderate increase in hemoconcentration.

        Quite similar changes, particularly in the plasma kinin
system, were observed in all other instances of isolated hind limb
perfusions in situ. This is shown in Table I, which presents in
summary form the effects in seven dogs of a single intra-arterial
injection of 5 ml. of pH 5.8 buffer on the arterial pressure in the
perfused limb and major components of the plasma kinin system. In
each instance the perfusion pressure declined by a mean value of
32.6 mm Hg, with a standard error of 6.6. Likewise, the kinin
levels rose in all instances, showing a mean increase of 9.5×10^{-9}
grams per ml. of plasma, with a standard error of 2.1. Kininogen
levels declined in all but one instance where no change at all was
registered. The mean decrease was 1.7×10^{-6} grams per ml. of
plasma, with a standard error of 0.7. Kininase activity likewise
decreased in most instances, while showing a 100% increase in one
animal, and no change at all in another. The mean decrease in kininase activity amounted to 61.7% with a large standard error of 65.3.

        In addition to these experiments two other in situ
hind limb perfusions were carried out following pretreatment
of the animals with the proteolytic enzyme inhibitor TRA-
SYLOL[*] with a dose of 25,000 units per kg. I.V. In both cases

_____

[*] TRASYLOL, product of Farbenfabriken Bayer AG, Germany.

CHANGE IN PERFUSION PRESSURE & KININ SYSTEM
20–40 secs. FOLLOWING I.A. INJ. OF 5 ml PHOSPHATE BUFFER, pH 5.8

Dog #	Perfusion Pres. (mm Hg)	KININ (g/ml Plas x 10^{-9})	KININOGEN (g/ml Plas x 10^{-6})	KININASE (% Cont. Act.)
333	− 35	+ 7	− 1.0	− 370
273	− 25	+ 1	not measured	− 50
871	− 10	+ 14	$\pm$ 0	− 20
737	− 38	+ 16.2	− 1.1	not measured
82	− 35	+ 4	− 4	+100
219	− 20	+ 12	− 0.13	$\pm$ 0
844	− 65	+ 12	− 3.8	− 30
Mean	− 32.6	+ 9.5	− 1.7	− 61.7
(S.E.)	(6.6)	(2.1)	(0.7)	(65.3)

Table I   Mean changes in hind limb perfusion pressure and the plasma-kinin system observed in seven dogs following injection of 5 ml. phosphate buffer, pH 5.8

repeated injections of the pH 5.8 buffer had a much diminished effect on the perfusion pressure and failed entirely to produce any of the aforementioned changes in the kinin-, fibrinolysin-, and blood coagulation systems. In still another animal 5 ml of TRASYLOL (25,000 units), adjusted to a pH of 8.5, was injected directly into the perfusion circuit. This stimulus caused no vasodilatation and no changes in the three biochemical systems.

b.   Perfusions of the Severed Hind Limb were carried out with artificially oxygenated autologous blood. This arrangement proved itself unsuitable for the intended purpose, since it became apparent that the oxygenation procedure employed (Fig. 4) was in itself capable of forming large amounts of kinin. Additional work is contemplated to investigate this phenomenon more fully, in view of its potential significance with respect to clinical heart-lung bypass procedures employing artificial oxygenating devices.

Conclusion

While the work here reported is of a preliminary nature and much still needs to be done to elucidate all the aspects of the phenomena described, evidence obtained so far is sufficiently strong to suggest a major role for the kallikrein - kinin system within the mechanism of peripheral vascular auto-regulation, at least in the muscle tissue. If such is the case, it would appear that a derangement of this mechanism, as might occur during peripheral vascular decompensation, could very well play an important role in the pathophysiology of various types of clinical shock. It is premature to think of kinin release as the possible initiating event in shock. The study would tend to ascribe to kinin a secondary role, wherein tissue hypoxia, as may be produced by extensive hemorrhage or a great variety of other causes, may act as the initiating event followed by the activation of the kinin system and related biochemical systems. Thus, the release of chemical mediators may contribute to the complex picture characteristic for progressive shock. Whether the presence of kinin, formed by proteolytic forces, under these circumstances is detrimental, is uncertain. Evidence obtained over the years by our own group with the use of potent proteolytic enzyme inhibitors clearly has shown increased survival rates in a variety of experimental shock models,(28) and thus tends to suggest a detrimental role. On the other hand, it was recently shown by us in experiments with perfused canine hind limbs, that the customary vasodilator action of bradykinin is reversed in the presence of histamine. (29)Histamine release during shock is a recognized occurrence. In summary, evidence has been presented, indicating a physiological role for kinin in the mechanism of tissue blood flow regulation. It has been suggested that kinin appears as a factor during the pathogenetic process of peripheral vascular shock. Whether the participation of kinin in shock is detrimental or perhaps even beneficial remains an unsolved problem.

REFERENCES

1.   Gaskell, T.W.A., J. Physiol., 1880, 3, 38.

2.   Bayliss, W. M., J. Physiol., 1901, 26, 32P.

3.   Krogh, A. , In: The Anatomy and Physiology of Capillaries.
          New Haven: Yale Univ. Press, 1922.

4.   Fleisch, A. et al. , Arch. Ges. Physiol. , 1932, 230, 814.

5.   Kester, N. C. , et al. , Am. J. Physiol. , 1952, 169, 678.

6.   Zsoter, T. , et al. , Am. Heart J. , 1961, 61, 777.

7.   Molnar, J. I. , et al. , Am. J. Physiol. , 1962, 203, 125.

8.   Kontos, H. A. , and J. L. Patterson, Jr. , Clin. Sci. ,
          1964, 27, 143.

9.   Ross, J. , Jr. et al. , Circulation Res. , 1964, 15, 473.

10. Rudko, M. , and F. J. Haddy, Physiologist, 1965, 8, 264.

11. Kontos, H. A. , et al. , Am. J. Physiol. , 1966, 211, 869.

12. Deal, C. P. , Jr. , and H. D. Green, Circulation Res. , 1954,
          2, 148.

13. Kontos, H. A. , et al. , Am. J. Physiol. , 1968, 215, 1403.

14. Frey, E. K. , Arch. Klin. Chir. , 1930. 162, 334.

15. Kontos, H. A. , et al. , Am. J. Physiol. , 1965, 209, 1106.

16. Kilburn, K. H. , J. Appl. Physiol. , 1966, 21, 675.

17. Bergan, J. J. , et al. , Clin. Res. , 1967, 15, 416.

18. Margolis, J. , Ann. N. Y. Acad. Sci. , 1963, 104, 133.

19. Back, N. et al. , In: Hypotensive Polypeptides, Springer
          Verl. , Germany, 1966, p. 495-505.

20. Frey, E. K. , et al. , In: Kallikrein - Padutin, F. Enke
          Verl. Stuttgart, 1950,   78-84.

21. Wilkens, H. & N. Back,   Unpublished data.

22. Fox, R. H. , et al. , J. Physiol. , 1961, 157, 589.

23.   Maxwell, G. M., et al., Circulation Res., 1962, 10, 359.

24.   Paldino, R. L., et al., Circulation Res., 1962, 11, 847.

25.   Kontos, H. A., et al., Circulation Res., 1964, 14, 351.

26.   Erdos, E. G., et al., Ann. N. Y. Acad. Sci., 1963, 104,
            222.

27.   Haddy, F. J., In: The Peripheral Blood Vessels, Williams
            and Wilkins, Baltimore, 1963, p. 92-105.

28.   Back, N. et al., Ann. N. Y. Acad. Sci., 1968, 146, 491.

29.   Back, N., and H. Wilkens, In: Pharmacology of Hormonal
            Polypeptides and Proteins. Plenum Publ. Co.,
            N. Y., 1968, p. 486-496.

30.   Cirstea, M., et al., Arch. Int. Pharmacodyn., 1966, 159, 18.

31.   Diniz, C. R. & I. F. Carvalho, Ann. N. Y. Acad. Sci.,
            1963, 104, 77.

32.   Habermann, F., et al. "Plasma Kinins: An International
            Symposium, Fiesole, Italy, 1969." Eds.
            Sicuteri, F., Back, N. and Rocha e Silva, M.
            Plenum Press, New York. In Press.

The authors acknowledge with appreciation the competent
technical assistance of the summer fellowship research
assistants, Miss Heidi Hanson and Mr. Efrem E. Back.

Supported by United States Public Health Service Grant Numbers
HE-11492 and HE-03784, National Heart Institute.

THE INFLUENCE OF SOME ENZYMES AND ENZYME INHIBITORS IN SHOCK

A. BERTELLI, L. DONATI

Institute of Pharmacology of the University of

Milan, Medical School, Italy

Basically events in shock pathogenesis are rather well
known to-day, and in some cases they are well known in
the very details. What is lacking is a clear understanding
of the mechanisms and reciprocal relations which join
between themselves the different and complex biological
phenomena.
As was the case for other problems raised by physiopathology, it has been attempted to interpret unilaterally
the series of pathological events characteristic to shock,
proposing a basal mechanism able to explain all the events,
as for example the theory of the generalized permeabiliza-
tion of capillaries, the neurogenic theory, the toxical
theory in all its nuances, and so on.
What is the clue in any case is the microcirculatory
response to different pathological events with inadequate
capillary perfusion of living tissues.(1).
In fact, the peripheric vascular failure could be initiated
by various factors and explain the physiopathological consequences of shock.
Among the agents that might cause or aggravate the shock
state there are, as is well known, the bacterial toxins,
hypoxia, lactacidemia, fibrinolytic substances, nucleotides, active polypeptides, histamines, tissue toxins,
coagulative alterations, lowering of blood pH and so on.
(2,3,4,5,6,7,8,9,10,11).
As some of these different co-factors are activated by
enzymatic systems or are activating them, the role that
enzymes, of hydrolasic and proteolytic type in particular,
play in shock has been especially considered and taken

215

under consideration.

An important increase of the proteolytic activity
has been in fact noted in traumatic, surgical, haemorrhagic, endotoxinic, anaphylactic and thermal shock.(11,12,
13,14,15,16).

The proteases are able in their turn to extend the
initial lesion, activating all the chemical mediators of
the phlogosis, with the metabolic consequences known (17,
18).
Fibrinolysis, blood coagulation and kinin formation are
among the most relevant phenomena, activated by proteases
and closely interrelated.(19).
It is supposed that mechanical, thermic, immunological,
nervous or bacterial stimuli are able to activate or induce the release of proteolytic enzymes and other hydrolases, either directly or indirectly. Following the release of these enzymes, there is an activation of the
chemical mediators of the flogosis and of the vasoactive
polypeptides with microhemodynamic alterations able to
induce by themselves a further activation of enzymes,
realizing the vicious circle of shock. Moreover shock
has been experimentally produced by trypsin and chymotrypsin, as well as a prolongation of survival in shocked
animals has been obtained by antitryptic substances (5,
20,21,22).

This interpretative scheme has been confirmed by
the studies on inflammation and by the studies dealing
with the characteristics of lysosomes.

These organelles are rich in hydrolasic enzymes which
are active under acid pH, able to be released under various
pathological conditions, especially those able to induce
shock, among which burns, immunological agents, bacterial
toxins, hypoxia and acidosis(23).

In various forms of shock it has been demonstrated
an increase of a typical lysosomal enzyme , acid phosphatase, and β-glycuronidase (24-25). Cytosegresomes,
lysosomes in a particular autophagic attitude , correlated
to an increase of hydrolases, has been seen in hepatic
cells following endotoxinic shock (26) and in hypovolaemic
shock (27). Furthermore a degranulation of lysosomal particles has been described in leucocytes after phagocytosis of antigen-antibody complexes, with an increased release of proteases and other hydrolases.(28-29-30).

This release of lysosomal enzymes from cells under pathological conditions may partly explain the characteristics
of progression and irreversibility that shock can induce.
The central function of the R.E.S. in the establishment
of the shock phenomena can also be interpreted considering
how rich in lysosomes the reticulo-endothelial cells are
and how the detoxicating action of these cells is conditioned by the integrity of these structures (31).

It has been proposed, for instance, that in hemorrhagic shock the lysosomes of the reticulo-endothelial
cells were disrupted and therefore not able to inactivate
endotoxin (32).
On the other hand, bacterial endotoxin is known to be
able to cause the release of lysosome proteases (25).

Hypothesizing a lysosomal mediation, the induced
tolerance to shock could also be interpreted, because
the pretreatment of animals, with,i.e., endotoxin, shows
a stabilizing effect on the lysosomal walls (33,34).
The most recent studies have for a large extent confirmed
these hypotheses, especially as far as the acid proteolytic enzymes are concerned, even if is not yet quite
clear the position or "Hierarchy" they are occupying in
the complex pathogenic mechanism of shock and whether
they are a primary or secondary phenomenon.
The use of some inhibitors of the proteases, among which
Trasylol and Epsilon-amino-caproic acid (EAC),has proved
useful in diminishing the gravity of hemorrhagic shock,
traumatic shock, thermic shock and anaphylactic shock.
The importance of the proteasic activation in shock is
thus indirectly confirmed(35-36).
In order to estimate better the efficiency of enzymatic
inhibitors in the treatment of shock, we have determined
the level of plasmatic proteasic activity in rats, at
pH3, under thermic and endotoxin shock.
Moreover we have determined the plasmatic activity of
an other enzyme of lysosomal origin : the acid phosphatase.
The increase of the acid phosphatase activity seems to be
predominant in the same strong organic reactions as
during rejection of organ homotransplantation.
These enzymatic activities have been determined in animals
submitted to shock and treated with various inhibitors of
the proteases; and the percentage of survival has also
been determined in animals protected by inhibitors and in
those not treated. The inhibitors used were the polypep-
tidic inhibitor of Frey (Trasylol) , epsilon -amino-
caproic acid (EAC), epsilon acetamido caproic acid (EAAC),
para-amino-methyl benzoic acid (PAMBA).
All these substances have a variable inhibiting capacity
towards the various proteasic and fibrinolytic systems

and have proved to possess a protective action in different reactions of inflammatory and anaphylactic type,
such as carrageenin , dextran, and white of egg oedema,
Sanarelli-Schwartzmann reaction, anaphylactic shock,
tuberculine reaction and survival time of skin allografts
(37,38).
In order to determine better whether the release of lysosomal enzymes is a determining moment in the establishment
of the irreversible shock in the experimental animal, we
have treated other animals in which shock had been induced with vitamin A, agent labilizing the lysosomal wall,
and prednisolone agent able to stabilize the lysosomal
wall (39-40).

MATERIAL AND METHODS

Thermic shock has been induced in male Sprague-Dawley
rats, weighing about 250 grammes, under anesthesia by
ether, through an 8" immersion in water at 80°C up to the
axilla level. Endotoxinic shock has been caused in male
Sprague Dawley rats, weighing 250 grammes, by the intraperitoneal injection of 2,5 mg of toxin of Salmonella
Enteritidis (Difco).
The rats, divided in groups of at least twenty animals
have been treated with solutions of Trasylol (100000 U.I./
Kg), EAC (1gr/Kg), EAA (1gr/Kg), PAMBA (1gr/Kg) and pred-
nisolone(50 mg/Kg) intraperitoneally and intramusculary
with vitamin A acetate (8000 U/Kg), an hour before the
burn or before the injection of toxin.
Enzymatic determinations have been done an hour after
the treatment effectuated on the plasma obtained from
the heparinated blood taken from the jugular vein.
The plasma has been maintained at 0°C and the determinations have been effectuated immediately.
The proteasic activity has been determined using hemoglobin as a substrate, incubating the plasma for 3 hours in
acetate buffer (pH3)and determining the optic spectro-
photometric density values at 260 μm (41).
The acid phosphatase has been determined with the method
of Bessey and Lowe, by measuring spectrophotometrically
the dinitrophenol (in millimoles) released in an hour.
The results of the percentage of mortality in rats submitted to various treatments and the cathepsinic and·
phosphatasic activities are exposed in tables Nr. I,II,
III,IV,V,VI.
As concerns the percentage of mortality in burned rats,
the reductions provoked by inhibitors, such as Trasylol,
EAAC, seem to us very important whereas EAC, PAMBA,pro-
ved being less efficient.

TABLE I THERMIC SHOCK IN RATS 24 HR. MORTALITY	
CONTROLS	—
SHOCKED	95 %
,, + TRASILOL	65 %
,, + EAC	75 %
,, + EAAC	70 %
,, + PAMBA	85 %
,, + PREDNISOLONE	60 %
,, + VIT. A	100 %

TABLE II ENDOTOXIN SHOCK IN RATS 24 HR. MORTALITY	
CONTROLS	—
SHOCKED	90 %
,, + TRASILOL	60 %
,, + EAC	70 %
,, + EAAC	65 %
,, + PAMBA	90 %
,, + PREDNISOLONE	55 %
,, + VIT. A	90 %

TABLE III

THERMIC SHOCK IN RATS
PROTEASIC ACTIVITY 1 HR.
AFTER SCALDING (pH 3)

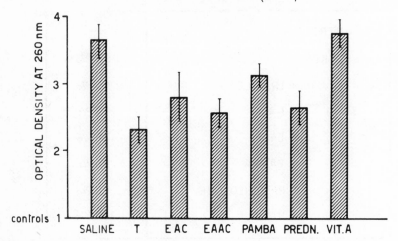

It is probable that the letal thermic shock caused to
the animals could be aggravated, as concerns mortality,
by other factors, which are not under the control of
inhibitors. These results are partly superposable as
regards Trasylol, with the precedent experiments of Back,
(42).
Worth being noted is the very important action of prednisolone, referable to the multiple pharmacological actions
of this substance. The increase of the mortality induced
by Vitamin A seems to confirm the role of lysosomal enzymes, if we consider the action labilizing the lysosomal
walls of this substance.
We obtained results rather similar concerning the mortality of animals submitted to endotoxinic shock.
The different vascular reaction of EAC and of its acetate
derivative can explain the less important action of these molecules in comparison with Trasylol.
In thermic shock, as well as in toxinic shock, the cathepsinic activity of the plasma is much increased and seems
to be much influenced by the treatment with inhibitors,
even if a strict parallelism does not exist. Between
plasmatic activity and mortality we must point out how
the most active substances, at the plasmatic level, are
also the most active in lengthening the life of the
animals.
The proceeding of the enzymatic activities, of the acid
phosphatase especially as regards the action of predniso-

TABLE IV

THERMIC SHOCK IN RATS
PA ACTIVITY 1HR AFTER SCALDING

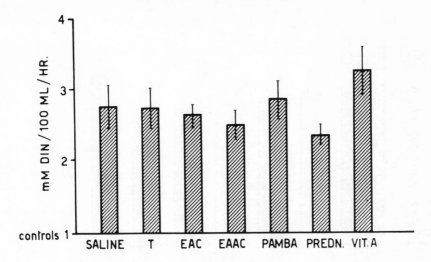

TABLE V

ENDOTOXIN SHOCK IN RATS
PROTEASIC ACTIVITY (1 HOUR AFTER) pH3

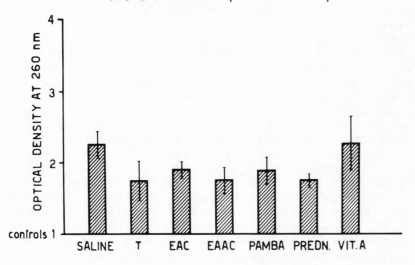

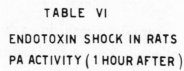

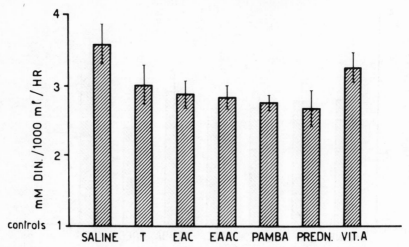

lone and of vitamin A, seems to confirm the lysosomal origin of the acid proteases.
The lacking action of the inhibitors of the proteases on
the phosphatasic activity seems to demonstrate that these
substances have no action at all on the lysosomal wall
and that a rupture of these membranes does not depend on
an endolysosomal activation of the peptidases.
An aspect which appears very important to us is the strict
parallelism which, from an enzymatic point of view, corre-
lates the two forms of shock and the univocal action of
prednisolone and vitamin A. The post-mortem exams of the
animals have shown less gastroenteric hemorrhages in the
treated animals than in controls.
These results confirm the importance of proteolytic systems in the shock appearance and of the important role
played by the anatomo-functional system of the lysosomes.
The use of the enzymatic inhibitors proves being promising
even if, for the present time, it is not yet completely
satisfactory. But, remembering what we have said at the
beginning of our report, about the tendancy of unilateral
approach in the attempt of understanding the basal moments
of the pathogenesis of shock, we think that in such a
complex syndrome, the approach can only be multilateral
and interdisciplinary.
Even if our research enable us to confirm the role
played by the lysosomal enzymes in these pathological

phenomena, we also consider as important other factors
which are not necessarily active with a mechanism mediated through lysosomal hydrolases.
In any case we believe that the clinical and pharmacological chapter on the use of enzymatic inhibitors in shock
deserves further and more thorough studies.

BIBLIOGRAPHY

1) Zweifach B.W. in "Microcirculation as related to shock"
   edited by D. Shepro and G.P. Fulton, p.247, Academic
   Press New York 1968.

2) Fine J., Rutenburg S.H., Schweinburg F.B.,
   J. Exptl. Medicine, 110,547,1959.

3) Rutenburg S.H., Rutenburg A.M., Smith E.E., Fine J.
   Proc. Symp. Inst. Microbiol. Rutgers, New Jersey,
   Quinn and Boden 1964.

4) Seligmen A.M., Frank H.A., Alexander B., Fine J.
   J. Clin.Invest. 26,536,1947.

5) Tagnon H.J., Lewenson S.M., Davidson C.S.
   Am.J.Med.Sci., 211,88,1946.

6) Green H.N., Stoner H.B.
   Biological actions of the adenine nucleotides, Lewis,
   London 1950.

7) Rocha e Silva M.
   Rend.Ist. Sup. Sanità,23,797,1960.

8) Schayer R.W.
   Am. Journal of physiology, 198,1187,1960

9) Allgöwer M. in"Shock Symposium"
   p.268,Springer Verlag 1962

10) Hardaway R.M., Husny E.A., Geever E.F., Noyes H.E.,
    Burns J.W.
    Ann. Surg. 154,791,1961

11) H. Green, Rapela C.E. in "Microcirculation as related
    to shock" edited by D. Shepro and G.P. Fulton .
    p.93, Academic Press New York 1968.

12) Beard E.L., Hampton J.K., Am. Journal of Physiology, 204,405,1963.

13) Ungar G.
    Lancet 1, 708,1947.

14) Back N. , Wilkens H., Steger R.
    Ann. N.Y. Acad. Sci. 146. 491,1968.

15) Mc Farlane R.G., Biggs R.
    Lancet 2,862,1946.

16) Bertelli A., Donati L., Cristofori G., Trabucchi E.Jr.,
    in "Pharmacological Treatment of Burns",
    Proceedings Int. Symposium on Burns edited by A.
    Bertelli and L. Donati; Excerpta Medica Amsterdam 1970.

17) Bertelli A.
    Proteases and antiproteasic substances in the in-
    flammatory response.
    Biochem. Pharmacol., 1968,suppl.p.229.

18) Bertelli A.
    Médicaments antipeptidasiques et activité anti-
    inflammatoire.
    Pathologie-biologie,1967,vol.15,N° 3-4,pp.163-167.

19) Rocha e Silva M.
    Ann. N.Y. Acad.Sciences, 146,448,1968.

20) Thal A.P., Sardesar V.M.
    Am. Journal Surgery 110,308,1965.

21) Gurd F.N.
    American Journal Surgery, 110,333,1965

22) Halpern B.N.
    Proc. Soc. Exp. Biol.Med., 115,273,1964.

23) De Duve C.
    in "subcellular particles", Ronal Press, New York 1959.

24) Irwin R., Ann. Surg.169,202,1969.

25) Janoff A., Weissmann G., Zweifach B.W., Thomas L.,
    J. Exptl. Med. 40,281,1962.

26) Boler R.K., Bibighaus A.J.
    Lab. Invest.17,357,1967

27) Blail O.M., Stenger R.J., Hopkins R.W.
    Simeone F.A.
    Lab. Invest. 18,172,1968.

28) Hirsch J.G.
    J. Exptl. Med.116,827,1962

29) Movat A.Z., Uriuhara T., Taichman N.S., Rowsell H.C.,
    Mustard J.F.
    Immunology, 14,637,1968

30) Astorga G., Bollet A.J.
    Arthritis Rheumat.(Abstract)7,288,1964

31) Straus W.
    J.Cell. Biol.17,597,1963

32) Bitensky L., Chayen J., Cunningham G.J., Fine J.
    Nature, Lond. 191,493,1963

33) Janoff A., Zweifach B.W.
    Proc.Soc. Exptl. Biol.Med., 114,695,1963.

34) Saito K., Suter E.
    J.Exptl.Med.121,739,1965

35) Sherry S.,
    Fed. Proc.20,9,209,1961

36) Back N., Ambrus J.C.,
    Handbook for Surgery and Specialities.
    Eds.A.W. Ulin and Gollub S.
    Mc Grow Hill, New York, 1966.

37) Bertelli A., Donati L., Marek J.
    in "Biochemistry of Inflammation" edited by A.Bertelli
    and J. Houck
    Excerpta Medica Amsterdam 1970.

38) Bertelli A., Donati L., Trabucchi E.Jr.
    Pharmacology 2, 223,1969

39) Dingle J.T., Sharman I.M., Moore T.
    Biochem.J.98,476,1966;

40) Weissmann G., Dingle J.T. 1961
    Exptl. Cell Res. 25,207,1961

41) Safia Wasi, Uriuhara T., Taichman N.S., Murray R.K.,
    Movat A.Z.
    Proteolytic activity in the serum of rabbits during
    anaphylaxis
    Experientia (Basel) 22/3, 195.

42) Back N., Wilkens H., Steger R.
    Annals N.Y. Acad.Sci.,146,2,491,1968.

PHARMACOLOGIC AGENTS IN SHOCK

Colonel Robert M. Hardaway, III, Medical Corps

Commanding Officer, US Army General Hospital,

Frankfurt, Germany

In recent years there has been increasing emphasis and interest in the use of drugs in the treatment of shock. A wide divergence of views exists as to the best method of treating shock, but this is characteristic in clinical medicine of any disease in which the pathophysiology is poorly understood and none of the available forms of therapy is fully satisfactory. It must be emphasized that any drug therapy in shock is secondary to adequate replacement of intravascular volume deficits with colloid and crystalloid solution, correction of hypoxemia with respiratory support, adequate surgical drainage and antibiotics in sepsis, and repair of acid-base and electrolyte abnormalities which exist. Indeed, the combined experience of the Walter Reed shock unit and the surgical research team in Vietnam with several hundred cases of shock has shown that the great majority of these cases represent solely a decreased effective circulating blood volume and respond well to adequate volume administration only.

The defect in shock, at which all therapy must be directed, is a derangement of the circulation resulting in tissue perfusion inadequate for normal cellular function. Although correctable at an early stage, insufficient perfusion, if inadequately treated, inevitably leads to death. In the laboratory animal, one may define an "irreversible" shock preparation in specific experimental situations. This term implies only that the animal is irreversible to the therapy utilized in that set of experimental conditions. In clinical medicine the term "irreversible" shock should not be used until the patient is pronounced dead. There is, however, a small group of patients who are "refractory" to conventional therapy. Such "refractory" shock patients continue to show clinical deterioration because of inadequate tissue perfusion in spite of the fact

227

that circulating volume has been restored, as measured by central
venous pressure and direct blood volume determinations, adequate
ventilatory function has been provided, hypoxemia corrected, vigorous measures have been instituted to combat sepsis and measurable
electrolyte and acid-base abnormalities have been corrected. It is
this group of refractory patients where drug therapy is of interest.
Innumerable types of therapy have been proposed for the treatment
of the refractory shock patient, but the present discussion will be
limited to those agents which have progressed to the point of having received clinical trials. The discussion will not be concerned
with the use of cardiac glycosides and antiarrhythmic drugs.

    Although it is generally accepted that the final common path-
way in shock is a failure of effective bloodflow in the microcirculation, there is no agreement regarding the basic etiologic factors which lead to this microcirculatory failure. Since the pharmacologic agents advocated for treating shock are primarily aimed
at the hemodynamic system, it must be pointed out, as emphasized by
Gilbert, that in the broadest sense there are three hemodynamic
abnormalities possible in refractory shock: 1) a volume deficit,
2) an abnormal state of the vascular bed, or 3) a deficit in the
work capacity of the heart. Drug therapy in shock is aimed at cor-
recting the second and third of these abnormalities since it is
assumed that provision has already been made to correct the first.

ADRENOCORTICAL STEROIDS

    The use of corticosteroids in the treatment of shock is cur-
rently the subject of lively discussion and of intensive laboratory
and clinical investigation. It has been proposed that adrenal cortical failure may be a common cause of death in severe trauma and
shock. This impression has been reinforced by several observations:
1) The adrenalectomized animal is extremely sensitive to the induction of shock by a variety of techniques. A small replacement
dose of adrenal steroid can increase the survival of these animals
significantly. 2) The addisonian patient is poorly able to with-
stand trauma or shock and frequently dies if his condition has not
been recognized at the time when trauma is inflicted. The fact remains, however, that the majority of people who die in shock show a
very high level of blood corticosteroid just before death and are
capable of responding to exogenous ACTH by a further increase in
the plasma level of steroids. The use of adrenal steroids or their
synthetic analogues, in treating shock must then be based on a pharmacologic, rather than a physiologic action.   ·

    The rationale for the clinical use of adrenal steroids is based
on experimental models, primarily canine, in which shock is induced
either by controlled hemorrhage or by the injection of an endotoxin
derived from gram-negative bacteria. Evidence of a protective action

by steroids in the treatment of endotoxin shock and hemorrhagic
shock has been reported, but the mechanism of this action remains
as much of an enigma as the pathophysiologic defects in shock itself.

A variety of mechanisms have been proposed for the observed
protective effects of pharmacologic doses of adrenal steroids in
experimental shock. It has been reported that such doses of glucocorticoids have an adrenolytic effect in canine endotoxin shock
and decrease systemic peripheral resistance while increasing regional flow. Extremely large doses (4 to 8 gm) are said to act as a
vasodilator with the same effect as phenoxybenzamine. This fact,
if confirmed, would be very helpful, since vasodilators such as
phenoxybenzamine are not generally available. A cardiotonic action
has also been demonstrated in isolated rat-heart preparations and a
third possible mechanism involves an intracellular stabilization of
lysosomal membrane integrity.

Studies at the Walter Reed shock unit and by the surgical research team in Vietnam aimed at delineating the hemodynamic effects
of pharmacologic doses (50 mg/kg) of glucocorticoids in patients
with a diagnosis of shock have failed to demonstrate any adrenolytic or cardiotonic effect. This is in contrast to the findings of
Sambhi et al. who reported a significant increase in cardiac output
while arterial pressure remained unchanged. These authors reported
a similar but less pronounced effect after administration of miner-
alocorticoid compounds. Certainly, the clinical investigator is at
a disadvantage when trying to define the pharmacological action of
steroids in shock. In addition to the problems of interpreting
therapeutic results in a heterogenous group of critically ill patients, evaluation of steroid therapy is complicated by the non-
specific effects of inflammatory suppression and euphoria which tend
to mask clinical findings.

If treatment with corticosteroids is of value in clinical shock,
it should be possible to demonstrate some beneficial effects. No
prospective study has been reported on the use of steroids in shock,
and the two largest retrospective studies differ widely in their
results. Weil et al. reported a significant decrease in mortality
from gram-negative bacteremia associated with shock when cortisol
was employed in doses greater than 300 mg daily, whereas McCabe and
Jackson reported a significant increase in mortality when steroids
were used in treating gram-negative bacteremia with shock.

In view of the conflicting data and opinions regarding the use
of adrenocortical steroids in shock, it would appear that the only
definite indication for their use is in those rare instances of shock
which are due to adrenal insufficiency. In other types of shock which
fail to respond to vigorous conventional therapy more specific agents
are available for use without the potentially hazardous ability of

steroids to suppress inflammatory processes and decrease resistance
to the spread of infection. If steroids are employed in pharmacologic doses to try to obtain a vasodilator effect, this use should probably be restricted to one large intravenous dose of 4 to 8 grams
followed for a close observation response.

DRUGS WHICH ACT AS VASODILATORS AND
CARDIAC STIMULATORS

The administration of vasopressor agents has been a popular
type of therapy in shock patients primarily because blood pressure
is one of the few quantitative clinical measurements available to
the clinician and because most patients show a transient improvement
in their clinical appearance when these agents are employed. The
enthusiasm for vasoconstrictor therapy in acute hypotensive states,
which was common a few years ago, has waned with an increased understanding of circulatory pathology, and a realization that flow rather
than pressure is the important determinant of survival. Pressure
is easy to measure; whereas tissue perfusion is not; but it is the
latter that is the important variable. A rise in pressure does not
necessarily imply an improved tissue perfusion.

The objection most frequently raised to the use of vasoconstrictors is that shock is usually characterized by intense sympathetic and adrenergic activity which redistributes blood from
parenchymal organs to the brain and heart. Since the vasopressor
agents act by further narrowing arteries and arterioles, the possibility exists that elevations of arterial pressure are obtained
at the cost of diminished tissue perfusion to essential viscera.
Thus, these agents may actually be detrimental.

Sympathomimetic Drugs

In 1948 Ahlquist concluded that most adrenergic receptors were
of either one or two types which he termed alpha and beta receptors.
It is obviously important in the choice of a vasoactive drug to
know whether the action is primarily on the blood vessels (alpha
activity) or whether there is also cardiac stimulation (beta activity). Vasoconstrictors usually affect both arteries and veins,
but the relative effects vary widely among drugs and are the results of many factors which interact in complex ways. Moreover,
individual differences in the responses to the various agents in
shock patients are to be expected. The type and duration of shock
may also affect the response to exogenous sympathomimetics.

The concept of alpha and beta receptor sites has helped simplify the classification of the sympathomimetic drugs and also the
adrenergic blocking agents. The direction of response to a given

sympathomimetic agent can be predicted on the basis of a knowledge of whether its alpha or beta action predominates. At one extreme is methoxamine, which has almost pure alpha action and raises blood pressure by contracting cutaneous and splanchnic vascular beds and has no inotropic or chronotropic activity. On the other end of the spectrum is isoproterenol, which acts entirely on beta receptors and increases heart rate and the force of cardiac action. Isoproterenol actually decreases total systemic peripheral resistance by stimulating beta receptors and dilating the blood vessels in skeletal muscle; this drug is therefore not a vasopressor in the usual sense of the word.

The action of norepinephrine falls between methoxamine and isoproterenol, since it acts on both alpha and beta receptors. This agent causes an increase in systolic, diastolic, and mean arterial pressure while cardiac output may fall or remain unchanged. Total peripheral resistance increases resulting in a decrease in blood flow through most vascular beds. Coronary flow increases only because of a rise in myocardial oxygen demand accompanying the increased metabolic activity. Norepinephrine is a potent vasoconstrictor as well, a fact of great clinical importance. On many occasions patients who become hypotensive have been started on norepinephrine or metaraminol immediately. When central venous pressure is subsequently found to be elevated, patient is deemed to be overhydrated; fluids are therefore withheld. In many of these patients, the mere discontinuation of the vasopressor results in a profound fall in central venous pressure uncovering large unreplaced fluid deficits. The administration of colloid and crystalloid solutions then suffices to restore the patient to hemodynamic normalcy and good tissue perfusion.

The generalized vasoconstriction initiated by norepinephrine and other sympathomimetics with alpha activity is usually accompanied by cardiac slowing and decreased cardiac output due to baroreceptor reflexes. If atropine is used to block reflex pathways, the infusion of norepinephrine is able to increase cardiac output slightly since reflex bradycardia is prevented. Another frequent complication associated with the administration of vasopressors having strong alpha adrenergic activity is renal vasoconstriction which results in anuria.

As previously stated, some of the sympathomimetic agents, isoproterenol and mephentermine, act entirely on beta adrenergic receptors resulting in both inotropic and chronotropic stimulation of the heart plus dilation of skeletal muscle and pulmonary vasculature. Isoproterenol has been studied quite extensively in the treatment of clinical shock of various etiologies. Here its direct cardiac effects augment heart rate and increase the strength and velocity of shortening of myocardial fibers. In all of these reports the authors have emphasized the frequent finding of diminished cardiac function in shock which appeared to be a limiting factor in recovery after adequate measures to correct volume deficits and measurable metabolic abnormalities had been carried out. Our own experience with isoproterenol in shock has been similar to that reported above. There is good physiologic rationale for using a drug in refractory shock states which stimulates the heart but does not compromise tissue perfusion by constricting vessels. It has been well documented that low cardiac output and high ventricular end-diastolic pressure may be reversed by judicious administration of isoproterenol. However, a note of caution must be sounded since the use of isoproterenol in critically ill patients is not without hazard, and undesirable effects may be disastrous. We have found that drug-induced tachycardias of 160 to 200 are not uncommon. Such rates interfere with diastolic cardiac filling and both stroke volume and cardiac output drop severely. In addition, myocardial irritability may result in rhythm disturbances, especially in the presence of hypoxia or excessive amounts of digitalis. For these reasons it is apparent that isoproterenol administration must be carefully monitored and minute-to-minute titration carried out as the hemodynamic status of the patient changes.

In conclusion, we have entirely abandoned the use of sympathomimetic agents with an alpha adrenergic component in their pharmacologic action. In the shock patient who is refractory to aggressive conventional therapy, there is often a deficit in cardiac function and the use of a cardiac stimulant such as isoproterenol is warranted. Proper precautions for the hazards associated with these agents must be observed however.

The use of vasoconstrictors in "neurogenic shock" due to spinal cord lesions, spinal anesthesia, or barbiturate poisoning is unnecessary since flow is well maintained even at the lower arterial pressures observed. Moreover, administration of fluids will generally restore blood pressure to normal levels suggesting that the basic problem is hypovolemia relative to the needs of the expanded intravascular space.

Angiotensin

Another vasoconstrictor which has been used to elevate blood pressure in shock is angiotensin. This drug is a nonadrenergic pressor polypeptide which causes intense constriction of vascular smooth muscle in normal subjects resulting in elevations in arterial pressures. The precise mode of action on smooth muscle is uncertain, but its direct effects are independent of adrenergic receptors and appears to be most pronounced at the precapillary region. Postcapillary vessels and veins are only mildly affected. In normal humans there appears to be no inotropic or chronotropic action on the heart and cardiac output falls because of a vagally mediated reflex

bradycardia. The renal vessels are extremely sensitive to angiotensin, and both renal blood flow and glomerular filtration rate
are sharply reduced by doses that have only negligible effects on
systemic blood pressure.

Clinical studies on the use of angiotensin in shock are limited. In one series of twelve hypotensive patients, angiotensin induced a marked elevation of peripheral resistance with diminished
urine flow without significant alteration in cardiac output. Although the action of this agent is not mediated through alpha adrenergic receptors, its vasoconstrictor action is very similar.
Consequently, the use of this agent in the treatment of shock is
without benefit and may be deleterious.

Vasopressins

The posterior pituitary antidiuretic hormone (vasopressin, ADH)
has cardiovascular effects which were first described by Oliver
and Schaffer. Vasopressin, when administered in a dose far exceeding that required for maximal antidiuresis, causes an initial rise
in blood pressure which tends to return toward resting levels after
five to ten minutes, even though the infusion is maintained. Vasopressin appears to act on all vascular smooth muscle, arterial and
venous. The resultant depression of coronary flow is a dangerous
side action of this drug and has been reported to cause myocardial
ischemia and death in humans.

Vasopressin causes constriction of splanchnic vessels in doses
which have little effect on systemic blood vessels. Because of
this marked splanchnic vasoconstriction, portal venous pressure
and hepatic blood flow fall. The agent has consequently found a
limited use as an adjunctive measure for the temporary control of
hemorrhage from esophageal varices. We have attempted to employ
this agent in several cases of septic shock which were associated
with generalized peritonitis. In these cases cardiac output was
elevated and peripheral resistance was very low. Since all other
therapy had failed to alter an inexorable downhill course, it was
felt that severe shunting through the area of intraabdominal inflammation might be diverting flow from other tissue. Unfortun-
ately the vasoconstrictive effects of vasopressin were not sufficiently localized to the splanchnic bed, and we have abandoned this
approach. Recently, a synthetic vasopressor analogue having a more
selective effect on mesenteric vessels has been reported, but its
value in the problem described above remains to be evaluated.

VASODILATOR THERAPY

Shock, regardless of the initiating factors, tends to progress

toward a final common pathway which is characterized by diminished
blood flow to vital organ structures. The opportunities to reverse
this downhill course by rational therapy should be aggressively
seized by the clinician. Immediate measures should be taken to restore fluid volume to effective levels, correct respiratory function, reinstate metabolic balances, treat infection, and aid the
failing myocardium. However, in spite of the appropriateness of
this kind of therapy, some patients are refractory to conventional
treatment and follow a course of progressive deterioration. Cardiac output remains inadequate relative to the increased requirements; tissue perfusion remains low; tissue anaerobiasis leads to
rising serum lactate levels; the blood pressure and urinary output
falls; central venous pressure climbs; respiratory dysfunction appears with consequent hypoxia; and coagulation abnormalities follow.

With increasing interest in the basic pathophysiology of shock
came the realization that as a result of the body's neurohumoral defense mechanisms a reflex vasoconstriction occurs which tends to
redistribute flow to the heart and brain at the expense of other
vital organ systems. Although this compensatory mechanism may be
necessary during the early phases of shock in order to compensate
for relative circulatory deficits, the prolongation or intensifica-
tion of these alterations by iatrogenic vasoconstrictor administration may further reduce an already insufficient peripheral and vis-
ceral blood flow. Even as blood pressure is maintained above normal levels by endogenously produced or exogenously administered catecholamines, vital tissue dies.

Increasing awareness of the importance of tissue perfusion and
maintenance of tissue capillary perfusion has stimulated interest
in a completely different concept of treating refractory shock.
This method employs adrenergic blocking agents to facilitate peripheral blood flow, a concept dramatically opposed to the use of vasopressor agents to maintain blood pressure by increased peripheral
resistance. Many experimental studies testify to the benefit of
vasodilators in cardiogenic, hemorrhagic and endotoxin shock. An
equal number of animal studies have discounted the value of vasodilators in the treatment of shock of various etiologies. Neither
set of studies, however, contributes information toward establishing
a basis for the clinical use of vasodilators. Certainly in a series
of hemorrhaged dogs or dogs given intravenous endotoxin, one would
hardly expect an improvement to occur due to administration of a
vasodilator unless the more obvious problems of fluid deficit, hypoxia, and metabolic abnormalities are first corrected.

The vasodilator agents which have been proposed as being of
possible benefit in the treatment of shock are primarily alpha
adrenergic blocking agents that selectively inhibit responses to
adrenergic sympathetic nerve activity and to sympathomimetic vasoconstrictors. These agents act at the effector cell and must be

distinguished from substances that prevent sympathoadrenal discharge
by blocking nerve impulse transmission within the cerebrospinal axis,
in autonomic ganglia, along peripheral neurons, or that interfere
with release of adrenergic mediators. The alpha adrenergic blocking agents of interest in the treatment of shock are phenoxybenzamine,
phentolamine and chlorpromazine. A fourth agent, hydralazine, has
been advocated as an effective vasodilator, and although many of its
cardiovascular effects are similar to the alpha adrenergic blockers,
the precise mechanism of its action remains unclear.

Phenoxybenzamine

Phenoxybenzamine is a haloalkylamine which produces a complete
and specific alpha adrenergic blockade at receptor sites and has no
demonstrable effect on beta receptor sites when complete, is persistent and unresponsive to exogenous stimulation by alpha adrenergic
agents such as methoxamine. The block develops slowly and is probably not complete for three to four hours following intravenous
administration. Once established the block may persist for up to
forty-eight hours, but we have usually found a limited response to
exogenous methoxamine twenty-four hours after administration of phenoxybenzamine to patients. This suggests that some of the alpha receptor sites are no longer effectively blocked and are capable of
responding to alpha stimulation.

In addition to its effects as an adrenergic blocking agent,
phenoxybenzamine has some antihistaminic and antiserotonin properties. The importance of these actions in the treatment of refractory shock may be considerable. Experimental evidence suggests
that the normal mechanism for opening and closing nutritive capillaries may be regulated by histamine. When mast cells become anoxic,
they produce histamine which causes that capillary to open. The
histamine is then destroyed in the general circulation and has no
systemic effects. In shock, due to capillary flow and sludging,
histamine exerts a continuous local effect and capillaries and
venules may remain open causing pooling of blood and increased intravascular capacity. Restoration of flow by relief of precapillary
arteriolar constriction allows destruction of accumulated histamine
and restoration of intravascular space toward normal.

Administration of therapeutic doses (1 mg/kg) of phenoxybenzamine to normovolemic recumbent volunteers has been shown to result in a rise in cardiac index of 66 per cent with a fall in total
peripheral resistance of 90 per cent two to three hours after administration of the drug. This rise in cardiac output probably
represents a reflex response to the diminished peripheral resistance
caused by vasodilation. Nickerson has also emphasized the differential effects on various vascular beds following adrenergic blockade
which results in an increased plasma volume and diminished pulmonary

blood volume. There have been few published studies on the use of
phenoxybenzamine in human cases of shock despite the extensive
philosophical discourse regarding the vasodilator-vasoconstrictor
controversy. Nickerson has reported several patients who were refractory to all therapy but responded to phenoxybenzamine with
prompt improvement in hemodynamic status and tissue perfusion. Eck-
enhoff and Cooperman reported on the use of phenoxybenzamine in.
seven patients all of whom were considered to have very little
chance of survival because of the prolonged course of their shock.
Improvement appears to have occurred in three; although only one
survived. No hemodynamic criteria were observed in administering
phenoxybenzamine to these patients, and in several cases the data
suggests that the patients were hypovolemic prior to administration
of the drug. Wilson, Jablonski, and Thal reported the results of
administering phenoxybenzamine to nineteen patients with advanced
clinical shock from a variety of causes. These authors concluded
that the overall effects of phenoxybenzamine were beneficial and
felt that improvement in myocardial performance might provide the
physiologic basis for the improvement seen in the cardiovascular
system after phenoxybenzamine. This study also pointed out that
alpha adrenergic blockade may be followed by sympathomimetic agents
such as norepinephrine -- thus restricting the response to the beta
adrenergic (cardiotonic) effects of these drugs.

In an attempt to evaluate vasodilator therapy under controlled
circumstances, a set of criteria for the selection of patients to
receive the drug were established in the Walter Reed shock unit.
The criteria were as follows:

1. Clinical picture of shock unresponsive to intravenous fluid
therapy sufficient to elevate the central venous pressure above normal range.

2. Clinical signs of sympathetic overactivity (pallor, cold ex-
tremities, low pulse pressure, and decreased capillary filling).

3. Low cardiac index relative to estimated needs with normal
or elevated peripheral resistance.

The absolute contraindications to the use of a vasodilator were
as follows:

1. Any evidence of hypovolemia.

2. Uncorrected electrolyte disturbance, acid-base disorder, or
respiratory dysfunction.

3. Evidence of acute myocardial infarction (now considered an
indication).

4. Inadequate facilities for monitoring changes in the patient's hemodynamic status.

Patients meeting these criteria were studied immediately prior to the administration of phenoxybenzamine and then serially after blockade was established. The results of our initial series of patients treated according to this protocol have been reported in detail. All patients in this series had a diagnosis of shock due solely to septicemia except for one, who had bilateral pheochromocytomas and whose clinical picture was characterized by myocardial failure and fulminant pulmonary edema. These patients demonstrated a dramatic improvement in clinical appearance following phenoxybenzamine administration and hemodynamically showed marked improvement in cardiac index and stroke volume with a fall in central venous pressure. No biochemical derangements were produced by the drug and evidence of increased cellular perfusion was inferred from the progressive return to basal levels of lactate and calculated excess lactate. On the basis of these studies we have reached similar conclusions to Wilson, Jablonski, and Thal that phenoxybenzmine, in addition to its vasodilating properties, appears to improve cardiac function which may be an important factor limiting recovery of these patients.

Recent studies have shown that there appear to be two general groups of patients in septic shock who can be segregated by different hemodynamic pictures. In one group (hypodynamic), cardiac output is appreciably reduced; in the other (hyperdynamic), cardiac output is normal or increased. After our initial gratifying results with the initial group of patients treated with phenoxybenzamine, it was decided to revise our criteria to include patients in low-output cardiogenic shock secondary to acute myocardial infarction. Our experience with this disease is admittedly small, but in those cases we have studied there has been significant improvements in circulatory hemodynamics, and we feel that as additional cases are studied we may be able to demonstrate increased survival.

A second group of septic shock patients have a measured cardiac index significantly higher than normal with a low total systemic peripheral resistance. A striking physiologic finding in patients with high output septic shock is the narrow arteriovenous oxygen difference which is associated with decreased oxygen consumption. In this group of patients it appears as though pathologic shunting through nonnutritive arteriovenous communications is far advanced and is the primary channel of flow. It is possible that nutritional capillaries are largely blocked by intravascular thrombi and no longer function in this stage of shock. These patients show no response to vasodilation by phenoxybenzamine and mortality has remained very high despite intensive therapy. Such patients may represent a more advanced state of septic shock since markedly

elevated arterial lactate values suggest an even poorer tissue perfusion than in the low output group. This finding is well correlated with the decreased arteriovenous oxygen and pH difference in
the high-output group and suggests that in addition to the myocardial dysfunction there may be peripheral vascular dysfunction.

In summary, the use of vasodilators appears to be of great
benefit in patients with a hypodynamic, low cardiac output, picture
of shock who have failed to respond to vigorous attempts at conventional therapy. Shock due to primary cardiac causes does not con-
traindicate the use of vasodilator therapy. In the hyperdynamic,
high cardiac output group of septic shock patients, the use of vasodilators appears to be of no benefit and may be contraindicated.
It must be reemphasized that the use of vasodilators without proper
monitoring of physiologic parameters is extremely hazardous and
should never be undertaken. These agents must never be administered
to hypovolemic patients since the rapid expansion of intravascular
capacity which they cause can result in complete cardiovascular collapse if adequate intravascular fluid support is lacking.

At the present time phenoxybenzamine is available only for
clinical research purposes as an investigative drug. However, this
need not be a deterrent. The use of vasodilator therapy is possible
for all physicians since phentolamine (Regitine) is clinically available and is also an alpha adrenergic blocking drug which differs
only in having a faster onset of action and being shorter acting.

Phentolamine (Regitine)

Phentolamine is a member of the two substituted imidazoline
family of agents and produces a moderately effective competitive
alpha adrenergic blockade that is relatively transient. This drug
also has antiserotonin properties and appears to be an effective
myocardial stimulant when administered in therapeutic doses. The
most disturbing clinical side effects of phentolamine are attribu-
table to cardiac and gastrointestinal stimulation. Because of the
short duration of the alpha adrenergic blockade produced by phentolamine, it is necessary that a continuous intravenous infusion of
the drug be given and that the rate of delivery be adjusted in order
to obtain the desirable alphalytic effects without causing untoward
side effects. In some respects the use of a short acting drug such
as phentolamine for treating shock is more desirable than the longer
acting and completely non-competitive alpha blockade which phenoxybenzamine produces. The hazards of administering a rapid acting
alpha adrenergic blocking agent such as phentolamine to a hypovolemic
patient must be emphasized. We have always withheld vasodilator
therapy until the patient's central venous pressure was maintained
above 10 mm Hg for at least thirty minutes even though the patient's
clinical appearance and hemodynamic status suggested he was a

candidate for vasodilation. Bradley and Weil have recommended the
intravenous infusion of phentolamine at a constant rate of approximately 0.5 mg/min to obtain optimal alpha blockade without limiting side effects. This appears to be a good starting dose, but each
patient must be carefully monitored and adjustments made to the individual's response to therapy. Although our clinical experience
with this agent has been limited, we have found it to be an effective vasodilator which appears to be safe when given with full awareness of the potential side effects.

Chlorpromazine (Thorazine)

Chlorpromazine, which may be taken as a prototype for the
phenothiazine derivatives, is one of the most widely used drugs in
medicine. Chlorpromazine has been employed primarily in the treatment of psychiatric patients, but it has been known for many years
that its actions were not limited to the central nervous system.
This drug appears to have strong adrenergic and weaker peripheral
cholinergic blocking activity and is capable of producing epinephrine
reversal similar to that produced by phenoxybenzamine. The clinical
significance of the peripheral adrenergic blockade produced by chlorpromazine is difficult to assess, but early reports of the French
in Indochina on the efficacy of the "lytic cocktail" have been sub-
stantiated by some animal experiments.

We have found that the response of the patient in shock to
chlorpromazine is extremely unpredictable and that better agents
are available which are capable of producing an alpha adrenergic
blockade under more controlled circumstances. For these reasons
we are no longer using this agent.

THE RETICULO-ENDOTHELIAL SYSTEM (R.E.S.) IN TRAUMATIC SHOCK

CARLO PALMERIO[*]

From the Department of Surgery, Harvard Medical

School and Beth Israel Hospital, Boston

Early in shock the Sympathetic Nervous System is hyperactive in response to deficient perfusion of tissues. This response maintains capillary hydrostatic pressure essential for exchanges between tissues and blood[1]. Prolonged sympathetic overactivity further reduces tissue perfusion and causes functional damage of all organs particularly in the liver and spleen which are very sensitive to hypoxia. Since these organs contain the largest fraction of the defense against bacteria and bacterial endotoxin, it is in such circumstances that endotoxin of intestinal origin can reach the systemic circulation in its still toxic state[2]. The resulting endotoxemia increases the ischemia of the tissues for endotoxin and catecholamines act sinergistically to damage the peripheral circulation[3]. Further decline of the peripheral flow causes generalized disorganization at the cellular level. The vascular smooth muscle cells develop structural changes[4] and consequently there is a loss of vascular tone and hyporeactivity of the vessels to catecholamines. A disproportionate amount of blood is retained in the peripheral bed so that progressive decline in venous return to the heart occurs. Cardiac output falls progressively. Death results when there is not enough blood

*Present Adresse: Via Venezia 4- Pescara- Italy

to sustain the minimal requiriments of vital organs.

Since surgical or chemical denervation of the coeliac plexus[5]prevents the loss in vascular tone,the splancnic organs play a central role in the pathogenesis of
vascular collapse.

If the ischemic loss of the detoxifying capacity of
the R.E.S. in liver and spleen that allows endotoxemia,
causes the peripheral circulatory insufficiency,therapy
must be directed toward the prevention of this loss or
if damage has already occurred, to substitution of the
damaged system with healthy donor reticulo-endothelial
cells until the hosts R.E.S. can recover normal antibacterial potential.

The data that follow support such hypothesis.
They show:
1- that the R.E.S. in the liver and spleen detoxify bacterial endotoxin.
2- that in non septic as well septic shock vascular integrity is dependent upon the endotoxin detoxifying capacity of the R.E.S., for when this function has been
depleted loss of vascular tone occurs.

The supporting experimental data were secured in
endotoxic, hemorrhagic and superior mesenteric artery
occlusion (S.M.A.O.) shock.

Toxic blood from animals dying in hemorrhagic
shock is no longer toxic if perfused through a normal,
denervated spleen[6],which is also able to rapidly extract
and detoxify bacterial endotoxin[7].

If the detoxification is due to the reticulo-endothelial elements of the spleen, then other organs with
such cells should have a similar detoxifying capacity.
This possibility was investigated for the liver in rabbits. Under nembutal anesthesia, the liver was isolated
from its vascular and nervous connections, except for
the hepatic artery and portal vein. 2000 ug of Cr 51

Salmonella Enteritidis Endotoxin in 10 ml of plasma was
injected in ten minutes into the portal vein via a
branch of the superior mesenteric vein. Venous hepatic
blood was collected from a catheter inserted into the
inferior vena cava just above di diaphragm. The volume
of blood lost in this fashion was replaced simultaneously via the left external jugular vein. Portal and
hepatic venous blood, tested for toxicity in Pertussis
treated Mice, showed that a single passage through the
liver was enough for a high degree of detoxification,
except in one rabbit with hepatic mycosis.

The intact liver does not prevent death when this
amount of endotoxin is injected into the systemic circulation, presumably because the liver becomes inaccessi-
ble owing to the vasoconstrictive action of the endotoxin. This was demonstrated to be the case in 9 rabbits
provided with a freshly excised donor liver, receiving
blood from a femoral artery and returning it to the external jugular vein by a pump at a speed sufficient to
maintain balance between supply and delivery. 7/9 rabbits in which perfusion was started immediately after
injecting a lethal dose of endotoxin, i.e. 2000 ug, did
not show hemodynamic deterioration and survived. These
observations confirm the view that endotoxin is promptly
destroyed by the liver and spleen, providing their R.E.
cells are fully accessible, as demonstrated in nembutalized rabbits which survived a dose which was lethal
when injected in a systemic vein, but not into the portal vein[7].

In 1964 we reported that denervation of the splenic
pedicle prevents the structural and functional changes
in the spleen caused by shock[8]. Recently we denervated
the spleen a week in advance in one series of dogs and
ewposed this series plus a control series to hemorrhagic
shock by the reservoir technic. In spite of the fact
that both series were bled to the same degree and to the
same level of hypotension (40 ml Hg), the course of the
event differed radically. The non-denervated series exhibited the hemodynamic deterioration typical of a re-

fractory state,with rapid loss of vascular tone, followed by death within 24 hours. The denervated dogs did
not show more than a minor loss in vascular tone: their
pressure response to transfusion was excellent and sustained and all survived,except one on which the spleen
was found to be infarcted[9]. Similar data were obtained
in dogs in S.M.A.O. shock. In this type the release of
the 5-6 hours occlusion is followed by shock that is in-
distinguishable from endotoxic shock. The hemodynamic
deterioration develops within an hour and is progressive until death. The gut mucosa ulcerates and bleeds pro-
fusely. The spleen constricts within 5 minutes after release of the legature, i.e. long before hypovolemia
from blood loss can account for it. The vasoconstriction
therefore, is caused by a circulating factor, which
seems to the liable of extraction by the R.E.S.: so the
splenic contraction is prevented by implanting a donor
spleen in the systemic circulation. If the vasoconstriction is prevented by blockade or denervation, the shock
is mild and transient, with little or no bleeding from
the gut and the survival rate is high[10]. The foregoing
observations warrant the conclusion that vascular integrity depends upon the accessibility of blood to the
R.E.S., which eliminates a substance that is responsa-
ble for the hemodynamic deterioration in all three types of shock. Testimony in support of the presence of
such a substance are data on splenic uptake and release
of red cells in dogs in S.M.A.O. shock[11]. Restoration of
flow in the mesenteric artery induces sympathetic stimulation which produces splenic contraction. Therefore the
spleen discharges red cells. But if the organ is denervated or a donor spleen is implanted there is a continous and large uptake of cells by the spleen, expecial-
ly in the latter. Since a normal animal with a denervated spleen does not extract RBC in significant number,
one suspects that survival in this experimental type of
shock is related to the degree of RBC extraction by the
denervated spleen, and consequently that the toxic substance which prevents recovery is attached to the extracted RBC, i.e. bacterial endotoxin which can attach

to RBC because they have structural components similar
to Group B substances[12].

COMMENT AND CONCLUSION
       The primary factor involved in the pathogenesis of
the irreversible state of the peripheral circulatory insufficiency is an endotoxemia due to the loss of the detoxifying function of the R.E.S. consequent to a prolonged ischemic damage by sympathetic overactivity.

       The experimental data supporting this hypothesis
are as follow: the liver and spleen are able to extract
and detoxify endotoxin. Hence the detoxification is a
function of the reticulo-endothelial cells since these
are the only cells common to the two organs. Since a
protection is achieved by implanting a liver in endotoxic shock or a spleen in S.M.A.O. shock and by splenic
denervation in the latter as well in hemorrhagic shock,
the function involved by the R.E.S. of both organs is
presumably concerned with the extraction of a vascular
toxin. There is a strong evidence that this toxic factor
is a vasoactive substance because it can not act upon
a denervated tissue. A large variety of vasoactive substances such as Kallikrein, Histamine, Serotonin, Catecholamines etc which can be identified in the blood of
dying shocked animals cannot be implicated in the genesis of the peripheral circulatory insufficiency,because
the R.E.S. is not known to be capable of clearing any
of them, nor any other known vasoactive substance,
except endotoxin.

BIBLIOGRAPHY
1- Palmerio,C.and Fine,J.-(1968)- La microcircolazione
splancnica nello Shock Traumatico.Minerva Medica 59,5323.

2- Fine,J.-(1954)- The bacterial factor in traumatic
Shock.
C.C.Thomas and Company, Springfield, Illinois.

3- Palmerio,C.,Ming,S.C.,Frank,E.and Fine,J.-(1962)-Car-
diac tissue response to Endotoxin.Proceedings of the Society for Experimental Biology and Medicine. 109, 773.

4- Ashford,T.,Palmerio,C.and Fine,J.-(1966)- Structural
Analogue in vascular muscle to the functional disorder
in refractory traumatic Shock and reversal by corticosteroid: Electron Microscopic Evaluation. Annals of surgery. 4, 575.

5- Palmerio,C.,Zettestrom,B.,Shammash,J.,Euchbaum,E.,
Frank,E.and Fine,J.-(1963)- Denervation of the Abdomi-
nal Viscera for the Treatment of traumatic Shock.
New England Journal of Medicine. 269, 709.

6- Palmerio,C.,Zettestrom,B.,Tudor,J.,Rutenburg,S.H.and
Fine,J.-(1964)- Further studies on the Nature of the Circulating Toxin in Traumatic Shock.Journal of the Reticu-
lo Endothelial Society. 1, 243.

7- Rutenburg,S.H.,Skarnes,R.,Palmerio,C. and Fine,J.,-
-(1967)- Detoxification of Endotoxin by perfusion of Liver and Spleen.Proceedings of the Society for experimental Biology and Medicine. 125, 455.

8- Zettestrom,B.,Palmerio,C.and Fine,J.-(1964)- Protection of functional and vascular integrity of the Spleen
in traumatic Shock by denervation.Proceedings of the Society for experimental Biology and Medicine. 117, 373.

9- Glass,K.,Palmerio,C.and Fine,J.-(1969)- Further Evidence of the role of the Reticulo-Endothelial System in
the Maintenance of Vascular Integrity.Surgery.In Press.

10- Fine,J.,Palmerio,C.and Rutenburg,S.H.-(1968)-New Developments in Therapy of Refractory Traumatic Shock.
Archives of Surgery. 96, 163.

11- Palmerio,C. and Fine,J.-(1969)- The Nature of Resistance to Shock. Archives of Surgery. 98, 679.

12- Springers, G.F., Wang, E.T., Nichols, J.H.and Smeat,
J.M.-(1966)- Relation between Bacterial Lipopolysaccha-
ride Structures and Those of Human cells. Annals of the
New York Academy of Sciences. 113, 566.

SECTION 4

CLINICAL AND THERAPEUTIC ASPECTS OF SHOCK

Problems of Clinical Research in Shock

L. Gallone, Milan, Italy

Istituto di Patologia Speciale Chirurgica,

Ospedale Maggiore "Ca'Granda"

The vascular pattern of hypovolemia with diminished cardiac output in the early stages of shock syndromes is well recognized and has been extensively studied by many investigators. However, with the development of techniques for rapid performing hemodynamic and respiratory measurements at the bedside, a new range of altered physiologic responses in shock syndromes has been observed. These recently recognized circulatory patterns consist of a hyperkinetic circulation with high cardiac output and rapid mean circulation time in the presence of arterial hypotension and progressive clinical deterioration (Mac - Lean et al. 1965; Khe and Shoemaker 1968; Duff et al. 1969).

It is well known, by this time, that several pathologic states are countersigned by an increased cardiac output, as liver cirrhosis, hyperthyroidism, beriberi, multiple myeloma, Paget's disease of bone and anoxia due to altitude. The vasodilation accompanying anoxia of mild degree and beriberi is, in part, related to increased flow of blood through arteriovenous shunts which short-circuits the capillary bed (Border et al. 1966; Cohn et al. 1968).

The compensatory increase in cardiac output may be viewed, in the presence of arteriovenous shunts, as waisted flow not contributing to tissue perfusion. From this point of view the greatest attention of clinicians is now given to that bacteriemic conditions which show a hyperkinetic circulatory pattern asso-

ciated with shock. In such patients, as a rule, the deep hypotension which almost immediately or within a few hours follows the
chills, the fever and the other common signs of a septic disease,
is characterized by abnormalities in the peripheral circulation,
such that at any given cardiac output the calculated vascular
resistance is low in comparison with the values observed in those
septic patients whose shock state is on the basis of hypovolemia
(Hopkins et al. 1965; Clowes et al. 1966; Desai et al. 1969).

Further, the septic patient can present with profound
hypotension and yet have a cardiac output which is either normal
or markedly increased over normal. In this hyperdynamic state
the septic shock patient may also show a reduction in total
peripheral oxygen consumption, in spite of the increased cardiac
output. In the septic patient a fall in oxygen consumption
frequently heralds clinical deterioration and is usually related
to the presence of a major undrained septic process which must
be resolved if the patient is to be cured. These abnormalities in
oxygen consumption are caused by a rise in the venous oxygen
content rather than by arterial hypoxemia, and appear to reflect
the presence of significant arteriovenous shunts.

It is not yet clear whether these vascular abnormalities
are on an anatomical or functional basis. Though the anatomical
research has demonstrated in several districts real anastomoses
between the arteriolar and the venular tree, the same conception
of arteriovenous shunting remains, at least in relation with the
disfunctioning microcirculation in shock, merely a hypothesis.
For instance, the well known model of microcirculation according
to Chambers and Zweifach shows the distribution of capillaries
along a "thoroughfare channel", with the so-called precapillary
sphincters. According to this scheme the vessel, to which belongs
the special function of giving a direct flow to the venular tree,
should be always open and only a functional shunt could be
realized provided the precapillary sphincters are closed. But
in other schemes a real anatomical shunt is considered, i. e.
a channel which occasionally functions as a by-pass, otherwise
it can be quite closed.

Now let us see the scheme designed by Poisvert
according to Lillehei's conception of microcirculation in the
splanchnic region (Poisvert et al. 1966). Here you see an
arteriovenous shunt, which is tight when the hydrostatic and
osmotic pressures are well balanced in the microcirculation

and no arteriolar spasm hinders the flow in the capillary bed.
But in the same scheme shunts begin to open during the initial
phase of shock, corresponding to hyperincretion of catecholamines,
together with arteriolar constriction and ischemic hypoxia.
Finally,the same shunts take part in the general overdilation of the
capillary net, when shock has become irreversible owing to
stagnant hypoxia.

Whatever may be the mechanism of microcirculatory
derangement in the hyperdynamic pattern of septic shock, it
seems undeniable that these patients, usually affected by a gram
negative septicemia or by peritonitis, behave as if they suffered
from a large arteriovenous fistula and frequently progress into
a high output cardiac failure. A cardiac index of more than 3
liters per minute and square meter, associated with hypotension
and clinical deterioration, should be considered as the most
typical sign of this syndrome. Considerable arterial hypoxemia was
also observed but it did not appear related to hyperventilation,
because arterial carbon dioxide tensions were not elevated (Cohn,
1968). In the same cases, however, a marked diminution in
arteriovenous oxygen difference reflected the low oxygen consumption, which has been already mentioned as a very important
character of gram negative speticemia.

As clinical deterioration is progressing, serial assessment
of circulatory function indicates that metabolic acidosis is
becoming more severe. This phenomenon is associated with a
myocardial failure; therefore central venous pressure increases
and stroke work decreases. If such a pattern of cardiac work
does not respond to drug therapy, stroke work continues to decrease,
with an increase in central venous pressure and a subsequent
decrease in cardiac index. One has also to consider that septic
and hyperpyretic patient is particularly inclined to a swift
dehydration. Hence, a shock which is initially hyperdynamic may
assume in a very short time the pattern of a hypovolemic one,
with a reduced cardiac index, if water and electrolytes are not
given in a sufficient quantity.

The following scheme shows how, during the course of a
septic and hyperdynamic shock, both cardiac index and central
venous pressure may change in relation with heart failure and
fluid losses. In the "hyperdynamic pattern" the cardiac index
may sometimes be of 4-5 litres or more, while the filling

pressure of the right atrium is rather high but still proportional
to the increased venous flow. When the shock pattern becomes
hypodynamic, with a decreasing of the cardiac index, then the
central venous pressure may go down on account of fluid losses
and hypovolemia, or may increase owing to heart failure. In
both these cases the calculated peripheral resistance will shift
to higher values.

Obviously, correction of hypovolemia and pharmacological
sustaining of the heart's work are both very important tasks,
whatever may be the pattern of shock. But in the special case of
a hyperdynamic shock the main point of the question is another.
In fact, all our efforts cannot be successful if we don't succeed
in restoring the microcirculation and to remove the impairment
in oxygen extraction by the tissues.

Therapy directed towards correction of a hyperdynamic
cardiovascular state leaves much to be desired. The use of
inotropic agents is frequently beneficial, but adequate physiologic
response in the peripheral circulatory beds is seldom obtained.

BIBLIOGRAPHY

Border, J. R. , Gallo, E. , Schenk, W. G. (1966): Systemic
arteriovenous shunts in patients under severe stress: a common
cause of cardiac high output failure? Surgery 60, 225.

Clowes, G. H. et al (1966): The cardiac output in septic
shock. Annals of Surgery, 163, 866.

Cohn, J. D. , Greenspan, M. , Golstein, C. R. , Gudwin, A.
L. , Siegel, J. H. , Del Guercio, L. R. M. (1968): Arteriovenous
shunting in high cardiac output shock syndromes. Surgery,
Gynecology, & Obstetrics, 127, 282.

Desai, J. M. , Kim, S. I. , Shoemaker, W. C. (1969): Se-
quential hemodynamic changes in an experimental hemorrhage
shock preparation designed to simulate clinical shock. Annals
of Surgery, 170, 157.

Duff, J. H. , Groves, A. C. , MacLean, A. P. , La Pointe,
R. , MacLean, L. D. (1969): Defective oxygen consumption in
septic shock. Surgery, Gynecology & Obstetrics, 128, 1051.

Hopkins, R. W., Sabga, G., Penn, I., Simeone, F. A. (1965): Hemodynamic aspects of hemorrhagic and septic shock. J. A. M. A., 191, 731.

Kho, L. K., Shoemaker, W. C. (1968): Evaluation of therapy in clinical shock by cardiorespiratory measurements. Surgery Gynecology, & Obstetrics 127, 81.

MacLean, L. D., Duff, J. H., Scott, H. M., Peretz, D. I. (1965): Treatment of shock in man based on hemodynamic diagnosis. Surgery, Gynecology, & Obstetrics 120, 1.

Poivert, M. et al. (1966): Journal de Chirurgie 92, 131.

THE RECOGNITION AND THERAPY OF PATHO-PHYSIOLOGIC PATTERNS IN HUMAN SHOCK

John H. Siegel, M. D., F.A.C.S.

Department of Surgery

Albert Einstein College of Medicine, New York, N. Y.

A variety of different patterns of deranged cardiovascular function can produce hypotension (1,2,5,8,9,15,16,20). Consequently, quantitative determinations of the specific set of physiologic abnormalities responsible must influence the physician's choice of a therapeutic program to support the failing circulation. In hypovolemic shock, produced either by hemorrhage or by a decrease in extra-cellular fluid secondary to a third space loss, appropriate replacement of the loss in circulatory volume is usually sufficient therapy and will generally result in an increase in both cardiac output and oxygen consumption reflecting an adequate peripheral perfusion (1,6,8,9). However, in many patients the presence of occult myocardial failure compounded by the hypoxemia brought about by the low flow state, may make the use of a cardiac inotropic agent mandatory if cardiovascular competence is to be restored. An example of this is seen in the case demonstrated of an 83 year old male who presented with an acute gastrointestinal hemorrhage and a long history of chronic duodenal ulcer (Fig.1). The patient when first seen had profound hypotension, and a pulse rate of 120 beats per minute despite attempts at massive transfusion. Even though his cardiac index was only 0.82 liters/min/m^2, the central venous pressure was noted to be elevated to 14 mm Hg. The determination of a Ventricular Function Index (19), derived from the normalized relationship between stroke work and mean right atrial pressure, demonstrated an extremely low level of ventricular function, and suggested that myocardial depression rather than over-transfusion accounted for the high central venous pressure. This may in part have been a combination of intrinsic myocardial disease, as well as decreased coronary perfusion, resulting from the low flow state (12,15). Since there was evidence of persistent bleeding from the gastrointestinal tract it became clear that continued volume

255

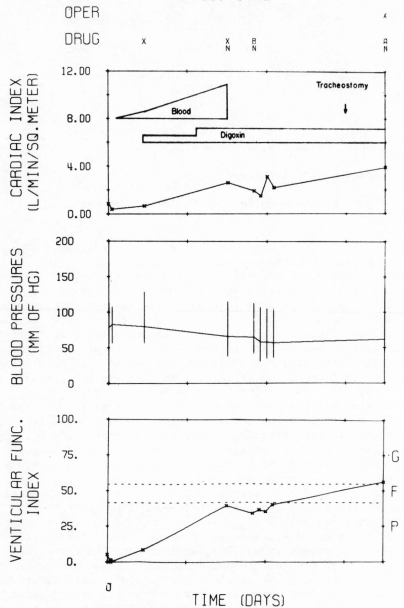

Fig.1 Summary time plot of course of 83 year old male with
       bleeding duodenal ulcer.

replacement would have to be given, and the use of an inotropic agent was decided upon to permit the obviously depressed myocardium to handle the necessary volume load. The administration of digoxin combined with further transfusion enabled a marked improvement in the ventricular function relationship and permitted an increase in the cardiac index to 2.60 liters/min/m^2, although the patient still lay within the Poor range of ventricular function curves. After digitalization had been completed, and with resumption of more normal systemic flow, and presumably more adequate coronary perfusion, the patient's ventricular function continued to improve. With the spontaneous cessation of bleeding, he progressed into the Good range of ventricular function relationships and was stable at this level permitting the later performance of a definitive surgical procedure. The details of this response are strikingly shown in Figure 2 in which the very marked increase in stroke work was accompanied by a progressively decreasing central venous (mean right atrial) pressure, demonstrating that a significant shift to the left in the patient's ventricular function relationship, and presumably therefore, a marked increase in myocardial contractility occurred during this period. This case clearly demonstrates the value in obtaining quantitative determinations of the cardiovascular function in the elderly high risk patient, as this permitted the rational utilization of a digitalis preparation and improved the patient's ventricular function enabling him to accept the necessary volume replacement. In our experience, the use of such inotropic preparations before the patient manifests overt cardiac failure, with the development of more classic physical diagnostic signs, has been of great value, since this type of patient already stressed by a major insult to the cardiovascular system, rarely survives the superimposition of myocardial distention and pulmonary edema.

In some patients, subjected to major trauma with considerable hemorrhage, excessive activity of the sympathetic nervous system may result in an inappropriate degree of vasoconstriction. This is especially true in the younger patient where the capacity for peripheral vascular activity may be greater than in the aged. This fact has been commented on by writers with a considerable experience in military and traumatic surgery (6,7). In these cases the net peripheral vascular resistance may be increased to a point where the impedance to ventricular ejection becomes a limiting factor permitting an adequate cardiac output response, and this increased after-load by further reducing stroke volume may further compound the peripheral hypoxemia produced by volume loss. In civilian practice this response is not uncommonly found in patients sustaining acute automotive trauma, or in the young patient undergoing a major operative procedure in which a considerable blood loss ensues. This is well shown in case No.2 (Fig.3a and 3b). This patient was a 39 year old obese female who underwent an abdomino-perineal resection for carcinoma of the rectum. The procedure was carried out with great difficulty because of the patient's

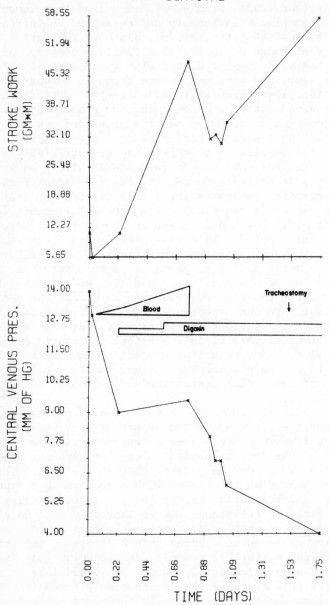

Fig.2 Evaluation of relation between left ventricular stroke work
       and central venous (mean right atrial) pressure in response
       to therapy. Patient is the same shown in Figure 1.

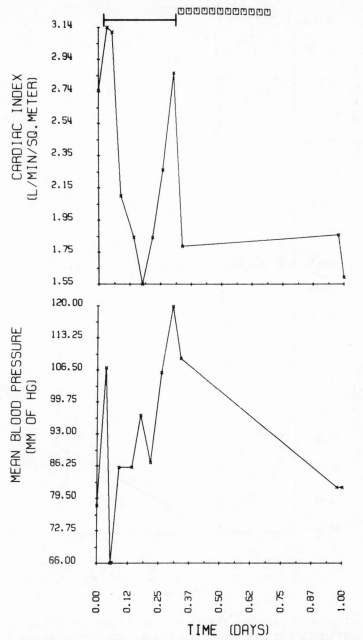

Fig. 3a   Effect of reflex vascular compensation to hemorrhage in 39
          year old female during abdominoperineal resection (black bar)

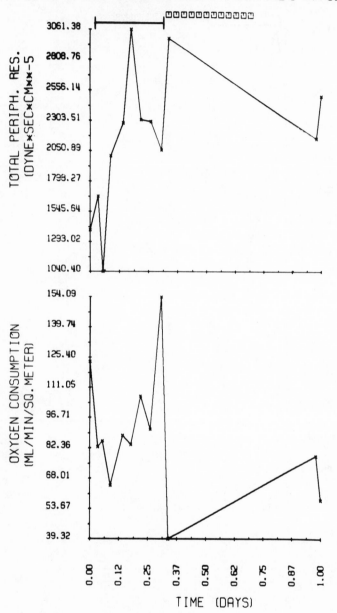

Fig. 3b   Relationship between vascular resistance and oxygen consumption in patient shown in Figure 3a.   From Siegel,
Goldwyn and Del Guercio (14) with permission of the
publisher.

obesity, and during the course of the operation there was a substantial blood loss requiring replacement of nearly 4,000 cc of
colloid and 1,000 cc of crystalloid solution. It is fortunately
rare that one has the opportunity to observe the physiologic response to such extensive blood loss in man. However, what we do
see is very revealing in terms of elucidating the compensatory
mechanisms which are brought into operation, and their occasional
pathophysiologic effect. As is shown in Figure 3a, after an initial
period of compensation for the progressive decrease in cardiac output, with the maintenance of a fairly steady level of mean blood
pressure, there ensued a sudden and major hypotensive episode,
undoubtedly related to the steady and continuing hemorrhage. It
is a tribute to the very great capacity for reflex compensation
manifested by this patient that there was a major drop in cardiac
output with virtually no significant change in blood pressure. Indeed, the patient compensated for an intra-operative fall in cardiac
index from 3.99 liters/min/m^2 to 2.21 liters/min/m^2, however, only
a small further decline in the cardiac index to 1.76 liters/min/m^2
was associated with the development of profound hypotension. As a
physiologic exclamation point to the ability of a progressive increase in vascular tone to impede ventricular volume ejection, is
the large increase in cardiac index to 2.85 liters/min/m^2 following
the sudden decline of vascular resistance which produced the hypotensive episode. This phenomenon has also been noted in other
conditions associated with sudden drops in vascular resistance,
when there is no major impairment in myocardial function (4,14,16).
That such over-activity of the sympathetic nervous system may result in a further impairment in peripheral oxygenation, which
compounds the decrease in perfusion already produced by the low
flow state, is suggested by the aspects of this case demonstrated
in Figure 3b, in which the progressive increases in total peripheral resistance during the period of reflex vascular compensation
are compared to the oxygen consumption. It can be seen that with
the increasing vascular resistance there was a tendency for a
further decrease in oxygen consumption during the compensated portion of the response to operative stress. However, at the time
that the major decrease in vascular resistance occurred, there
was a large increase in oxygen consumption. This increase occurred
at the point of maximum hypotension at a time when the decline in
cardiac index had reached its nadir. As can be seen in this Figure,
the dimensions of this increase in oxygen consumption were quite
remarkable, and suggest that this decrease in peripheral vascular
resistance and vascular tone, occurring during a period of decompensation, is caused by sudden vasodilatation. In association
with a previous period of profound reduction in oxygen consumption
further suggests that its etiology may be on the basis of hypoxemia
at the peripheral tissue level. Even more important is the fact
that this resultant hypoxemic vasodilatation, by further reducing
coronary perfusion pressure, may produce an additive myocardial
depressant effect, especially when the patient is receiving

general anesthesia which may also produce intrinsic myocardial
depression (13). In a similar fashion, a reduction in perfusion
pressure may also materially influence circulation to the brain
and kidney, and may be an important factor in the development of
acute tubular necrosis in the post-operative period. It is in
this sort of patient that the use of agents with mild alpha adrenergic blocking activity may be of some value in that they permit
more adequate tissue perfusion at any given level of cardiac output (7) and prevent the anesthesiologist or surgeon from being
lulled into a false sense of security by the maintenance of an
adequate blood pressure in spite of a large decrease in systemic
flow. Since after even minimal impairment of sympathetic reactivity,
because reflex compensation mechanisms are interfered with, the
blood pressure and cardiac output responses are more nearly parallel. The caveat, however, in the use of blocking agents is the
fact that reductions in perfusion pressure may be much more
dangerous in the elderly patient with significant athereosclerosis
of the coronary or cerebral arteries, where vasodilatation in
response to either alpha adrenergic blockade or beta adrenergic
sympathetic activity, and to increases in pCO_2 may be impaired
(5,13). In patients with demonstrated myocardial depression, as
in the first case, volume replacement may have to be accompanied
by the use of cardiac inotropic therapy.

     In patients whose shock process is due to severe sepsis, the
hypotension is characterized by abnormalities in the peripheral
circulation such that at any given cardiac output the septic
patient manifests a lower vascular resistance (decreased vascular
tone), than does the patient whose shock process is on the basis
of hypovolemia. This is demonstrated in Figure 4, which shows the
relationship between cardiac index and total peripheral resistance
in two groups of patients in shock. When one compares the vascular
tone relation in septic and non-septic shock, it can be clearly
seen that the two groups have entirely different mean pressure-
flow relationships, which in fact are on opposite sides of the
group of similarly aged control patients who were neither septic
nor hypotensive. Furthermore, as this Figure shows, the septic
patient can present with profound hypotension and yet have a cardiac
output which is either normal or markedly increased over normal.
This "hyperdynamic" state seen in the septic shock patient is
frequently accompanied by a reduction in total peripheral oxygen
consumption, in spite of the increased cardiac output. This is
well demonstrated in Case No.3, a 31 year old woman who developed
intra-abdominal abscesses following caeserean section, culminating
in the development of a right sub-diaphragmatic abscess (Fig.5).
As is shown in this Figure, when this young woman was first evaluated early in the course of her septic illness 36 hours after
drainage of the sub-diaphragmatic collection, she was profoundly
hyperdynamic with a cardiac index of 7.98 liters/min/m^2. Her pulse
pressure was wide with an acceptable mean pressure, but the

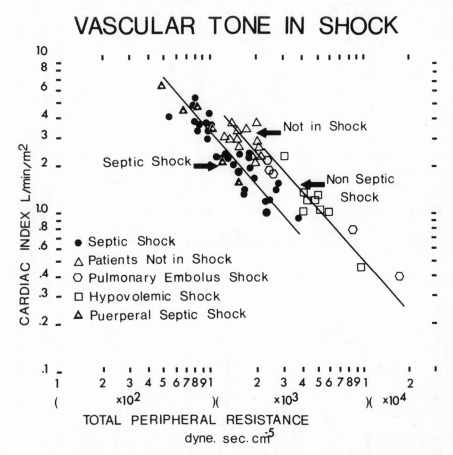

Fig.4 Vascular tone in different shock states compared to patients
not in shock. Mean lines are for all patients with shock
due to sepsis (Septic Shock) and for all patients in whom
shock was due to a non-septic process (Non-Septic Shock).
From Siegel, Greenspan, and Del Guercio (16) with permission
of the publisher.

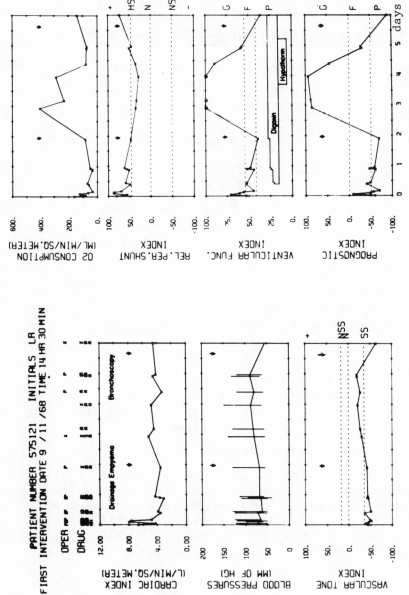

Fig. 5. Summary time plot of course of 31 year old female with intra-abdominal sepsis following cae-
sarean section. In Vascular Tone Index NSS = non-septic shock, SS = septic shock mean. In Relative
Peripheral Shunting Index HSS = hyperdynamic septic shock mean. In Ventricular Function and Prognostic Indices G = Good, F = Fair, and P = Poor ranges. From Siegel, Loh, and Goldwyn (18) with
permission of the publisher.

Vascular Tone Index (19) revealed a reduced pressure-flow relationship which was lower than the mean value seen in untreated patients
with septic shock (SS). Similarly the index of Relative Peripheral
Shunting (19)(which reflects relationship between oxygen consumption
and vascular tone) was increased to a value greater than the mean
level seen in patients with hyperdynamic septic shock (HSS). However, she manifested a good level of ventricular function, and
only a slight reduction in oxygen consumption. An ominous sign,
however, was the Prognostic Index (18)(relating the abnormalities
in vascular tone, oxygen consumption, and ventricular function)
which lay at the junction of the Fair and Poor range, indicating
a relative disparity between the alterations in the peripheral
circulation and the level of myocardial function. As the septic
process progressed, there was a slow but steady decline in oxygen
consumption, in spite of the continued increase in cardiac output,
and in the face of an adequate arterial pO_2. This fall in oxygen
consumption frequently heralds clinical deterioration, and is
usually related to the presence of a major undrained septic process
which must be resolved if the patient is to be effectively treated.
This was, indeed, the time history of this patient, the offending
purulent collection was found in the right pleural space, and a
thoracostomy tube was inserted. The resultant hemodynamic changes
were dramatic. Within 18 hours of drainage of the empyema there
was a striking increase in oxygen consumption, which was caused
not by an increase in arterial oxygen tension, but by a fall in
the mixed venous oxygen content.

These abnormalities in oxygen consumption appear to reflect
the presence of significant arteriovenous shunts, although it also
appears that the septic process may be associated with some abnormalities in the oxyhemoglobin dissociation curve. It is not clear
whether the vascular abnormalities are on an anatomic or functional
basis, but septic patients behave as if they had a large arteriovenous fistula and frequently progress into a high output cardiac
failure (15,16). This did occur in this patient early in her
clinical course, when it was noted that in spite of the increased
cardiac output the level of ventricular function was declining
toward the Poor range. Even though there was no evidence of overt
failure, digitalization with digoxin was begun as a prophylactic
measure just before the drainage of the empyema, and the combination
of the prophylactic digitalization and the drainage of the septic
process was associated with a striking improvement in the index of
ventricular function and the related Prognostic Index, mainly as a
consequence of better cardiac contractile function. This case
makes the point that it is important to recognize the potential
for the development of myocardial failure in patients with septic
shock, and to treat aggressively for it before the occult decreases
in myocardial contractility are manifested by overt cardiac failure.

Patients with major trauma and patients with severe sepsis

frequently manifest an increased degree of pulmonary veno-arterial admixture (Table I) (14). This abnormality in pulmonary function most probably is the result of at least three factors which have been very elegantly discussed by Moore et al (10); 1) the presence of abnormal anatomic or physiologic connections between the pulmonary arterial and pulmonary venous beds, 2) abnormalities in the relationship between alveolar ventilation and pulmonary capillary blood flow, and 3) alterations in the diffusion of oxygen across the blood-gas barrier. It can be exaggerated by increases in pulmonary capillary permeability because of inflammatory exudates secondary to infection (3), by overhydration with non-colloid containing fluids (10), and possibly by immunologic phenomena related to blood transfusion (11). It is important to emphasize that the net product of the effect of these abnormalities is to increase the percent of systemic venous blood which bypasses the blood-gas interface and that the resultant reductions in arterial oxygen tension may have a further deleterious effect on an already depressed myocardium as is commonly found in patients with a severe septic process (16). This phenomenon was dramatically shown in this patient in whom, as the pulmonary veno-arterial admixture increased from 35% to 45%, there was a second decrease in both oxygen consumption and ventricular function. Both of these responded only minimally to removal of secretions by bronchoscopy suggesting that the pathophysiologic processes affecting the microvasculature of the lung noted by Clowes (3) and Moore (10), rather than retained bronchial secretions, may have been largely responsible for the increasing physiologic pulmonary shunt (16). At the time of the last study shown in this sequence, when the ventricular function index had decreased to its lowest value, the arterial pO_2 was noted to be 67 mm Hg. The simple therapy of increasing the arterial pO_2 to 122 mm Hg, by raising the inspired oxygen tension, resulted in return in ventricular function relationships to the levels which approached those seen earlier after the initial response to digoxin.

In this regard it is important to stress that altering the level of arterial oxygen tension is one more way to influence both the level of myocardial function and the state of peripheral vascular tone. As with any drug having powerful cardiovascular effects, the inspired oxygen concentration and the resultant arterial pO_2 levels must be carefully manipulated for maximum therapeutic effect. On the one hand, when the abnormalities in pulmonary function causing the increased pulmonary veno-arterial admixture become very great, they may result in arterial hypoxemia which can further contribute to the reduced oxygen consumption seen in various forms of shock. Conversely, however, maintenance of excessively high levels of arterial oxygen tension has been shown to be associated with progressive respiratory insufficiency due to direct toxic effects on pulmonary capillary endothelium, and if maintained, 100% oxygen can of itself produce fatal respiratory insufficiency (10).

TABLE I

PULMONARY VENOARTERIAL ADMIXTURE[**]

	N	MEAN % V-A	RANGE
NORMAL YOUNG MEN	[*]	7.0	
AGED PRE-OPERATIVE PATIENTS	34	10.9	5-18
POST-OPERATIVE: MODERATE VOL. REPLACEMENT	7	17.0	8-31
POST-OPERATIVE: MASSIVE VOL. REPLACEMENT	6	22.9	8-34
HYPOVOLEMIC SHOCK	10	21.0	7-30
POST-CARDIAC SHOCK	10	31.0	17-52
SEPTIC SHOCK	15	38.4	15-78
FAT EMBOLUS SHOCK	2	60.5	48-72

[*] From Comroe et al.
in The Lung, Clinical Physiology and Pulmonary Function Tests
Chicago, Year Book Medical Publishers, Inc.
1965 pp. 145, 305, 325

[**] From Siegel, Goldwyn, and Del Guercio (14) with permission of the publisher.

Finally, it is important to emphasize that cardiovascular support of the patient in shock, and especially patients in septic shock, frequently requires the use of several drugs in concert (digitalis preparations, isoproterenol, steroids, glucagon, and oxygen) to achieve the proper balance between peripheral and cardiac effects (2,5,6,7,9,15,16,17). An example of the synergistic use of two drugs whose inotropic action is effected through different receptor sites is shown in the last case (Fig.6). This patient, also a 31 year old woman, with multiple intra-abdominal abscesses following total hysterectomy, illustrates how the action of the inotropic vasodilator, isoproterenol, can be potentiated by a continuous infusion with intravenous glucagon (17). This patient was severely septic although not hypotensive. Because of inadequate ventilation she suffered a respiratory and cardiac arrest from which she was immediately resuscitated without central nervous system injury. In spite of the continuous infusion of the beta adrenergic agent, isoproterenol, the patient showed only a moderate improvement in cardiac output and ventricular function. however, the simultaneous infusion of glucagon resulted in a marked increased in cardiac index associated with an immediate improvement in the Ventricular Function Index. This improvement persisted and increased during combined isoproterenol and glucagon infusion. However, the dependence of this patient's myocardial function on the synergistic action of these two agents was clearly demonstrated when the glucagon infusion was stopped. Even though continuous inotropic support with isoproterenol was continued, it became clear that the patient's cardiovascular status was deteriorating. A repeat determination of the hemodynamic parameters showed that the cardiac index had decreased to a level near that at which the patient had previously suffered her cardiac arrest, and that the Ventricular Function Index was again in the Poor range. The glucagon infusion was reinstituted and there was an immediate return of cardiac index to the level previously associated with glucagon administration. The Ventricular Function Index also returned into the Fair and finally into the Good range of function.

In concluding, the major point which all of these illustrative cases serve to make is that it is the physician's responsibility to establish not only the proper qualitative therapy, but also to determine the optimal dose of each agent needed to achieve the desired net cardiovascular effect in a particular patient. The development of quantitative techniques for the bedside evaluation of cardiovascular function (5,6,8,9,15,19,20) permits an individualized approach to the therapy of shock based on an "as often as necessary" evaluation of the patient's response to a given therapeutic program. It is important to emphasize that while there are general rules which may be useful as clinical guide lines, nevertheless, the very best patient care requires that the therapeutic program be exactly tailored to fit the specific pattern of the patient's disease process.

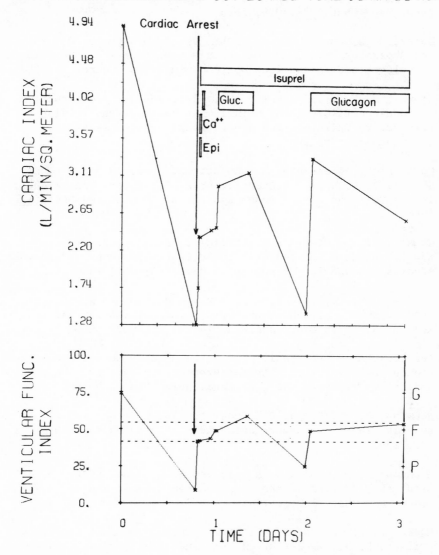

PATIENT NUMBER 579206   INITIALS EG
FIRST INTERVENTION DATE 11 / 21 /68 TIME 15 HR 30 MIN

Fig.6   Synergism between isoproterenol and glucagon in 31 year old
        female with intra-abdominal abscesses following total
        hysterectomy.   From Siegel et al (17) with permission of
        the publisher.

REFERENCES

1. Carey J. S., Brown, R. S., Woodward, N. W., Yao, S. T., and
   Shoemaker, W. C. Comparison of hemodynamic responses to whole
   blood and plasma expanders in clinical traumatic shock.
   Synec. and Obst. 121:1039, 1965

2. Carey, J. S., Brown, R. S., Mohr, P. A., Monson, D. O., Yao, S.T.,
   and Shoemaker, W. C. Cardiovascular function in shock. Responses
   to volume loading and isoproterenol infusion. Circ. 35: 327, 1967

3. Clowes, G. H. A., Zuschneid, W., Slobodan, D., and Turner, M.
   The non-specific pulmonary inflammatory reactions leading to
   respiratory failure after shock, gangrene, and sepsis.
   J. Trauma 8: 899, 1968

4. Cohn, J. D., Greenspan, M., Goldstein, C. R., Gudwin, A. L.,
   Siegel, J. H., and Del Guercio, L. R. M. Arteriovenous shunting
   in high cardiac output shock syndromes. Synec. and Obst. 127:282,
   1968

5. Gunnar, R. M., Cruz, A., Boswell, J., Bun, S., Pietras, R. J.,
   and Tobin, J. R. Myocardial infarction with shock. Hemodynamic
   studies and results of therapy. Circ. 33: 753, 1966

6. Hardaway, R. M., James, P. M., Jr., Anderson, R. W.,
   Bradenberg, C. E., and West, R. L. Intensive study and treatment of shock in man. J.A.M.A. 199: 779, 1967

7. Hermreck, A. S. and Thal, A. P. The adrenergic drugs and their
   use in shock therapy. Current Problems in Surgery. Year Book
   Medical Publishers, Inc., Chicago, July 1958

8. Hopkins, R. W., Sabga, G., Penn, I., and Simeone, F. Hemodynamic aspects of hemorrhagic and septic shock. J.A.M.A. 191:
   127, 1965

9. MacLean, L. D., Duff, J. H., Scott, H. M., and Peretz, D. I.
   Treatment of shock in man based on hemodynamic diagnosis.
   Synec. and Obst. 120:1, 1965

10. Moore, F. D., Lyons, J. H., Pierce, E. C., Morgan, A. P.,
    Drinker, P. A., MacArthur, J. D., and Dammin, G. J. Post-
    traumatic Pulmonary Insufficiency. W. B. Saunders Co.,
    Philadelphia, 1969

11. Nahas, R. A., Melrose, D. G., Sykes, M. K., and Robinson, B.
    Post-perfusion lung syndrome: Effect of homologous blood.
    Lancet 2: 254, 1965

12. Sarnoff, S. J., Case, R. B., Waithe, P. E., and Isaacs, J. P. Insufficient coronary flow and myocardial failure as a complicating factor in late hemorrhagic shock. Am. J. Physiol. <u>176</u>: 439, 1954

13. Siegel, J. H. The myocardial contractile state and its role in the response to anesthesia and surgery. Anesthesiology <u>30</u>: 519, 1969

14. Siegel, J. H., Goldwyn, R. M., and Del Guercio, L. R. M. Hemodynamic alterations following massive fluid replacement in man. Proc. Symposium on Fluid Replacement in the Surgical Patient, Grune & Stratton, N. Y. (In Press) 1970

15. Siegel, J. H., Greenspan, M., Cohn, J. D., and Del Guercio, L. R. M. A bedside computer and physiologic nomograms: Guides to the management of the patient in shock. Arch. Surg. <u>97</u>: 480, 1968.

16. Siegel, J. H., Greenspan, M., and Del Guercio, L. R. M. Abnormal vascular tone, defective oxygen transport, and myocardial failure in human septic shock. Ann. Surg. <u>165</u>: 504, 1967

17. Siegel, J. H., Levine, M. J., McConn, R., and Del Guercio, L.R.M. The effect of glucagon infusion on cardiovascular function in the critically ill. Synec. and Obst. (In Press) 1970

18. Siegel, J. H., Loh, L., and Goldwyn, R. M. An application of computer techniques to the assessment of the circulation in the critically ill. Submitted for publication. 1969

19. Siegel, J. H., and Williams, J. B. A computer based index for the prediction of operative survival in patients with cirrhosis and portal hypertension. Ann. Surg. <u>169</u>: 191, 1969

20. Udhoji, V. N., Weil, M. H., Sambhi, M., Mohinder, P., and Rosoff, L. Hemodynamic studies on clinical shock associated with infection. Am. J. Med. <u>34</u>: 461, 1963

Supported in part by grant HE 10415 from the National Institutes of Health and GM 16709 from the National Institute of General Medical Sciences.

THE EFFECT OF TRASYLOL IN SHOCK

Gert   L.   Haberland

Prof. Dr. med. Bonn University

Forschungszentrum, Bayer Wuppertal, Germany

The casual observer finds the ever increasing number of indications for Trasylol too numerous to survey easily and it has
become even more difficult to associate the variety of indications
for this drug. For this reason we would like to emphasise that
the action of Trasylol can and should be explained only in terms of
its inhibitive action on esteroproteinases, because so far no other
enzymes have become known to us which are - in reasonable concentrations - inhibited or directly altered in their action by this
compound. Esteroproteinases which include trypsin, chymotrypsin,
plasmin and leucocytal proteinases, are ubiquitous. They are
found in active form in excess in many pathophysiological processes. In these processes certain aspects of the pathophysiology
of inflammation and shock play a role, the perpetuation of which
is closely associated with protein metabolism.

Almost all the indications for Trasylol, commencing with
simple or primary hyperfibrinolysis by way of secondary hyperfibrinolysis based on consumption coagulopathy, to the local biochemical processes which are seen in degenerative changes in the
joints, can be demonstrated occurring as fragments during the
course of shock.
In the f ollowing, therefore, we have attempted to draw a picture of
the different pathophysiological sequelae which turn up once a shock
has been initiated and, in doing so, show those fragments where
Trasylol is effective or, to put it more precisely, indicate in which
shock fragments an effect of Trasylol can be demonstrated.

At the same time we shall try to demonstrate that, although there are different forms of shock such as haemorrhagic, toxic, burn shock, endotoxine shock etc. , there are certain basic mechanisms that are common to all these forms of shock. If one looks at these various parameters as an entity, it can be seen that they may be arranged in the form of a vicious circle. Once this vicious circle is established it is only of secondary importance at which site the shock process is evoked, since the circle perpetuates itself, providing the counter-regulatory mechanisms are inadequate or fail completely.

In order to demonstrate this, we will examine for example the course of events in the haemorrhagic shock in some detail, using a modified illustration by Ahnefeld/Francke (1968) and Rein/Schneider (1969) (see Fig. 1).

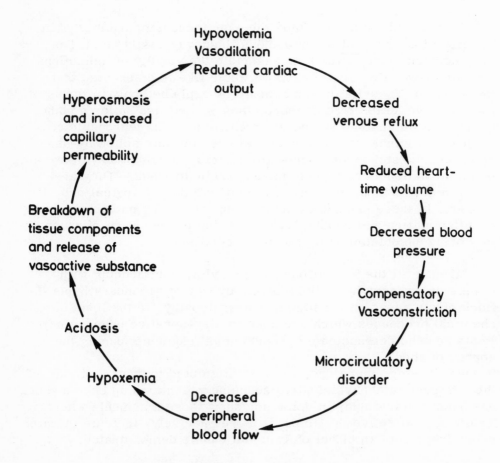

The loss in volume caused by haemorrhage, when exceeding a certain amount, results in a fall in venous return and thus to a reduction in cardiac output and to a fall in blood pressure.

The body attempts to compensate this event by constricting the
medium and small vessels (reactive vasoconstriction). This
reactive vasoconstriction results, in certain areas, in disturbances
of the microcirculation, which are manifested as a fall in tissue
oxygen supply.

This oxygen deficiency disturbs carbohydrate metabolism,
pyruvic acid is no longer properly metabolised and lactic acid is
formed in increased quantities, which contributes to the formation
of acidoses. Acidosis among others, causes tissue decomposition
which has a whole series of consequences:

First of all decomposition of acid mucopolysaccharides results
in liberation of heparin and histamine. Furthermore, hyperosmosis develops in the tissue resulting in the passive transfer of liquor
and plasma into the tissue. This process is enhanced by leuco-dia-
pedesis. Proteinases are liberated from the leucocytes and these
potentiate the degradation of the fragments and contribute to an increasing hyperosmosis at the tissue level. Through the pH shift,
as well as through other factors, tissue proteinases are activated
which further aggravate this process.

Finally, in the train of this degradation process, other vasoactive polypeptides - to which the kinins also belong - are liberated
and which in their turn have an increasing permeability effect. These
two main components, hyperosmosis and increased vasculary permeability lead to intensified loss of circulating volume, where-
upon the circle is completed.

At the same time a number of side reactions take place which
add to the basic events of the circle (Fig. 2).

The reactive vasoconstriction is evoked by an emergency reaction
of the adrenals resulting in the liberation of catecholamines. The
action of the catecholamines not only causes vasoconstriction but
also an increase in free fatty acids. The latter after forming fat
globules activate the coagulation factors which in turn results in a
partial closure of the microcirculation due to the formation of micro-

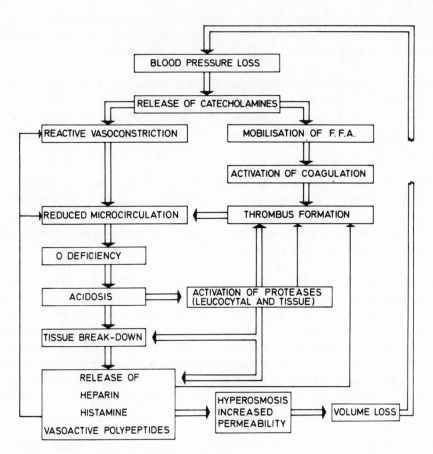

thrombi. This in combination with the reactive vasoconstriction
still further increases the oxygen deficiency with all its sequelae.
It is well known that these sequelae, to which amongst others one
can place hyperfibrinolysis, which again enhances also the liberation of vasoactive substances; are not always catastrophic. This
is because at every stage substances are liberated which have a
compensatory function. As mentioned, the reactive vasoconstriction with its attendant oxygen deficiency and subsequent acidosis
produces a degradation of mucopolysaccharides resulting in liberation of heparin and histamine. Histamine is a vasodilator and
heparin acts as an thrombin inhibitor. Besides this, inactivators
which neutralise the proteinases are liberated by the pH shift at
tissue level into the acid region.

The capacity of these compensatory mechanisms is variable and to an extent limited. Therapeutic measures should, therefore, be primarily aimed at supporting the body's own counter-regulators, where this is desirable, and to shorten them where an over-active counter-regulation which exceeds its function produces deleterious consequences.

What therapeutic possibilities are open to us:

a)   Substitution of the loss of volume

b)   Inhibition of the superfluous reactive vasoconstriction, as well as an inhibition of a superfluous vasodilatation produced by histamine e. g.

c)   Inhibition of the early phase of coagulation by the use of Trasylol or in the late stages by using heparin.

d)   Enhancement of the inhibitor potential by using Trasylol.

What is meant by an enhancement of the inhibitor potential? It means to enable the organism to cope with the surplus quantities of deleteriously active esteroproteinases. The following groups belong to these esteroproteinases:

1.   Kininogenases i. e. enzymes which liberate kinins from inactive precursors. Their main representatives are kallikrein and trypsin. The inhibitory effect of Trasylol within this field has become so universally known that I do not need to mention names other than those of Frey, Kraut and Werle (1968).

2.   Plasmin, the inhibition of which by Trasylol was first described by Marx (1959) and later confirmed by numerous authors.

3.   Early phase of coagulation. The effect of Trasylol within this group of enzymes was first described by Olsson, Francken and Norström (1963) and then further analysed by various teams (see Haberland, Matis, Pauschinger, Thies and Vinazzer (1969). Finally,

4.   Leucocytal proteinases, the inhibition of which by
        Trasylol was reported on by Barnhart, Quintana, Lenon
        and Bluhm (1968) by Janof and Zeligs (1968) and by
        Spilberg and Osterland (1969).

Especially the last mentioned group which has long been neglected in discussions, deserves, in our opinion, special attention.

Because, while the indications for Trasylol in the coagulation
and lysis region can easily be developed from the inhibited enzymes,
the interpretation of the antioedematous effect of Trasylol is really,
according to our present knowledge, only possible via the inhibition
of the kinin liberation and the inhibition of tissue proteinases and of
leucocytal proteases. The investigations by Habermann (1969) on
the significance of the kinin system in experimental inflammations
give rise to justified doubts on a greater pathogenetic significance
of the kinins so that the inhibition of the tissue and the leucocytal
proteases stands, at the moment, in the foreground for us as the
explanation for the efficacy of Trasylol on oedematous processes.

That Trasylol has such an anti-oedematous effect was first
described by Kaller (1966) and later confirmed experimentally as
well as clinically by other teams. (Eigler (1969), Eigler/Stock
(1968), Pauschinger (1969), Haberland et al. (1969), Blümel (1969),
Spilberg (1969), Ludwig (1969).

Circulatory and metabolic disturbances which we see in inflammatory oedema are qualitatively essentially the same as those
we see as shock fragments - like disturbance of the peripheral
micro-circulation, oxygen dificiency, acidosis and their sequelae.
From this alone it is justifiable to consider these processes together. As a matter of fact the shock cycle as drawn in Fig. 1 can
be divided into two halves, the one representing mainly the circulatory and the other the tissue side of events taking place during the
disease. Basing on this model the anti-oedematous action of Trasylol resulting from an inhibition of proteolysis in the tissue, can
well explain the action of Trasylol which could be demonstrated in
other shock fragments. To these belong the positive influence on
the venous return (Pauschinger 1969) Haberland et al (1969) as well
as the positive influence on the oxygen content in the blood, acidosis, pyruvate and lactate levels (Hollmann, Liesen (1969) also the

influence on the lipoid metabolism (Heller, Mayer, Mörl (1969), and
Mörl and Heller (1969), Gurd (1969), Blümel (1969), Huth (1969). The
prevention of the fall in blood pressure or its therapeutic influence
by Trasylol could be verified by numerous findings in experimental
shock models as well as clinically.

The clinical results obtained with Trasylol in recent years in
the various forms of shock as, for example, in haemorrhagic shock
(Ludwig 1968), peritonitis shock, lung and fat embolism (Haberland
and Matis (1967) and Mörl 1968), burn shock but also pancreatitis,
for which Creutzfeldt very early on attached more importance to
the circulatory action of Trasylol than to its direct action on organ,
should be viewed in the light of these experimental results.

It is important that the action of Trasylol in these forms of
shock can clearly be seen from a decrease in the mortality rate by
half or more (Marx, Imdahl, Haberland (1967) and Haberland, Matis
(1969).

Naturally, in trying to explain the action of Trasylol in these
different forms of shock one has, as regards the individual inhibited
enzyme systems, to allocate the factors of importance proportionately to the original cause.

This applies, however, more to the quantitative and to a lesser
degree to the qualitative aspects which, according to the circle of
events shown above, are all incorporated in the course of the shock
process. It now only remains to be said that if we are to fix the
measures to be taken in the treatment of shock in order of importance, they would in our opinion fall as follows:

Volume substitution, Trasylol and Heparin, whereby the first
two measures should be taken together.

In the late forms of shock the picture is largely determined by
the peripheral vascular obstruction. In this case it would be appropriate to discuss whether objective short term application of
fibrinolysis activators (streptokinase) according to Lasch firstly
achieve the reopening of the circulation before in the second phase
of therapy the other above mentioned measures are applied, or
whether the sequence should be reversed. There are good arguments for both possibilities and experiments which are under way
now should clarify this still open question.

From the shock cycle we have just shown, one can in our opinion clearly see that all forms of shock can be observed together and that it is merely a question as to which parameter is first influenced from where the shock is perpetuated in the first place. In shock caused by endotoxins or snake bite or by a local burn, local processes are taking place which result in an inner loss of volume. Shock from asphyxiation likewise involved a volume loss. Basically, however, it may be said that all processes once initiated proceed with participation and mutual support of all the parameters indicated in the circle.

BIBLIOGRAPHY

Ahnefeld, F. W., and Francke, W. (1968): Der Schock in der operativen Gynäkologie. Der Gynäkologe 1, 1.

Barnhart, M. I., Quintana, C., Lenon, H. L., Bluhm, G. B., and Riddle, J. M. (1968): Proteases in Inflammation. Annals for the New York Academy of Sciences 146, 527.

Blümel, G. (1969): Experimentelle Untersuchungen aufgrund klinischer Beobachtungen. Neue Aspekte der Trasylol Therapie 4, Schattauer Verlag, Stuttgart. (In print).

Eigler, F. W., Stock, W. (1968): Verminderung des postischämischen Extremitätenödems an der Ratte durch einen Proteinasehemmer. Klinische Wochenschrift 46, 1283.

Eigler, F. W. (1969): Experimentelle Untersuchungen zur Behandlung des Torniquet-Syndroms mit Trasylol. Neue Aspekte der Trasylol Therapie 3, 151. Schattauer Verlag, Stuttgart.

Frey, E. K., Kraut, H., Werle, E. (1968): Das Kallikrein-Kinin-System und seine Inhibitoren. Ferdinand Enke Verlag, Stuttgart.

Gumrich, H. (1969): Klinische Befunde zum posttraumatischen Ödem an den unteren Extremitäten. Neue Aspekte der Trasylol Therapie 4, Schattauer Verlag, Stuttgart. (In print).

Gurd, A. (1969): Treatment of fat embolism in experimental
animals. Neue Aspekte der Trasylol Therapie 4,
Schattauer Verlag, Stuttgart. (In print).

Haberland, G. L. , Matis, P. (1967): Trasylol, ein Proteinasen-
inhibitor bei chirurgischen und internen Indikationen.
Medizinische Welt 18, 1367.

Haberland, G. L. , Matis, P. (1969): Neue Aspekte der Trasylol
Therapie 3, Schattauer Verlag, Stuttgart.

Haberland, G. L. , Matis, P. , Pauschinger, P. , Thies, H. A. ,
and Vinazzer, H. (1969): Zur Beeinflussung postoperativer Zir-
kulations- und Gerinnungsveränderungen durch den Proteinasen-
inhibitor Trasylol. Medizinische Welt 20, 1270.

Habermann, E. (1969): Probleme der Pathophysiologie des Kinin-
systems. Neue Aspekte der Trasylol Therapie 3, 37.
Schattauer Verlag, Stuttgart.

Heller, W. , Mayer, W. , Mörl, F. K. (1969): Experimentelle
Studien zur Fettembolie. Neue Aspekte der Trasylol Therapie
3, 173. Schattauer Verlag, Stuttgart.

Hollmann, W. , Liesen, H. (1969): Der Einfluß von Trasylol auf
kardio-pulmonale Parameter bei dosierter Arbeit. Neue Aspekte
der Trasylol Therapie 3, 75. Schattauer-Verlag, Stuttgart.

Janof, A. , Zeligs, J. D. (1968): Vascular Injury and Lysis of
Basement Membrane in vitro by Neutral Protease of Human
Leukocytes. Science 161, 702.

Kaller, H. (1966): Die Beeinflussung experimentell erzeugter
Ödeme durch Trasylol. Neue Aspekte der Trasylol Therapie 1,
152.

Ludwig, H. (1968): Mikrozirkulationsstörungen und Diapedese-
blutungen im fetalen Gehirn bei Hypoxie. S. Karger, Basel;
Fortschritte der Geburtshilfe und Gynäkologie, 33

Marx, R. , Clemente, P. , Werle, E., Appel, W. (1959):
Zum Problem eines Antidotes in der internen Thrombotherapie
mit Fibrinolytika. Blut - Zeitschrift für Blutforschung V , 367.

Marx, R. , Imdahl, H. , Haberland, G. L. (1967): Neue Aspekte
der Trasylol Therapie 2.   Schattauer Verlag, Stuttgart.

Mörl, F. K. , Heller, W. (1969): Zur Pathogenese und Therapie
der Fettembolie.   Neue Aspekte der Trasylol Therapie 3, 161.
Schattauer Verlag, Stuttgart.

Mörl, F. K. (1968): Klinik der Proteinaseninhibitoren in der
Chirurgie, Ergebnisse einer alternierenden Applikation des Pro-
teinaseninhibitors Trasylol.   Schattauer Verlag, Stuttgart.

Olsson, P. , Francken, I. v. , Nordström, S. (1963):
Antithrombin Activity (Heparin Co-Factors) in Plasma after Major
Surgery in Heparinized Patients.   Acta Chir. Scand.

Rahmel, R. (1969): Klinische Befunde zum posttraumatischen
Ödem an der Hand.   Neue Aspekte der Trasylol Therapie 4
Schattauer Verlag, Stuttgart. (In print).

Rein, H. , Schneider, M. (1956): Einführung in die Physiologie
des Menschen. Springer Verlag, Berlin, 12.

Spilberg, I. and Osterland, C. K. (1969): Anti-inflammatory
Effect of Trasylol in Acute Experimental Arthritis Induced by
Urate Crystals.   Neue Aspekte der Trasylol Therapie 4,
Schattauer Verlag, Stuttgart.   (In print).

TREATMENT OF ACUTE RENAL FAILURE AND CHRONIC RENAL INSUFFICIENCY WITH ADDITIONAL TRASYLOL THERAPY

G. Stötter - S. Thune

Medical and Neurological Clinic I
City Hospitals
"Städt. Krankenanstalten",Augsburg

Despite improved dialysis techniques, in combination
with balanced infusion therapy, early regulation of
the water, electrolyte and acid/base metabolism and
specific antibiotic therapy, acute renal failure (ARF)
has 29-69 % mortality rates. During the last 1 1/2
years, patients in ARF received in addition to the
mentioned standard therapy, Trasylol by continuous drip
infusion of usually 1 million KIU in 24 hours. Trasylol
inhibits besides trypsin, chymotrypsin, plasmin and the
kallikreins which are responsible for the liberation of
kinin, as well as leukocytic lysosomal proteinases;
these enzyme systems are mainly held responsible for
the tubular damage to the kidneys, and in conjunction
with oxygen deficiency and other noxae such as bacterial toxins, endogenous poisons and bilirubin, they
induce ARF.

The ARF in the patients had a variety of causes.

There were 7 cases of liver disease, 3 patients with
leptospirosis, 3 cases of a necrotic episode in chronic
liver disease and 1 chronic cholangiohepatitis in pregnancy, 1 urosepsis with endotoxin shock. In 8 other
patients ARF occurred after a surgical or gynaecologi-
cal intervention. 3 cases in endotoxin shock in peritonitis and ileus, in 3 cases in haemorrhagic shock,
in 1 post-renal urinary tract obstruction by blood
clots in the renal pelvis. The mechanical impedement
to urinary flow was removed by inserting a catheter

Fall	Alter	Ursache des ANV	Harnstoff	Kreatinin	Harnsäure	Serumkalium in mval	B.E. in meql	HCO₃ in meql	Hämodialyse	Peritoneale	Oligoanurie vor Therapiebeginn	Oligoanurie nach Therapiebeginn	D. Polyurie in Tagen	Norm. der Harnfixa Woche	End.Kreat.Clearance nach Wochen	End.Kreat.Clearance nach Monate	Phenolrot nach Wochen	Phenolrot nach Monate
1	22 J. ♂	Indurierte Fettleber (nekrotischer Schub) (Histologisch gesichert)	216	8,1	20,1	6,2	-9,7	16,9	0	0	3	2	12	1,1	3:75	4:69	3:22	4:53
2	35 J. ♂	Hepatonephritis (Leptospirosis)	233	6,4	25,6	5,4	+5,3	29,0	0	0	3	1	18	1,0	3:72		3:30	
3	31 J. ♂	Kreislaufschock nach Polamidonintoxikation Indurierte Fettleber	314	12,8	18,6	6,4	-4,0	21,0	0	0	0	1	14	2,0		4:69		4:23
4	39 J. ♂	Chron. persist. Hepatitis (akuter Schub) (Histologisch gesichert)	413	26,0	24,0	6,0	-15,2	13,6	1	0	3	3	23	2,1		4:93		4:21
5	25 J. ♂	Hepatonephritis (Leptospirosis)	213	21,3	12,7	6,2	-9,6	16,3	0	1	2	5	24	2,6	3:131		3:20	
6	31 J. ♀	Rezidiv. cholangiohepatitis in Graviditate (tox. Leber- und Nierenschaden)	229	15,6	25,1	4,7	-6,7	17,2	0	0	2	3	14	2,0	2:73		2:24	
7	35 J. ♀	Hepatonephritis (Leptospirosis)	293	8,8	18,6	4,5	-4,5	21,0	0	0	2	1	14	2,0	2:93		2:27	
8	48 J. ♂	Urosepsis Endotoxinschock	355	15,5	13,8	6,5	-15,4	13,6	0	1	2	1	24	2,5				
9	33 J. ♀	Verschlußikterus Operationsschock (Cholezystektomie)	132	6,0	16,3	3,5	-6,8	17,4	0	0	1	2	37	2,1	5:69		5:18	
10	29 J. ♂	Gicht mit Uratstein li. Ureter ANV nach Cholezystämie	445	12,3	39,4	5,5	-7,3	13,2	2	0	5	3	16	1,8	3:85		3:22	
11	27 J. ♀	Zustand nach Billroth II Subileus. Op.-Revision mit Resektion der Anastomose. Postoperativer Endotoxinschock	240	5,4	8,6	3,8	+3,0	26,0	0	0	3	3	16	1,0	5:80		5:34	
12	44 J. ♀	Appendektomie. Lokale Peritonitis. Endotoxinschock	690	19,2	25,4	6,1	+3,0	26,1	1	0	9	1	26	1,6	5:81		5:10	
13	49 J. ♀	Appendektomie. Lokale Peritonitis. Endotoxinschock	319	14,8	11,4	4,4	+2,3	24,5	0	0	2	2	16	2,1				
14	33 J. ♀	Postpartaler Entblutungsschock bei Zervixruptur	337	13,2	21,0	6,3	-11,8	15,5	1	0	3	5	19	3,2	5:76		5:20	
15	36 J. ♀	Entblutungsschock bei Sektio Caesarea (Vorzeitige Plazentalösung)	118	4,6	9,1	5,4	-8,7	13,0	0	0	2	3	16	1,5		2:85		2:24
16	50 J. ♂	Rektumresektion mit Anus praeter. Intraoperative Blutung. Postrenale Harnwegsobstruktion durch Blutkoagula in Nierenbecken	130	8,2	8,3	4,8	-15,6	11,5	1	0	3	3	18	1,2		4:82		4:22
17	38 J. ♂	Akute Pankreatitis	255	13,8	17,9	3,7	+3,8	29,0	0	1	2	5	In der 3. Woche Exitus letalis infolge profuser Blutung aus dem Magen-Darmkanal Ulcus ventriculi und Schleimhauterosionen					
18	15 J. ♀	Sublimatvergiftung	493	13,9	20,5	7,2	-20,0	9,3	1	0	3	2						
19	62 J. ♀	Hautverbrennung (> als 40% Oberfläche)	244	4,6	15,2	5,4	-7,5	18,2	0	0	4	1	22	2,3		2:107		2:26
ANV bei vorgeschädigten Nieren																		
20	46 J. ♂	Chron. Pyelonephritis (Anurischer Schub)	152	5,5	10,2	5,9	-5,7	19,6	0	1	2	6	18	2,1	4:65		4:20	
21	68 J. ♂	Chron. aszend. Pyelonephritis Prostataelektroresektion (intravasale Hämolyse durch Spüllösung)	200	10,4	14,3	5,1	-5,9	19,5	0	1	3	6	14	2,5	5:70		5:18	

into each renal pelvis and irrigating with streptase.
In 2 instances ARF was connected with cholecystectomy,
in 1 case with shock due to burns and in 2 with mercuric
chloride poisoning. One of the corrosive sublimate
poisonings, in a 42-year-old man, is not included in the
review table. This patient received immediately infusions of glucose with 1 million KIU Trasylol in addition to the conventional treatment (BAL, EDTA - 5.0 g
EDTA Na$_2$, glucose 50.0 g in 500 ml, and metal captase -
150 mg D-penicilliamine HCl). ARF did not become manifest, although the patient had ingested the same preparation and approximately the same quantity of mercury
as the other, and signs of mercury kidney, erythrocytes
and granulated casts were already found in the sediment.
The patient was treated for 11 days, receiving a total
of 4 million KIU Trasylol. Urea values remained in the
normal range, uric acid increased to 10.3 mg%, creatinine to 1.9 mg%. The latter values both decreased with
the treatment within 5 days to within normal limits. -
One patient with pancreatitis and ensuing pancreatic
necrosis was lost in ARF despite the high dosage intravenous and intraperitoneal Trasylol treatment. On the
2nd treatment day, peritoneal dialysis was started.
Insertion of the catheter was followed by a bilious
and turbid serious discharge as in bilious peritonitis.
Trasylol was added to the washing fluid at the rate of
100,000 KIU per 1 litre. Intravenous Trasylol treatment was continued with 1.5 million KIU. The washing
fluid soon became clean. Abdominal pains subsided. The
blood pressure remained about 130/90 mm Hg and only
finally fell to below measurable values. Diuresis did
not start again. The patient died with cardiac and
circulatory failure on the 5th treatment day. Pathological anatomic changes comprised extensive, not very
recent, haemorrhagic necrosis of the pancreas and wide
spread foci of fat necrosis of retroperitoneal tissue
on both sides and in the mesenteric root. The irrigat-
ed space showed only a few chalky white spots and was
free of fatty tissue necroses. The jelly-like oedema
extended retroperitoneally to the groin. The liver
showed marked fatty degeneration, partly with beginning fat cirrhosis. Changes of the kidneys were re-
markably slight. In 2 cases ARF occurred in pre-existing renal damage, in chronic pyelonephritis and after
electroresection of the prostate with intravascular
haemolysis.

All patients showed an extremely critical pattern of
disease despite the non-homogenous composition of the
case material. In the great majority of cases the

electrolyte, water and acid/base metabolism had broken
down. A proportion of the stated dialyses were only
carried out as a safety measure after the break through
the ARF had already been achieved by the combined
treatment with Trasylol.

The average duration of the anuric and the polyuric
phase, the number of dialyses which were necessary
with conventional therapy according to literature data
(1, 2, 3, 4) and in our case material until 1967 are
demonstrated and compared in a diagram with 21 cases
ARF in which Trasylol was additionally administered.
The comparison clearly shows that with additional
Trasylol treatment the duration of the oligo-anuric
phase was shortened to 2.7 days even in cases in which
it had been persisting for up to 9 days.

Additional Trasylol therapy achieved in our opinion in
19 patients in ARF without and in 2 patients in ARF
with pre-existing renal damage, a more rapid break
through the oliguric-anuric phase, a shortening of the

Durchschnittlicher Krankheitsverlauf des ANV ohne Zusatztherapie
von Trasylol (Literaturangaben sowie eigene Fälle bis 1967)

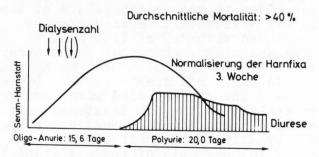

Durchschnittlicher Krankheitsverlauf des ANV unter Zusatztherapie
mit Trasylol (21 Fälle)

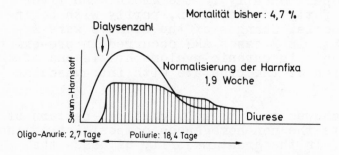

polyuric phase and, especially, an accelerated decrease
of the fixed urinary constituents (urea, creatinine,
uric acid) in about 2 weeks instead of otherwise 3
weeks. The rate of necessary dialysis was reduced to
less than 1 dialysis per patient. The mortality rate
was substantially reduced.

Uraemic decompensation in chronic renal insufficiency
was treated with apparently good success in 35 patients
with Trasylol in smaller doses of 400,000 - 600,000 KIU
for 4-6 weeks, in addition to standard therapy.

The success of treatment was assessed by the criteria:

1. Decrease of the period of persistence of accompani-
   ments of uraemia, such as twitchings, vomiting, agi-
   tation, insomnia, etc.

2. The time required for compensated retention to be
   achieved.

3. The rate of necessary dialysis.

In chronic kidney disease when anatomical renal lesions
are already marked, additional Trasylol treatment cannot
be expected to lead to the same good results as in ARF
when the kidneys are healthy.

The therapeutic success was in our opinion very good
in 10 cases, good in 7, moderate in 10 and poor in 8
cases. Altogether 43 haemodialyses or peritoneal dialyses were carried out. Comparatively better results
were obtained in chronic pyelonephritis in the stage
of compensated retention.

Discussion

Truss (5) has recently presented comparative experimental studies of the behaviour of the renal enzyme
system in various forms of shock (shock in burns, haemorrhagic shock and renal ischaemia after 2 hours
arterial ligations). Only in the last case was it that
a rapid tissue destruction occurred, otherwise there
were only very slight histological changes of the kidneys.

Nevertheless, substantial changes of some tissue enzymes were present within only 1 hour to 1 day after
the shock and continued for up to 3 weeks. Normally,
the enzyme pattern of cells is maintained because the

enzymes are bound to the cell structure, or the cell
membrane prevents their passage into the blood and
urine. When the cell membrane is damaged it is for the
large-molecular enzymes possible to escape, and the
intracellular enzyme content decreases in the presence
of normal formation rates. This is especially remarkable for the fact that enzyme changes already occur at
a time when histological alteration of the cell structure is barely discernible. A multitude of factors are
held responsible for the renal damages. Most of them
induce, directly or indirectly, local circulatory disturbances in the kidney and thereby provide for tissue-
damaging hypoxia. By the agency of the liberated enzymes
also the mitchondria of the tubular cells and the cells
lining the glomeruli are damaged, the cellular metabolism is switched to anaerobic glycolysis. Sodium absorption in theproximal tubules distinctly decreases.
Thus develops a sodium overload of the distal tubules
or the macula densa. Hyperosmolarity against peritubular
plasma occurs, and due to enhancement of the renin-
angiotensin activity the vas efferens is closed with
resultant impairment or arrest of the glomerular blood
flow and glomerular function (6).

After the early administration of Trasylol we observed
clinically almost always a rapid increase of diuresis
which sometimes reached excessive proportions. Therefore, we assume that proteinase inhibitors already prevent or lessen the initial damage to lysosomes and mitochondria. The normal sodium gradient in the course of
the nephron is restored and spastic occlusion of the
vas efferens removed. In pathological circumstances the
intrinsic inhibitor systems do not apparently suffice
to prevent an increase of the liberation of kinin.
Back and Wilkens (7) studied the action on the microcirculation. The result of a prolonged kinin action on
the microcirculation can lead to a shock-like state.
The mechanism of the inhibition of the proteolytic,
esterolytic and kinin-liberating activity of the enzyme
is by engagement of the "inhibitor area" of the inhibitor molecule with the "active centre" of the enzyme
molecule, by which an inactive enzyme-inhibitor complex forms. The blood concentration of the inhibitor
rapidly decreases after it has been injected. After
3 minutes only 20 % of the injected dose is still
found in the blood. The rapid escape from the blood is
superseded, with delay, by a substantial rise of the
inhibitor concentration in the kidneys. One hour after
an injection, more than 60 % of the administered inhibitor quantity is already present in the kidneys and

after 4 hours almost 90 %. Thus, the kidneys possess
a selective capacity for the storage of Trasylol. The
accumulated inhibitor is stored in the kidneys for a
prolonged period of time and converted by splitting
off both terminal amino radicals, by which it does not
lose its inhibitor potency for the mentioned enzymes.
Only after 12 to 24 hours the inhibitor concentration
in the kidneys slowly decreases and after 5 - 6 days
reaches the threshold at which the possibility to demonstrate it ceases. Why Trasylol is stored in the
kidneys to such a degree is not yet known (Werle 8).

Proposals for Therapy

Despite the differences between the primary renal noxa,
renal insufficiency is initially of a functional nature.
Only after a certain space of time develops from the
functional condition an increasing degree of morpholo-
gically evident organic damage, mainly of the tubular
epithelial cells, and this progresses until a chiefly
or entirely organic renal insufficiency has become
established. Therapy with an essentially prophylactic
action is thus only possible before, during and shortly
after the impact of the noxa which induces the ARF.
Renal damage up to the degree of ARF is not very rare
in diseases associated with jaundice and after operations on the gall-bladder and biliary tract in the presence of jaundice.

Recent experimental investigations by Wolf, P. (San
Francisco) have revealed that renal lesions are less
after jaundice alone and after moderate renal ischaemia,
but that the tubular mitochondrial enzymes of the kidney are severely damaged by ischaemia and jaundice.

Concomitant damage of liver and kidney is often found
in non-surgical diseases of the liver, for example in
viral hepatitis, leptospirosis and chronic persistent
hepatitis. Therefore, in icteric diseases, monitoring
should, from the outset, not be limited to the usual
hepatic parameters but extended to fixed urinary constituents and renal function. If in acute liver disease
a simultaneous increase in urea, perhaps connected with
oliguria, is observed, then the conventional measures
should be immediately supplemented with balanced infusion therapy, administering 1 million KIU Trasylol in
24 hours, and continuing according to urinary volume
and fixed urinary constituents. In these cases we continued the Trasylol therapy also in the compulsory polyuric phase.

If in surgical cases which have led to ARF, an impairment of renal function is already present prior to the intervention (case 21), then prophylactic Trasylol infusion treatment should be started before or during the operation. If, as also happens in a series of surgical cases, any shock syndrome develops before or during the operation - embolic shock (case 14), surgical shock (cases 9, 11, 15, 16), shock following intravascular haemolysis (case 21) - then the control of the shock state takes first place.

In such cases it is not enough to observe the arterial pressure and venous filling pressure; more more significant criteria of the shock state are a decrease of the urinary output below 30 ml/hour, the rise of transaminases as a result of deficient hepatic perfusion, and the appearance of arrhythmia (case 14) and blocks which indicate "protraction of the shock" due to microcirculatory disorders in organic systems. With the onset of disorders of the microcirculation and, especially, intravascular clotting, the peripheral uptake of oxygen decreases, tissue acidoses and anoxaemia increase.

Conventional therapy was guided by the concept to overcome shock by replenishing the circulatory volume and raising the blood pressure. This symptomatic treatment is very important but does not take account of more recent biochemical insights, among which the influence of proteinase inhibitors can have a decisive therapeutic effect.

It is becoming more and more evident that the primary shock stimulus begins locally and affects both cell function and the cell structure by changes which cause the release of biologically active chemical substances.

In order to safeguard against a microcirculatory disorder or its sequelae in the tissues, it would be advisable to institute additional high-dosage Trasylol infusion therapy at the latest when, after relief of the shock, the fixed urinary constituents begin rising and the 24-hour urinary volume decreasing.

In the oliguric-anuric phase, Trasylol is indicated for the still existing functional renal insufficiency. We have also observed a good effect of Trasylol in the anuric state and therefore wish to submit the hypothesis that even in this advanced stage a more rapid improvement of kidney function may be obtainable with Trasylol.

Therefore, in all cases of shock and beginning impairment of renal function, infusion treatment with added
Trasylol doses should be attempted as early as possible.
It is hoped that this suggestion will incite further
trials, as the number of cases which we have so treated
is still relatively small. I trust that we shall obtain
similarly good results in future.

References

(1) Dittrich, P., H.J. Gurland, M. Kessel, M.A.Massini,
     E. Wetzels: Haemodialysis and Peritoneal Dialysis.
     Pages 243, 272, and 277.
     Edited by E. Wetzels - Springer, Berlin-Heidelberg-
     New York, 1969.

(2) Braun, L.: For Prognosis of Acute Renal Insuffic-
     iency. IN: Peter v. Dittrich and Klaus F. Kopp:
     Actual Problems involved with Dialysis Procedures
     and Renal Insufficiency. Pages 172, 174 and 177.
     II. Symposium Innsbruck, 1967. Friedberg, 1968.

(3) Hoeltzenbein, J.: The Artificial Kidney. Pages 212,
     213, and 214. Edited by F. Enke, Stuttgart, 1969.

(4) Braun, L.: The Acute Kidney Failure. Pages 3, 4, 5.
     Edited by F. Enke, Stuttgart, 1968.

(5) Truss, F.: Medical World, 1968, pages 1845 - 1851.

(6) Thurau, K.: The intrarenal roll of the Renin-Angio-
     tensin system in the regulation of the Glomerulu-
     min filtrate and of sodium excretion. In: Actual
     Problems of Nephrology. Pages 75-87. IV. Symposium
     Saarbruecken and Homburg/Saar, 1965. Springer,
     Berlin-Heidelberg-New York, 1966.

(7) Back, N. and H. Wilkens: The Effects of Trasylol on
     Microcirculatory Phenomena. IN: G.L. Haberland and
     P. Matis: New Aspects of Trasylol Therapy, pages
     61-73. Symposium Munich, 1968. Edited by Schattauer,
     Stuttgart-New York, 1969.

(8) Werle, E.: To the Biochemistry of Trasylol.
     In: G.L. Haberland, P. Matis: New Aspects of
     Trasylol Therapy, pages 49-59. Symposium in
     Munich, 1968. Edited by Schattauer, Stuttgart-
     New York, 1969.

THE TREATMENT OF ORTHOSTATIC SHOCK

M. NEUMAN

Hosp. COCHIN - PARIS

The regulation of the blood pressure is assured essentially through two mechanisms :

1) a rapid regulation through the CNS and neuro-vegetative system ;
2) a second and more slowly regulation - of hormonal origin.

The first one only interesses us in the pathogeny of the orthostatic shock.

If we simplify in the extreme, we may say that in the orthostatic shock there is a venous stasis in the legs and the splanchnic territory ; this venous stasis provokes a diminution of the venous return to the right heart, a diminution of the cardiac ejection and of the blood pressure. This fall of the blood pressure stimulates the cardio-accelerators and vasoconstrictor centers ; the conjugated and simultaneous effects of tachycardia, peripherical vasoconstriction and venous hypertonia, increases the blood pressure to its initial level.

Every process liable to inhibit one of these corrective mechanisms can provoke an orthostatic shock, especially in predisposed people : old persons, prolonged immobilisation, during gestures provoking thoracic hypertension, and so inhibiting the venous return to the heart, and so on ...

In fact there are two main forms of shock according to the presence or absence of compensatory reflexes (fig. 1).

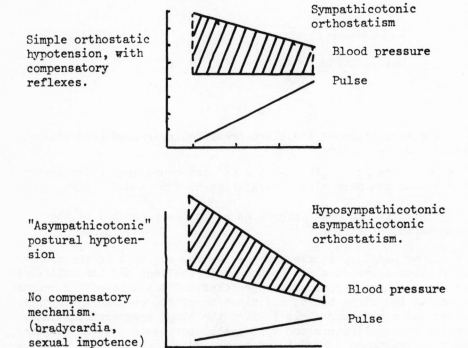

FIGURE I

Simple orthostatic
hypotension, with
compensatory
reflexes.

Sympathicotonic
orthostatism

Blood pressure

Pulse

"Asympathicotonic"
postural hypoten-
sion

No compensatory
mechanism.
(bradycardia,
sexual impotence)

Hyposympathicotonic
asympathicotonic
orthostatism.

Blood pressure

Pulse

Blood pressure and pulse in orthostatic syndromes

This is the reason why the orthostatic shock, contrary to what it is generally thought, is very frequent in the general practice, in very different situations, each time the venous return to the right heart is inhibited.

Table 1 shows the promoting circumstances and the etiologies associated with the orthostatic syndrome.

We wish to insist particularly upon the very important role of the venous tonus ; it is sufficient to look at figure 2 to see that the venous extra-thoracic sector contains by himself more than 50 p. cent of the total blood volume.

It is, by reflex increases in venous "tone" that a promptly acting, and, in acute situations, very adequate, compensation for loss of blood can be achieved. This capacitance response of the veins form a "first line of defense", acting in synergism with a pump adjustment for maintaining an adequate supply of blood to the tissues.

Before discussing the treatment we would do well to consider the more detailed analysis of orthostatic shock of drug origin shown in table 2 and the level of action of drugs provoking orthostatic hypotension (table 3). Whatever the etiology, the preventive and curative treatment of orthostatic shock include the following measures:

- correction or suppression of propicious factors ;
- measures intended to increase the venous return :
  . compressive bandages around the legs, elastic stockings (especially in the varicose legs) ;
  . motor reeducation, gymnastic in the water (due to the hydrostatic realised in the bath) ;
  . treatment by drugs.

As a rule we dispose of 3 categories of products in the treatment of orthostatic shock :

- sympathomimetics amines
- ergotamine and especially DHE (better tolerated)
- corticosteroids with salt retainin action : hydrocortisone, fludrocortisone.

DHE has not these disadvantages ; it provokes bradycardia, tachyphylaxis is not observed, its main action is exerced on the venous sector having a direct phlebotonic action (increase of the tonus of the venous wall) on non adrenergic receptors. It possesses a central sedative action, it can be used when the orthostatic shock is provoked by M.A.O.-inhibitors. DHE possesses also an alpha-sympathicolytic action but of a secondary importance : the direct phlebotonic effect being its main action.

TABLE 1

THE DIFFERENT ETIOLOGICAL FACTORS ASSOCIATED
WITH THE ORTHOSTATIC SYNCOPE

1) Temporary rise of the intrathoracic pressure impending the
   venous return to the heart especially in certain favorable
   backgrounds (aged, arteriosclerotic patients) : Valsalva manoe-
   ver, blowing strongly in a musical instrument, defecation, mic-
   turition, sneezing, coughing access, overventilation, large
   enemas, pregnancy and parturition period, etc...

2) Syncope after excessive effort especially when after the effort
   the subject is forced to remain immobile in the erect state
   (static muscular effort).

3) Voluminous varices in the situations sited in 1) and 2).

4) Prolonged immobilisation, squattering followed by a sudden re-
   dressing, hemiplegia, paraplegia.

5) Conditions provoking a generalised vasodilatation :
   hot baths (Sauna), hot season, floor central heating, especially
   in the conditions sited in 1), 2) and 3).

6) Hypokaliemia.

7) Anemias.

8) Conditions provoking hypovolemia : deshydratation, haemorrhages.

9) Dumping syndrome - after gastrectomy.

10) Adrenal insufficiency, hypopituitarism, phaechromocytoma in the
    initial stage.

11) Degenerative deseases of the SNC : tabes, Parkinson, multiple
    sclerosis, syringomyelia, diabetic and alcoolic neuropathy,
    Guillain-Barre syndrome, and so on ...

12) Idiopathic orthostatic hypotension (Shy and Drager syndrome).

13) Iatrogenic hypotensive shock provoked by various drugs : MAO
    inhibitors, tricyclic antidepressive drugs, phenothiazinic neu-
    roleptics, ganglioplegics, hypotensive and vasodilator drugs
    (alpha and bêta-blocking drugs), local anesthesics and espe-
    cially the association of two drugs of these categories (poten-
    tialisation).

FIGURE 2

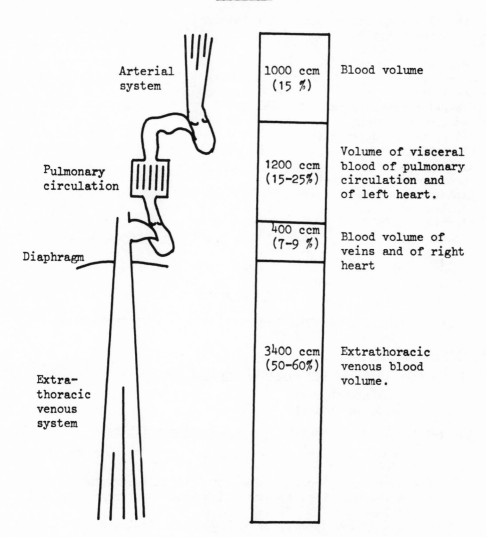

	1000 ccm (15 %)	Blood volume
	1200 ccm (15-25%)	Volume of visceral blood of pulmonary circulation and of left heart.
	400 ccm (7-9 %)	Blood volume of veins and of right heart
	3400 ccm (50-60%)	Extrathoracic venous blood volume.

Arterial system

Pulmonary circulation

Diaphragm

Extra-thoracic venous system

Total blood volume : 5000 ccm
(100 %)

Repartition of total blood volume

The capacitance function of extra-thoracic venous
blood is about 60 % of total blood volume.

TABLE 2

ORTHOSTATIC SHOCK PROVOKED BY DRUGS

- Central analgesics : morphine, pethidine, dextromoramide
- Alpha-adrenolytics
- Beta-adrenolytics
- Terminal sympatholytics
- Ganglioplegics
- Local anesthesics
- Central sympatholytics
- Sedative neuroleptics
- Tricyclic antidepressives
- MAO-inhibitors
- Hypotensive drugs
- Coronaro-dilating agents
- Alpha-methyl-para-tyrosine
- Disulfiram
- Nicotinic acid
- Associations of two or more of drugs of these categories.

TABLE 3

LEVEL OF ACTION OF DRUGS PROVOKING ORTHOSTATIC HYPTENSION

A/ Sympatholytics

1 - At the level of the sympathic ganglionic split :

    - local anesthesics
    - M.A.O. inhibitors.

2 - At the level of sympathic post-ganglionic fibers :

    a) through blockade of the synthesis of endogenous catecho-
       lamines :
       - alpha-methyl-dopa (inhibitor of dopa-decarboxylase)
       - alpha-methyl-p. tyrosine (inhibitor of tyrosine hydro-
         xylase)
       - disulfiram (inhibitor of dopamine hydroxylase).

    b) impermeabilisation of the presynaptic vesicles membrane
       of the sympathetic nerve ending, leading to an inhibi-
       tion of the releasing of endogenous catecholamines :

       - bretylium.

    c) depletion of catecholamines from the storage depots (the
       presynaptic vesicles) :

       - reserpine
       - guanethidine

d) substitution of catecholamines - at the level of presynaptic vesicles - by "false mediators" :

- guanethidine
- alpha-methyl-dopa
- alpha-methyl-p. tyrosine.

3 - At the level of the synaptic neuro-effector split :

a) inhibition of physiological catecholamine re-uptake into
the storage depots (the presynaptic vesicles of the
sympathic nerve endings) :

- cocaïne
- reserpine
- tricyclic antidepressives
- antihistaminics
- adrenolytic alpha
- adrenolytic beta

b) inhibition of enzymatic catabolism of catecholamines :

- M.A.O. - inhibitors.

B/ Adrenolytics at the level of receptors :

Substitution through competition of catecholamines at the level
of adrenergic receptors :

- alpha-adrenolytics including :
  . neuroleptics (except reserpine)
  . and thymoanaleptics, both possessing an alpha-blocking action
  . phenoxybenzamine (Dibenzyline)
  . phentolamine (Regitine)
  . tolazoline (Priscol)
  . ergotamine and derivatives
  . yohimbine
  . azapetine (Ilidar).

- beta-blocking agents (beta-adrenolytics) :
  . propranolol
  . alprenolol (Aptin)
  . oxprenolol (Trasicor)
  . practolol (Eraldin)
  . sotalol
  . betadrenol
  . butidrin.

The associations of 2 or several drugs of categories A/ and
B/ (exemple figure 3) show the complexity and the risks which may
result from this.

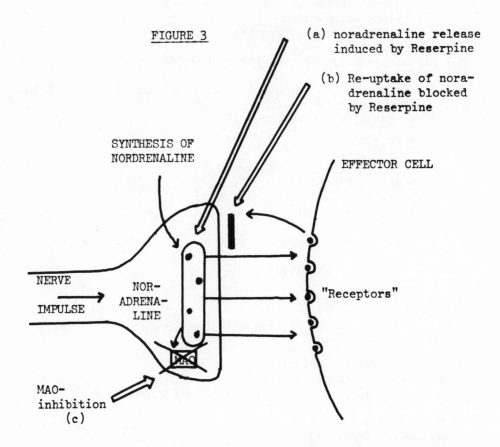

FIGURE 3

(a) noradrenaline release
    induced by Reserpine

(b) Re-uptake of nora-
    drenaline blocked
    by Reserpine

SYNTHESIS OF
NORDRENALINE

EFFECTOR CELL

NERVE
IMPULSE

NOR-
ADRENA-
LINE

"Receptors"

MAO-
inhibition
(c)

A simplified theoretical model of an adrenergic nerve ending
to illustrate the "reserpine-reversal" effects of an MAO-
inhibitor used with reserpine.

Reserpine causes depletion of the noradrenaline from the
nerve ending pool (a) causing its release and (b) by preventing its re-uptake. This results in transmission loss.

In the presence of a MAO-inhibitor (c), newly synthetised
noradrenaline can accumulate once again within the pool thus
restoring and possibly potentiating transmission.

FIGURE 4

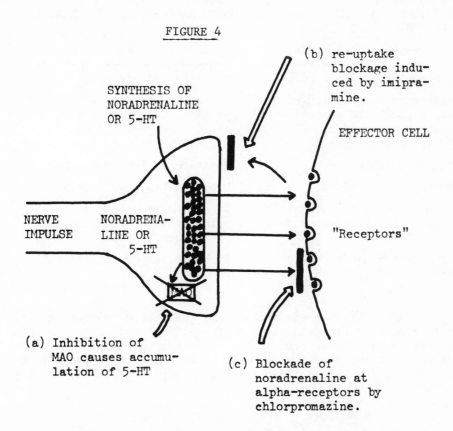

(b) re-uptake blockage induced by imipramine.

EFFECTOR CELL

SYNTHESIS OF NORADRENALINE OR 5-HT

NERVE IMPULSE

NORADRENA-LINE OR 5-HT

"Receptors"

(a) Inhibition of MAO causes accumulation of 5-HT

(c) Blockade of noradrenaline at alpha-receptors by chlorpromazine.

A theoretical model of an adrenergic (noradrenaline-releasing) nerve ending within the brain illustrating the possible mechanism of interaction between the imipramine compounds and the MAO-inhibitors.

The MAO-inhibitor (a) allows the accumulation of noradrenaline at the nerve ending. Noradrenaline released by the nerve impulse accumulates at the receptor sites, further increased by the re-uptake blockage induced by the imipramine. (b) Reversal by chlorpromazine could occur by blockade at receptors and general CNS depression (c).

TABLE 4

COMPARATIVE PHARMACOLOGY, WITH ADVANTAGES AND INCONVENIENTS OF SYM-
PATHOMIMETIC AMINES AND DIHYDROERGOTAMINE (DHE) IN THE TREATMENT
OF ORTHOSTATIC SCHOCK.

Sympathomimetic amines	D H E
Tachyphylaxis	No tachyphylaxis.
Vasoconstrictor action exclusively through the sympathic stimulation and predominantly on the arterial sector.	Predominantly direct parietal phlebotonic action (on non adrenergic receptors of smoogh fibers), especially on the venous sector.
Stimulant action on the CNS.	Sedative action on the CNS.
Provokes tachycardia.	Provokes bradycardia.
Cannot be used to correct the orthostatic hypotension action of M.A.O.-inhibitors.	It can be used to correct the orthostatic hypotension of M.A.O.-inhibitors.
Very short vascular action	It has a longer-lasting vascular action.

The sympathicomimetic amines have been rather disappointing in
the treatment of orthostatic shock for all these different reasons :
they have a very short action, they increase the tachycardia, the
vasoconstriction action is predominant in the arterial sector, they
are contre-indicated in the orthostatic shock provoked by M.A.O.-
inhibitors.

The ordinary dosage we have used in our cases is 6 to 12 mg/
day.

During the treatment with the drugs able to provoke orthostatic shock, DHE can be used prophylactically, associated during the
first few weeks of treatment, especially with neuroleptics. As a
matter of fact, after this period a tolerance for this kind of side
effect is appearing.

Finally, some cases of orthostatic shock can benefit of the
association of DHE with a salt retainin corticosteroids.

THE TREATMENT OF SHOCK WITH BETA ADRENERGIC BLOCKADE

James L. Berk, M.D.

Assistant Clinical Professor of Surgery, Case Western

Reserve University School of Medicine.

Hemodynamic inconsistencies in the Vasoconstrictor Theory of Shock and the unsatisfactory results of the treatment of shock founded on this concept, led to experimental studies designed to re-evaluate and clarify the role of adrenergic stimulation in shock. (1, 2) Based on these findings we suggested that in shock of various causations beta adrenergic stimulation with the opening of multiple arteriovenous shunts in the pulmonary and splanchnic areas was of major importance in the pathogenesis of late refractory shock and that excessive alpha adrenergic stimulation with arteriolar vasoconstriction was only of secondary importance. (3) It was suggested that the beta adrenergic stimulation causes a rapid arterial runoff with a fall in peripheral resistance and a lowering of the arterial pressure. The arterialized blood enters the thin walled venules causing dilatation and pooling. The resultant increase in capillary hydrostatic pressure and stagnant anoxia causes a loss of plasma and blood and a further decrease in the effective blood volume. In addition, in the lungs the bypassing of the alveolar capillary bed due to anatomical shunting leads to arterial unsaturation. The transudation of plasma can wash away pulmonary surfactant causing alveolar collapse. The hypoperfusion of the type II alveolar cells leads to a decrease in the biosynthesis of pulmonary surfactant resulting in more alveolar collapse. The pulmonary edema, hemorrhages, and atelectasis cause physiological shunting and a further increase in arterial unsaturation. The other effects of adrenergic stimulation are compensatory at this stage, beta stimulation resulting

in an increased heart rate and increased myocardial contractility
and the alpha stimulation resulting in compensatory arteriolar
vasoconstriction in the renal and cutaneous areas. As shock progresses the pooling continues but due to the increasing metabolic
acidosis of cellular hypoperfusion the catecholamines become less
effective and there is a progressive loss of the compensation and
the development of irreversible shock and death.

To test this thesis beta adrenergic blockade with propranolol
was produced in dogs in hemorrhagic and endotoxin shock. (3, 4)
There was a statistically significant increase in the survival rates
in the treated dogs. In addition the treated dogs showed markedly
improved hemodynamic patterns consistent with the closure of
arteriovenous shunts, and lacked microscopic findings of excessive beta adrenergic stimulation in the pulmonary and splanchnic
areas present in the untreated dogs. These findings supported
the Beta Theory of Shock in animals.

We then turned our attention to the treatment of shock in man
with beta adrenergic blockade. (5, 6) Thirteen consecutive pa-

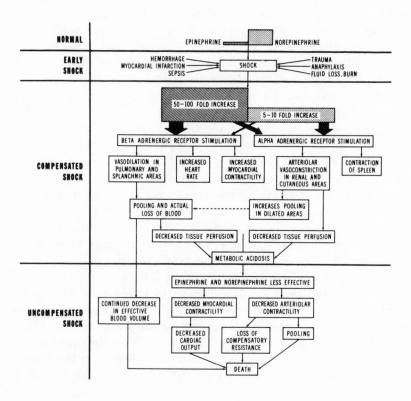

tients who remained in deep septic shock despite conventional
methods of treatment were studied. Aggressive treatment with
additional intravenous fluids, therapeutic doses of corticosteroids,
digitalis, and respiratory assistance, resulted in survival in 8
patients. Five patients remained in shock and were given intravenous propranolol. One patient with uncompensated acidosis
and a low cardiac index became worse. In four patients following
beta blockade there were improved hemodynamic patterns consistent with the closure of arteriovenous shunts with a progressive
increase in the arterial pressure, the PaO_2, and the urinary
output; and a decrease in the pulse rate, the central venous
pressure, and the cardiac index. Survival resulted in the three
with an initially increased cardiac index. Because of a suspected
intra-abdominal emergency in the fourth patient, surgery was
planned but the patient died of a cardiac arrest during anesthetic
induction. These observations support the thesis that beta adrenergic stimulation is also important in the pathogenesis of shock
in man.

It is concluded that beta blockade with propranolol is effective
in the treatment of hyperdynamic shock in man, such as septic
shock. Shock of other causations has responded in animals, and
if the cardio-depressant effects of propranolol can be prevented,
beta blockade should be effective in man in these situations with
microcirculatory failure. We are currently evaluating the effec-
tiveness of glucagon in reversing the cardio-depressant actions
of propranolol, and in a limited number it shows great promise.
Improved beta blocking agents capable of a microcirculatory block
with less cardio-depressant effects are becoming available and
should be evaluated.

REFERENCES

1. Berk, J. L. , Pecic, I. , Shields, E. and Natwick, R. (1964):
   The Role of Multiple Arteriovenous Anastomoses in the Patho-
   genesis of the Dumping Syndrome. Surgery, Gynecology &
   Obstetrics, 119, 817.

2. Berk, J. L. , Hagen, J. F. , Beyer, W. H. and Niazmand, R.
   (1967): The Effect of Epinephrine on Arteriovenous Shunts in
   the Pathogenesis of Shock. Surgery, Gynecology & Obstetrics,
   124, 347.

3. Berk, J. L. , Hagen, J. F. , Beyer, W. H. , Dochat, G. R. and
   LaPointe, R. (1967): The Treatment of Hemorrhagic Shock by
   Beta Adrenergic Receptor Blockade. Surgery, Gynecology &
   Obstetrics, 125, 311.

4. Berk, J. L. , Hagen, J. F. , Beyer, W. H. , Gerber, M. J. and
   Dochat, G. R. (1969): The Treatment of Endotoxin Shock by
   Beta Adrenergic Blockade. Annals of Surgery, 169, 74.

5. Berk, J. L. , Hagen, J. F. , Dunn, J. M. (1969): The Treatment
   of Septic Shock with Beta Adrenergic Blockade. Circulation
   (Supplement), 40, 44.

6. Berk, J. L. , Hagen, J. F. , Dunn, J. M. (1970): The Treatment
   of Septic Shock. Surgery, Gynecology & Obstetrics. To be
   published.

SHOCK IN ACUTE PANCREATITIS

G. C. Castiglioni, L. Lojacono, F. Spinola

The Surgical Clinic of the Catholic University

of the S. Heart. Rome, Italy

Shock in human acute pancreatitis is a serious prognostic sign. The average mortality of 14% in the cases of acute pancreatitis increases to 71% when features of shock are present in the early stages of the disease (4, 5, 6, 10).

Not considering the hypovolemic secondary shock, which can be treated with large infusions of liquids and antitryptic agents (8, 9, 12), we have observed a fulminating shock five times in 52 patients with acute pancreatitis. This represents a problem both for genesis and treatment. It dominates the course of the disease from the very beginning simultaneously with the onset of pain. Most cases fail to respond to treatment and fatality occurs in the course of few (3-24) hours.

The purpose of this study was to investigate the haemodynamic changes in induced acute pancreatitis in the canine model with the aim of clarifying the interpretation of pancreatic shock in man.

MATERIALS AND METHODS

Acute fulminating pancreatitis was induced in 12 adult mongrel dogs (I group) following Hureau's method (11) (5 ml of mixture of bile and Trypsin introduced in the major pancreatic duct left pervious), without further treatment. To compare the haemodynamic behavior of this situation with that of a hypo-

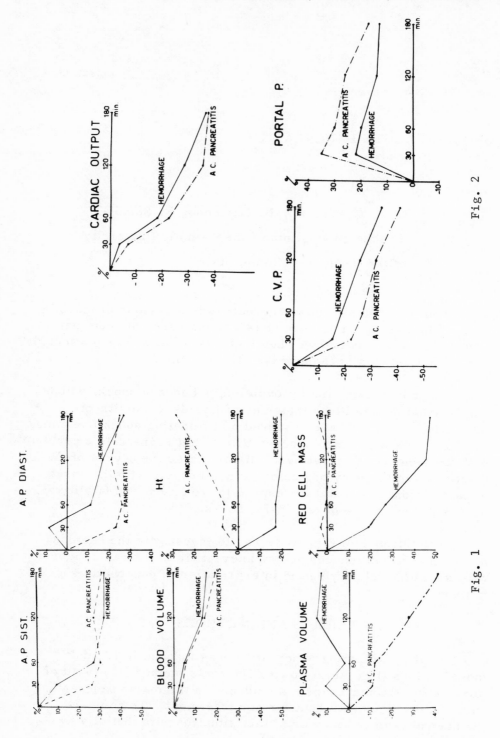

Fig. 1

Fig. 2

volemic shock, a haemorrhagic state was induced in 5 adult
mongrel dogs (II group), by continuous blood subtraction of
percentages of the blood mass corresponding in quantity and
rates to the volemic losses in the first group of animals
(haematic losses were determined at short intervals with
the radio-iodinated serum albumin (RISA) method).

Central venous pressure, cardiac output (flowmeter on
ascending aorta), total and femoral vascular resistances,
hourly diuresis, total and fractionated blood volume (RISA
method), blood flow (Nycotron flowmeter) and pressure of
right femoral, superior mesentheric, hepatic arteries and of
portal vein were determined at short intervals in both groups
of dogs.

At the end of the experiment pathology of the pancreas
was obtained in each dog.

RESULTS

Immediate and evident circulatory phenomena were
observed in experimentally induced acute pancreatitis, associated with intense pancreatic alterations.

The comparison between these phenomena and those
observed during haemorrhagic shock with corresponding
hypovolemic states (group II) has shown that blood pressure
falls more rapidly in pancreatic shock (Fig. 1).   The initial
diastolic pressure relative increase present in dogs in haemorrhagic shock (increase of 9% after 30' of bleeding) was lacking in
pancreatitis (reduction of 23% at 30' from the induction of the pancreatic damage). Later on, the fall in blood pressure was slower and
similar in both situations.   Although the experimentally
induced blood losses were both similar for quantity and times,
arterial pressure values were initially lower in acute pancreatitis.   The phenomenon is not simply related to the blood
loss (arterial pressure decrease of 30%, with volemia loss of
5% after 30').   Later on, from three hours after the induction
of the pancreatic damage, the hypotension curve may be ascribed
to blood volume reduction (loss over 20%) (Fig. 1).

In the acute pancreatitis, plasma volume was more
reduced, and haematocrit values increased, while in the
haemorrhagic state the reduction was mainly of red cell mass,

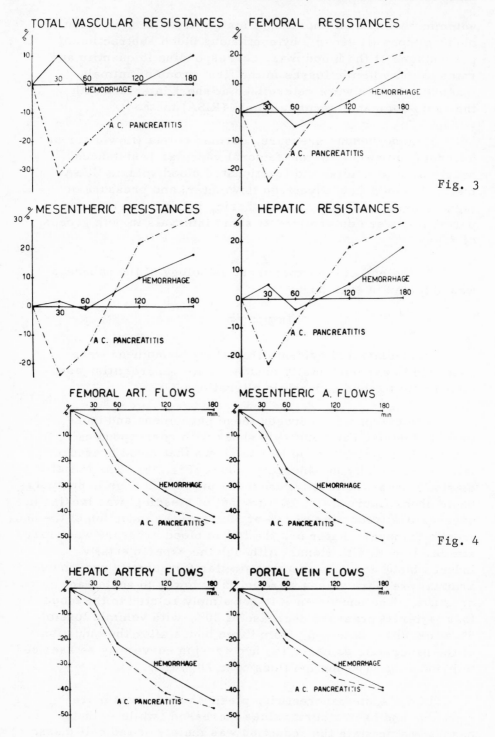

Fig. 3

Fig. 4

and consequently haematocrit values were reduced (Fig. 1).

Values of cardiac output and central venous pressure
were progressively decreasing in both circumstances, but
more evidently in acute pancreatitis (Fig. 2). Total and
femoral vascular resistances were intensely reduced in the
first stage of acute pancreatitis, while they increased in the
haemorrhagic situation. Starting from the second hour, the
vascular resistances in acute pancreatitis showed a tendency to
increase (Fig. 3), mainly in the femoral artery.

Portal pressure (Fig. 2) increase was more prominent
- especially in the first stage - in the pancreatic condition.
Correspondingly, portal flow was decreasing from the beginning
(Fig. 4).

The mesentheric and the hepatic arterial flows (Fig. 4)
decreased progressively and rapidly in both circumstances,
more than the femoral flow. The relative vascular resistance
in the splanchnic area (Fig. 3) after an initial drop, increased
both in pancreatitis and in the hemorrhagic condition.

DISCUSSION

The haemodynamics of shock in acute pancreatitis has
been studied both experimentally and clinically (2, 3, 6, 7, 8, 9,
10, 12, 13, 14). The opinion of many authors leads to an
interpretation of a primary hypovolemic (plasmorrhagic) shock.
Our results show significant differences between haemodynamic
patterns in shocks from acute pancreatitis and from haemorrhagic
conditions similar in degree and times to hypovolemia. Particularly in experimental acute pancreatitis the data indicate an
initial haemodynamic stage in which there occurs a) a rapid
drop of mean arterial pressure not explained by the severity of
hypovolemia without a relative increase in the diastolic blood
pressure, b) a tendency to plasma loss with high haematocrit
values, c) a lower cardiac output, d) a decreased central
venous pressure value, e) a reduction of peripheral
vascular resistance, f) a tendency to lower flows, and g)
an increased resistance in hepatic and superior mesentheric
arteries and in portal vein.

A second haemodynamic stage follows, in which arterial
pressure and flow values decrease more gradually, hypovolemia

becomes severe with an intense and progressive loss in the
plasmatic component, and an increase in peripheral vascular
resistances in both systemic and splanchnic areas.

The lack of proportion between hypotension and hypovolemia in fulminating pancreatitis has been noted experimentally (2, 3) and probably exists also in the human condition,
where the blood loss is considered 19-20% after 2-3 hours of
hypotension (2, 12, 13).

This indicates in the first stage of pancreatic shock
an extrahypovolemic factor of the shock, responsible of
the peculiar hemodynamic pattern here described. It seems
possible to determine from the very beginning a paresis and a
permeation of peripheral vessels with a mesentero - hepatic
"pool", especially in canine species (1). Only in the second
stage, the increased vascular space, the plasma loss and red
cell loss (intravascular pools) may stimulate a relative
arteriolo-constriction and realize a hypovolemic pattern
of shock. We believe in an initially and determinating action on
the microvessel walls of vasoactive substances of polypeptide
type (bradykinin) (6, 9, 10, 13, 14) produced through the action
of trypsin, present in blood during acute pancreatitis.

This interpretation is also confirmed by the results
of early treatment of acute pancreatitis with plasma-expanders
and antitryptic agents in high dosages (4, 5, 6). In the same
experimental condition it leads to lower haemodynamic changes
and a longer survival.

REFERENCES

1.   Anderson, M. C.   Hepatic morphology and function:
          Alteration associated with acute pancreatitis
          Arch. of Surg. <u>92</u>: 664, 1969.

2.   Anderson, M. C., Schoeneeld, F. B., Iams, W. B., and
          Suwa, M.   Circulatory changes in acute pancrea-
          titis. Surg. Clin. N. Am. <u>47</u>: 127, 1967.

3.   Anderson, M. C., Schiller, W. R., Gramatica, L.   Altera-
          tions of portal venous and systemic arterial pressure
          during exp. acute pancreatitis.   Am. J. of Surg.
          <u>117</u>: 715, 1969.

4.   Castiglioni, G. C.   La pancreatite acuta: suggerimenti
            dell'esperimento alla clinica.. Chir. e Pat.
            Sperim. 12: 357, 1964.

5.   Castiglioni, G. C.   Alcuni aspetti dell'attuale terapia
            delle pancreatiti acute.   Gazzetta Sanitaria 36:
            97, 1965.

6.   Castiglioni, G. C. , Lojacono, L. , Tamborini, G.
            Alterazioni emodinamiche nella pancreatite
            dell'inibizione triptica e callicreinica nella
            pancreatite acuta.   Arch. It. de Chir. 91: 365, 1965.

7.   Dos Reis, L.   Importance of blood volume changes in
            acute pancreatitis. Am. Surgeon 29: 605, 1963.

8.   Facey, F. L. , Weil, M. H. and Rosoff, L.   Mechanism
            and treatment of shock associated with acute
            pancreatitis.   Am. J. Surg. 111: 374, 1966.

9.   Haig, T. H. B. and Thompson, A. G.   Experimental
            acute pancreatitis.   Canadian J. of Surgery, 7,
            97, 1964.

10.   Hollenberg, M. J. , Kobold, E. E. , Pruettur, and Thal,
            A. P.   Occurrence of circulating vasoactive
            substances in human and exp. pancreatitis.
            Surg. Forum 13: 302, 1962.

11.   Hureau, J. , Vayre, P. , Martin, E.   La pancreatite
            aigue hemorragique avec necrose chez le chien.
            Mise au point d'une technique experimentale.
            La Presse Med. 71: 710, 1962.

12.   Keith, L. M. and Watman, R. N.   Blood volume deficits in
            acute pancreatitis. Surg. Forum 5: 380, 1955.

13.   Ryan, J. W. , Moffat, J. C. and Thompson, A. G.   Role of
            bradykinin system in acute hemorrhagic pancreatitis.
            Arch of Surg. 91: 14, 1965.

14.   Thal, A. P. , Kobold, E. E. , and Hollenberg, M. J.   The
            release of vasoactive substances in acute
            pancreatitis.   Am. J. Surg. 105: 708, 1963.

KININS IN THE PATHOGENESIS OF CARDIOGENIC SHOCK AND PAIN *

Sicuteri F., Del Bianco P.L. and Fanciullacci M.

Department of Medicine, Division of Clinical Pharmacology

University of Florence

One usually speaks of cardiogenic shock when, as result of myocardial infarction, a severe arterial hypotension with symptoms of nervous hypoxia occurs. In some cases it actually is shock; in others the term is used incorrectly, as it is merely a failure in arterial pressure, with consequent brain hypoxia. The distinction is subtle but important both from a practical and theoretical point of view.

Shock is often confused with causes that may but do not necessarily provoke it. Shock is a syndrome conditioned by an hypoxic damage of the capillaries. The causes of this condition are multiple as the term "syndrome" indicates.

Hypoxia which injuries the capillaries must be dosed in term of entity and duration. A condition which provokes shock if it acts with adequate intensity and duration, will not provoke shock if it acts too lightly or too intensely. If for instance one considers hemorrhagic shock, it is evident that, if hemorrhage is mild or of short duration, there will be no hypoxia damage to the capillaries; on the other hand if the hemorrhage is too severe capillary damage will similarly not take place, since the patient will die from acute cerebral hypoxia. Yet, in this last case one usually speaks of hemorrhagic shock.

The term shock is often improperly used and this is perhaps a result of the wide and generic value given to the word. The improper use of the word "shock" has passed into several fields of pathology and medicine. For instance, one speaks of anaphylactic shock in guinea pigs when the animal, few minutes after the inducing injection, loses consciousness. It is evident that the indispensable conditions for shock have not had time to set in, since an intense bronchospasm, with acute cerebral hypoxia occurs. We should therefore speak of reaction or of anaphylactic phenomenon. If however this reaction is classified as shock one must look for another term to define the condition under discussion. A too generic use of term, the number of causes able to provoke acute phenomena resembling shock; the difficulty in determining

* With the help of Consiglio Nazionale delle Ricerche - Rome - Italy

the exact moment of onset of shock have all added to the confusion in the clas -
sification of the syndrome.

All researchers agree that shock is a single pathologic state determined by different causes. A single pathologic condition usually has a single pathogenesis, i. e.
hypoxia, of intensity and duration that will not directly kill the animal but will cause
organic damage to the capillaries.

Among the various attempts to classify the causes of shock we suggest the following, which has the advantage of being simple and the disadvantage, perhaps, of being
too schematic (fig. 1)

ETIOLOGY OF SHOCK

1) **Hematogenic shock** { *(hemorrhage)*

2) **Dynamogenic shock** { *(cardiac insufficiency)*

3) **Autogenic shock** {
(burns
necrosis
trauma
antigen-antibody reactions)

Fig. 1

Hemorrhagic shock is the most typical example of the hematogenic group: it
can be achieved experimentally, but withdrawal of blood, which must be regulated
in time and quantity according to arterial pressure, presents considerable technical
difficulties. (Crowell 1961).

Dynamogenic shock includes those conditions that induce asphyctic damage to
capillaries and tissues by a decrease in the work of the heart, or its substitute, for
instance the pump used for the extracorpored circulation in surgery.

Cardiogenic shock from infarction is essentially a dynamogenic shock, but
recently it has been suggested that it is also autogenic (Sicuteri et al.1967).

In autogenic shock asphyctic damage is caused by a suffecently prolonged
hypotension, provoked by biological hypotensive substances. The concept of auto -
genesis recall that of autopharmacology, namely all those reactions induced by
active biological substances released in the organism, as result of pharmacological
or spontaneous conditions. The release of histamine, bradykinin and serotonin
induced, for example, by 48/80 B.W., kallikrein, reserpine, are all examples of
condition charaterized by a high release of hypotensive substances in blood. Shocks
from burns, crushing, ischemia, antigen-antibody reaction, endotoxin, pancreatitis

and peritonitis are all autogenic. The released substances are principally kinins, histamine and serotonin: all of which affect arterial pressure and permeabilize the capillaries, thus inducing edema.

Shock is reversible but if prolonged becomes irreversible. The causes of the irreversibility of shock are not clear: it is probable that the capillary damage of some areas is extended to certain parenchimas such as brain and myocardium. It has been noted that hemorrhagic shock becomes irreversible, i.e. no longer con - trollable by blood transfusion, when lesions of myocardial enzymes appear (Hackel 1955, 1963). With regard to myocardial infarction, the term shock is also used for what are simply acute nervous disorders due to failure of the left ventricle. Hypotension, in myocardial infarction as well, must be of a given entity and duration to damage the capillaries by hypoxia. If the hypotension is too marked, the subject dies of acute cerebral anoxia, before the capillaries are damaged and therefore before shock has time to set in.

Cardiogenic shock is at present classified as dynamogenic shock. Recently, it has been suggested that cardiogenic shock is also autogenic and therefore has a mixed etiology (fig. 2), (Sicuteri et al. 1967, Massion et al. 1969, Pitt et al. 1969).

SHOCK OF MYOCARDIAL INFARCTION

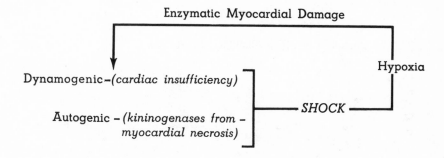

Fig. 2 - Double etiology of myocardial infarction shock.

It is in fact known that proteases and more specifically kininogenase, are released in blood from the injured area of myocardium. These enzymes having entered the circulation carry out a kinin release. In the pathogenesis of hypotension and collapse from myocardial infarction, the autogenic mechanism, that is kinin release, is joined to the dynamogenic one. The autogenic mechanism is accepted in the genesis of other types of shock, such as acute tissue damage, pulmonary infarction, pancreatitis and crush syndrome.

From the earliest stages of infarction a decrease in level of plasmatic kininogen has been noted, sometimes associated with the failure of the arterial pressure (fig. 3 -

fig. 4). These results have been confirmed by recent studies on spontaneous infarction in man and on experimentally induced infarction in dogs by ligature of a coronary
branch (Massion 1969). In the plasma of blood collected from the coronary sinus,
only a few minutes after the ligature of the coronary branch, a significant decrease
in the level of kininogen is observed, followed by an increase and subsequent further
decrease.

The possibility of an autogenic etiology in the genesis of cardiogenic shock is
also important from a practical point of view, since it can justify the very early use
of those drugs which antagonize kallikrein, thus preventing the release of kinins.
Therefore in the etiopathogenesis of shock from myocardial infarction the heart is
involved twice. Further, if enzymatic lesions of myocardium are important in the
severity of shock, heart is again concerned in the mechanism of the irreversibility
of shock (Edwards et al. 1954). It is conceivable that the non injured myocardium,
already overworked owing to the failure of the injured zone, is particularly vul-
nerable to hypoxia from systemic hypotension, which also affects coronary flow.

Precordial pain is a frequent, though not indispensable, symptom in myocardial
infarction. The pain has nothing to do with circulatory failure. Cases of myocardial
infarction with pulmonary edema or serious circulatory failure without pain are
observed. The mechanism by which cardiac pain is generated is not clear. Researches
on man (Sicuteri 1964; Pitt 1969) and animals (Massion 1969) suggest that kinins
play a part in the pathogenesis of coronary pain; however, kinins do not seem to have
a physiological role in the control of the coronary flow (Bassenge et al. 1969). In

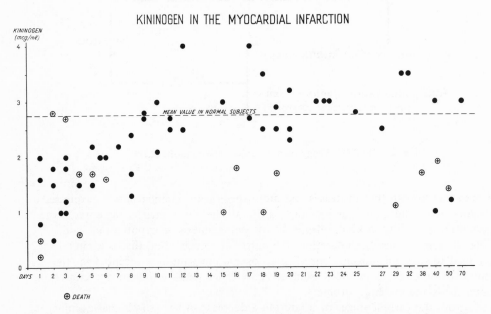

Fig. 3 - Kininogen levels in 14 cases of myocardial infarction; values are low in the first week
of disease; point with cross are cases where death occurred.

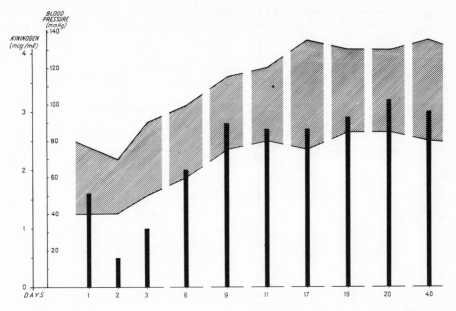

Fig. 4 - Comparison between kininogen values and blood pressure in a case of myocardial infarction.

cardiac infarction it is very likely that pain is provoked by a concentration of pain-producing substances in the injured or necrotic area or, more probably, in its periphery.

The most important chemical mediators in myocardial infarction seem to be 5-hydroxytryptamine, bradykinin and potassium (Sicuteri 1967). 5HT does not posses pain producing capacity, but is able to sensitize pain receptors to the action of kinins, of potassium and of other pain mediators for a long period (Sicuteri et al. 1965; Sicuteri 1967).

The serotonin coming from the intravascular clot, more precisely from the disgregation of blood platelets, concentrates just below the coronary occlusion and sensitizes pain receptors to the action of kinins and potassium (Fig. 5).

Kinins are released whenever an ischemia of a certain importance takes place and this can also be demonstrated in man (Bavazzano et al. 1969). Kinins in the ischemic area have a longer life not only because they are diluted and not carried away by blood flow, but also because the lowering of pH, induced by ischemia, notably reduces the activity of carboxypeptidase B (Edery and Lewis 1962), enzyme which inactivates kinins (Erdos and Sloane 1962). On the contrary, potassium is released in a considerable amount when a muscle is made to work and it is assumed that has relevance in the mechanism of hyperemia by muscolar exercise (Kjllmer 1965, b). A significant observation on the aminoacid taurine should be emphasized: suggested as an antianginal agent (Sicuteri et al 1969), it also influences the adrenaline provoked output of potassium from the cells (Welty and Read 1964), and antagonizes the local decrease of plasmatic kininogen, induced by ischemia (Bavazzano A. et al.

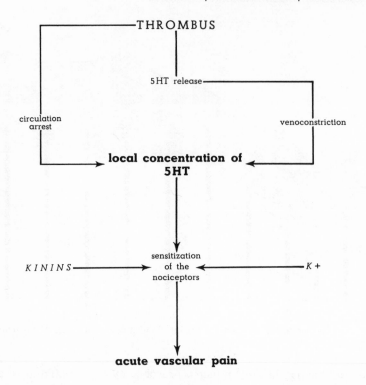

Fig. 5 -   Relationship between ischemia, 5HT, kinins and potassium following to coronary
           thrombotic occlusion.

1969). However, kinins can be released and concentrated in the infarcted myocardium
not only as a result of ischemia but also of reactive and inflammatory processes which
take place very early at the periphery, that is at the limit between the injured and the
normal myocardium. Actually in inflammatory processes, both septic and aseptic, an
important role of kinins is assumed (Rocha y Silva 1964). In addition the circulatory
arrest, impeding the dilution and the removal of these substances, prolongs the duration of their action on pain receptors .

     Even in absence of a controlled therapeutical investigation, it is our impression
and that of other authors (Sotgiu 1964; Palma e Brusadelli 1969; Massion et al.1969)
that the administration of Trasylol has an advantage in cases of shock from myocardial
infarction. Further morphine resistant acute pain from infarction seems to be relieved
by Trasylol. This observation, if confirmed, may furnish indirect evidence of the
implication of kinins in the pathogenesis of shock and pain from myocardial infarction, particularly if one considers that Trasylol, besides its principal activity as kalli-
crein and plasmin inhibitor, appears to have no other pharmacological activity relating to the present problem.

SUMMARY

Shock is a syndrome and therefore it assumes on the one hand a single pathogenic mechanism, the hypoxic damage of the capillaries, and on the other numerous causes.

On the basis of etiology the authors propose to distinguish three kinds of shock: hematogenic, dynamogenic and autogenic shock.

Shock by myocardial infarction constitutes a unique case in that there is a dynamogenic cause, insufficiency of the left ventricle, and an autogenic cause, release in the circulation of proteases from the necrotic area able to liberate kinins.

Some biochemical data support the hypothesis of an implication of the kininogen-kinin system in cardiogenic shock. Kinins together with other pain-producing chemical mediators, such as potassium and serotonin, seem to take part in the mechanism of pain.

The favourable action of the pharmacological inhibition of kinin release on shock and pain further supports the evidence of an implication of kinins in the pathogenesis of some phenomena which follow the infarction of myocardium.

REFERENCES

Bassenge E., Werle E., Holtz J. and Fritz H.: "Significance of kinins in the coronary circulation". Int. Symp. on "Cardiovascular and Neuro-Action of Bradykinin and related kinins." Fiesole-Florence, July 1969 (in Press).

Bavazzano A., Sidell N., Michelacci S. and Sicuteri F.: "Local ischemia as a kininogen depressant: effect of cortisone, taurine and kallikrein inhibitor". Int. Symp. on "Cardiovascular and Neuro-Action of Bradykinin and related kinins" Fiesole-Florence, July 1969.

Crowell J.W. and Guyton A.C.: "Evidence favoring a cardiac mechanism in irreversible hemorrhagic shock."Am. J. Physiol. 201, 893, 1961.

Edery H. and Lewis G.P.: "Inhibition of plasma kininase activity at slightly acid.ph." Brit. Pharm. Chemother. 19, 299, 1962.

Edwards W.S., Siegel A. and Bing R.J.: "Studies on myocardial metabolism. III. Coronary blood flow, myocardial oxygen consumption and carbohydrate metabolism in experimental hemorrhagic shock". J. Clin. Invest. 33, 1646, 1954.

Erdös E.G. and Sloane E.M.: "An enzyme in human blood plasma that inactivates bradykinin and kallidins. Biochem. Pharm. II, 585, 1962.

Hackel D.B. and Goodale W.J.: "Effects of hemorrhagic shock on the heart and circulation of intact dogs". Circulation II, 628, 1955.

Hackel D.B. and Breitenecker R.: "Time factor in reversibility of myocardial metabolic changes in hemorrhagic shock". Proc. Soc. Exp. Biol. and Med., 113, 534, 1963.

Kjellmer I.: "Studies on exercise hyperemia". Acta Physiol. Scand. 64, 244, 1965. a

Kjellmer I.: "The potassium Ion as a vasodilatator during the muscolar exercise". Acta physiol. Scand. 63, 460, 1965 b

Massion W.H., Blumel G. and Peschl L.: "The role of the plasma kinin system in cardiogenic shock and related conditions". Proceed. Int. Symp. on "Proteasi e antiproteasi in cardiologia", Vietri, Italy June 1969 (in press).

Palma G. e Brusadelli S.: "Prospettive terapeutiche con inibitori enzimatici nell'infarto miocardico". Proceed. Int. Symp. on "Proteasi e antiproteasi in cardiologia". Vietri, Italy June 1969 (in press).

Pitt B., Mason J. , Conti C.R. and Colman R.W.: "Activation of the plasma kallikrein system during myocardial ischemia". Int. Symp. on "Cardiovascular and neuro-actions of Bradykinin and related kinins". Fiesole - Florence, July 1969 (in press).

Rocha y Silva M.: "Chemical mediators of the acute inflammatory reaction". Ann. N.Y. Acad. Sci. 116, 899, 1964.

Sicuteri F.: "La mediazione chimica del dolorè coronarico". Mal. Cardiovasc. suppl. 2, 37, 1964.

Sicuteri F.: "Vasoneuroactive substances and their implication in vascolar pain" on Res. Clin. Stud. Headache. S.Karger I, 6, 1967 .

Sicuteri F., Fanciullacci M., Franchi G. e Del Bianco P.L.: "Serotonin-bradykinin potentiation on receptors in man". Life Science 4, 309, 1965.

Sicuteri F., Franchi G., Del Bianco P.L. e Del Bene E.: "A contribution to the interpretation of shock and pain in myocardial infarction" Mal. Cardiovasc. 8, 3, 1967.

Sicuteri F., Franchi G., Fanciullacci M., Giotti A.. e Guidotti A.: "Sulla azione antianginosa di un aminoacido solforato non coronarodilatatore". Clin. Terapeutica 49, 205, 1959.

Sotgiu G.: "Azione dell'inibitore delle proteasi (Trasylol) nell'infarto miocardico". Boll. Sci. Med. 136, 279, 1964.

Welty J.D. Jr. and Read W.O.: "Studies on some cardiac effects of taurine". J. Pharm. Exp. Ther. 144, 110, 1964.

DIAGNOSIS AND TREATMENT OF SHOCK IN INTERNAL MEDICINE

ALVISE BERENGO

Istituto di Patologia Medica I, University of Milan

Medical School, Italy

The present status of diagnosis and treatment of shock in internal medicine will be discussed here in front of pathogenetic, bioche-
mico-pathological and pharmacological progress in shock research.
The report will be grounded on the clinical experience got in two
decades in several Medical Clinics (Istituto di Patologia Medica
and Istituto di Clinica Medica Generale, University of Modena;
Istituto di Patologia Medica, University of Siena; Istituto di
Patologia Medica I, University of Milan, Italy). Further data have
been obtained courtesy of several colleagues (University of Milan)
and, with reference to septic and allergic shock of Prof. C. Zanussi
(Head of the Institute for Infectious Diseases, University of Milan).

Twenty years of clinical practice are however not sufficient
for a reliable evaluation of pharmacological agents in clinical
shock. This because of lack of technical facilities in the first
period and because there are remarkable difficulties in statistics,
due to heterogeneity in types, depth and duration of shock, underlying
diseases, age groups. Clinical methods are moreover not standardized
to collect and correlate data. The clinical approach to shock is
therefore far from satisfactory.

I think that to-day we can try to agree about a definition
including all the types of shock we are concerned with. Shock is
mainly a clinical entity of acute circulatory hypoxia, sometimes
relative to increased metabolic requirements, with a life-threatening
damage of parenchymatous cells leading to failure in circulatory,
ventilatory, cerebral and reticulo-endothelial functions. This
definition is very similar to the one suggested by Thal et al. (1967)

It appears misleading to collect into shock both syncopes, which are so acute to result only in a transient cerebral ischemia, and more chronic forms of hypotension.

DIAGNOSIS

Several approaches to the patient in shock may be considered.

Causes and Clinical Features of Shock are Obvious

Direct diagnosis both of shock and of type of shock are easy in front of a patient exhibiting hypotension, pallor, cold clammy skin, increased heart rate, thready pulse, poor capillary filling, increased respiratory frequency and tidal volume following hemorrhages, severe loss of water through vomiting and diarrhea, burns, traumas, administration of an antigen (usually penicillin in our experience), serum or other, acute surgical abdominal diseases, myocardial infarction, congestive heart failure in terminal stages, sepsis, chronic urinary or biliary infection.

Causes of Shock Obvious, Clinical Features not Significant

Following the insults listed above, a diagnosis of early shock may be considered if a trend towards hypotension is recorded when the recumbent patient sits up and in front of oliguria (urine output less of 25ml per hour). Blood pressure may be quite normal. Beads of cold sweat on the forehead, a pale clammy skin, restlessness, increased respiratory frequency, increased tidal volume may support an early diagnosis.

The early treatment following an early diagnosis may prevent the parenchymatous damage and an irreversible shock. This might explain the sentence of MacCannel et al.(1966) : "One is faced with the paradox that the better a center is organized to study and treat shock, the fewer patients there are to study".

Causes of Shock not Obvious, Clinical Features Obvious

Cardiogenic and hypovolemic shock should be differentiated at first, looking for signs of congestive heart failure (gallop, dyspnea, pulmonary rales, swollen cervical veins, cardiac arrhytmias) and of hypovolemia (collapsed cervical veins). A further support to the diagnosis of cardiogenic shock might result from an electrocardiogram (myocardial infarction, right ventricular strain pattern) and a chest X-ray film (pulmonary congestion), while a decrease of blood volume attaining 20 to 30% points to the hypovolemic shock (this sign is particularly valuable for internal hemorrhages). At present a very important procedure to differentiate cardiogenic and hypovolemic shock is the determination of central venous pressure. An increase is recorded in cardiogenic, a decrease in hypovolemic shock. Under fluids load the increase is emphasized in cardiogenic shock while in the hypovolemic type the venous pressure reverts to normal. Cohn (1967) has recently reviewed these topics.

If a hypovolemic shock is shown, a further differentiation must be done between dehydration (dry anelastic skin, mainly following diarrhea, polyuria, sweat losses) and internal hemorrhage (anamnesis, previous treatment with anticoagulant drugs which represent an important present cause of internal bleeding). A low content of hemoglobin in blood supports hemorrhage. Packed red cell volume is low in hemorrhage, normal in hypertonic dehydration and high in isotonic and hypotonic dehydrations. An unrecognized diabetes must always be borne in mind when dehydration is observed.

In our patients hypovolemic non-traumatic shock was more often due to hemorrhages from gastric ulcus or esophageal varices. In nephrosic syndrome 2 cases of hypovolemic shock were recorded.

Causes of Shock not Obvious, Clinical Features Obvious but Allied to Other Signs

Itching, urticaria, abdominal pain, bronchiolar constriction suggest allergic shock (we could observe sporadic cases of spontaneous burst of an echinococcus cyst).

Fever, chills, warm skin suggest septic shock. I had not many opportunities of observing septic shock, not even in hematologic malignancies and immunosuppressive treatments which are often assumed to favorize it. Following urologic instrumentation, which is rather common in this Institute because of hypertension studies, no septic shock was recorded. A few cases were observed in meningitis and one in a sepsis from Aerobacter.

Skin hemorrhages suggest acute adrenal failure (Waterhouse-Friderichsen syndrome).

Causes not Obvious, Clinical Features of
Intense Sympathetic Activity

Thready pulse due to a low pulse pressure, pallor, cold clammy
skin, increased heart rate, oliguria, poor capillary filling are
signs of intense sympathetic activity which may be observed in
patients who received sympathomimetic amines with vasoconstrictor
activity. This iatrogenic syndrome has been called "pseudo"-shock
by MacCannell and Goldberg (1966). Their patients usually had never
been in shock and amines were administered because of incorrect
readings of blood pressure or sometimes because of a non-shocking
hypotension.

Further Diagnostic Studies

Every patient, with particular reference to the elderly, must
be investigated for parenchymatous damages antecedent to shock
(heart,lungs, kidneys), which may be emphasized later on by the shock
itself.

Liver cirrhosis appears also in my experience to introduce or
to facilitate shock. Artero-venous shunts have been investigated
and possibly this condition promotes tissue typoxia.

TREATMENT

Though the general therapeutic measures are always the same,
including shock position, ventilatory assistance, comfortable
temperature, suppression of pain and anxiety, fluid replacement
possibly under central venous pressure monitoring, see Cohn (1967),
vasopressors and hydrocortisone, important differences in emphasis
and specific cautions emerge in different forms of shock.

In cardiogenic shock norepinephrine or angiotensin, intravenous
infusions, usually associated with strophantin, are in my experience
the treatment of choice. Metaraminol has been administered too, more
frequently per os, mainly in patients with collapsed veins to allow
a further venous infusion. Low molecular weight dextran, dextrose
solutions and also saline may be valuable, but caution is imperative
to prevent pulmonary edema. Hydrocortisone is useful, while chlorpromazine gave us discouraging results.
The shock position should not be adopted in these patients. Mannitol
15% may prevent acute tubular necrosis if remarkable oliguria is
recorded.

In hypovolemic shock the patient must lie in shock position. Immediate fluid replacement is required : blood in hemorrhages (while awaiting for blood use plasma expanders or even saline when nothing else is available), standard replacement solutions in dehydration with particular care for electrolyte and pH abnormalities. Hydrocortisone is valuable unless ulcus is present or diabetes. Vasoconstrictors are usually unnecessary.

In septic shock blood and urine must be sampled for cultures and antibiotics immediatly started. We have always used hydrocortisone, more than 300 mg per day, supporting the usual procedures.

In acute adrenal failure a massive treatment will be performed with antibiotics and all the general measures. In allergic shock particular emphasis was put on epinephrine instead of norepinephrine and on large doses of corticosteroids.

A very peculiar form of surgical shock with which an internist may be concerned results from clamping the vessels of the tumor while removing pheochromocytoma. Norepinephrine is imperative. I wonder if all the arguments against cathecolamines in the treatment of shock were correct and if their beneficial effect might really be referred to the beta-stimulation of the heart. See about this controversy Corday et al. (1969) and for general information Mills et al. (1967) : the 12th Hahnemann Symposium.

Bibliography

Cohn J.N. (1967) : Central venous pressure as a guide to volume expansion (Editorial). Annals of internal Medicine, 66,1283.

Corday E., Lillehei R.C. (1969) : Pressor agents in cardiogenic shock. The American Journal of Cardiology , 23, 900.

MacCannell K.L. and Goldberg L.I., (1966) : The evaluation of drug therapy in shock and hypotension. International Encyclopedia of Pharmacology and Therapeutics, Section 6, Volume II, 405.

Mills LLC. , Moyer J.H. (1967) : Shock and hypotension. The twelfth Hahnemann Symposium, 2nd printing, Grune and Stratton, New York and London.

Thal A.P., Kinney J.M. (1967) : On the definition and classification of Shock. Progress in cardiovascular Diseases, 9,527.

POLY-N^5-(2-HYDROXYETHYL)-L-GLUTAMINE

A NEW PLASMA EXPANDER

Gerola A., Antoni G., Benvenuti F., Cocola F., Neri P.

Istituto di Patologia Medica, Università di Siena

Research Centre, I.S.V.T. Sclavo, Siena, Italy

Together with many distinguished contributions on the biology of shock at molecular and at cellular level, quite a few speakers at this symposium have emphasized that, in the treatment of shock, monitoring of arterial blood pressure is important; more than that, cardiac output is important; and more even than that, total circulating fluid volume is important.

Increasing rates of casualties as well as the extension of surgical procedures with the aid of extracorporeal circulation, have tremendously increased our needs for blood, blood derivatives, plasma and plasma substitutes. We believe that it is not unfair to state that some plasma substitutes at present available on the market are not entirely devoid of undesirable side-effects. Therefore research for new plasma expanders is justified.

Some time ago, Sodium Poly-glutamate (SPG) was proposed as a plasma expander, because of elevated oncotic power and apparent lack of antigenic properties. This macromolecule resulted in being highly toxic, however (4).

Since SPG toxicity has been attributed to elevated electrical charge at physiological pH, we proposed to block SPG carboxylic groups with ethanolamine, a substance hydrophylic enough in order to maintain water solubility. The proposed polymer is identified as Poly-N^5-(2-hydroxyethyl)-L-glutamine (PHEG).

CHEMISTRY

PHEG can be synthesized from glutamic acid.

Glutamic acid gamma carboxyl is esterified with methanol
in the presence of acetyl chloride; later on, the aminic
group is acylated with carbobenzoxy chloride.

Carbobenzoxy-δ-methyl-L-glutamate, so obtained, is reacted with phosphorus pentachloride and heated; the resulting
N-Carboxyanhydride, after repeated crystallization with ethyl
acetate, is polimerized in dioxane; polimerization is initiated by 0.4 N Na hydroxide in methanol with an anhydride/
initiator concentration ratio equal to 250.

Poly-δ-methyl-L-glutamate is then treated with ethanolamine (10 ml/g) at 70-80°C. for 20-30 hours; the resulting
thick gel, treated with chloroform, gives a water-soluble
precipitate; the solution is neutralized with diluted hydro-
cloric acid; finally the solution is dialized and liophylized.
This synthetic material appears as a white, solid substance,
water-soluble up to very high concentrations at any pH.

We are certainly dealing with homogeneous PHEG, since
we have proved that no expected intermediate or side products
can be found in appreciable amounts.

We can state, first of all, that in our product, no
carboxyls either free or esterified with methyl groups,
are present. The infrared spectrum of the solid film shows,
indeed, no absorption bands in the $1750-1700$ cm^{-1} region.
Moreover, no methyl alcohol has been found after alkaline
hydrolysis of PHEG.

The absence of glutamic acid-free residues can also be
inferred from an enzymatic approach. Pepsin, in fact, is inactive (being unable to hydrolize glutamine-like bonds) while
it can downgrade SPG (by hydrolizing glutamic acid bonds). On
the other hand, papaine (active on glutamic acid bonds when
gamma carboxyl is blocked or non-ionized) can split our product on a large pH range, while it is active on SPG at acidic
pH only. Good correlation between theoretical and experimental
content of PHEG can be taken as a further confirmation that
all gamma carboxyls of glutamic acid have been blocked with
ethanolamine by our procedure.

Oncotic pressure developed by PHEG water solutions is
as high as for SPG: 20 g of PHEG equals I00 g of B.S.A.
Osmotically, in other words, relative B.S.A. oncotic power
being made equal to I, PHEG gives 3.75/g of water solution
and I.72/g of colloid.

Average molecular weight of PHEG calculated on the above
physico-chemical data is 40,500 (B.S.A. is 69,000). On the
other hand, calculations based on viscosity measurements
have given a value of 45,000. For this calculation we have
taken advantage of the observed relation between viscosity and
molecular weight of PHPG (poly-hydroxypropyl-glutamine)(6)
as well as of the demonstration that PHPG and PHEG, with a
similar degree of polymerization (experimental conditions
being similar) have identical viscosity values; obviously
in the final calculation we have considered the different
molecular weight of the two monomers.

Sterilization in autoclave decreases viscosity of 3%
PHEG solutions in saline at pH 7.0. In terms of molecular
weight this reduction appears to be minor. The titration of
aminic groups liberated by heat has given constant results
over a period of time.

In conclusion, our procedures for synthesis of Poly-
N⁵-(2-hydroxyethyl)-L-glutamine from glutamic acid give
highly homogeneous material with predictable physico-chemical
properties.

TOXICOLOGY AND PHARMACOLOGY

Acute and subacute toxicological observations made after
i.v. exhibition of PHEG have given satisfactory results.

Acute Observations

Mortality. No death has been recorded among the 5 groups
of male mice (8 animals each) 24 hours after i.v. injections
of 2 ml of five different saline solutions of PHEG (total
amount injected : 78.5, I22.4, I9I.2, 300.0 and 460.0 mg,
respectively).

Plasma Volume, measured with Evans Blue in rats, rises
following a good dose-response curve. Doses, injection procedures and results are shown in fig. I.

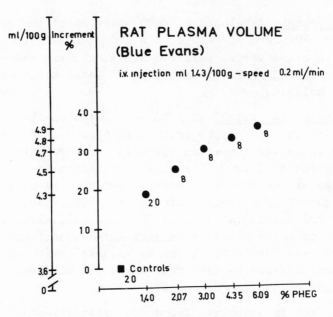

In two additional groups, of 5 cats each, treated with 3% and
6% solutions of PHEG, (14 ml/kg of body weight), plasma
volume rose significantly 10 ml above the controls
(34.6 ± 2.8 ml/kg).

Erythrosedimentation rate in the same groups of cats rose
significantly 70 mm above the controls (4.48 ± 0.81 mm/Ist.hour)

Hematocrit, accordingly decreased slightly but significantly
below the controls after i.v. injection of 3% PHEG solution in
cats (36.80 ± 2.13%).

Subacute Observations

As the PHEG turnover rate is as yet unknown, our subacute observations on rats have been prolonged up to the 15th
day, a time interval usually requested when tested drugs are
proposed for acute exhibition. All control animals have been
tested with saline (I ml/rat/day).

Experimental animals have been treated with PHEG at three
different concentrations (C_I = 2.07%, C_2 = 3.00%, C_3 = 4.35%,
respectively). Equal numbers of males (M) and females (F)
have been treated with each concentration. The six groups will
be indicated as M_I, M_2, M_3 and F_I, F_2 and F_3 respectively.

Mortality. None of the 60 animals treated with PHEG died during the observation period.

Body weight. No group among the 60 animals treated showed significant variation in comparison with the controls (♂ 283.6 g ± 4.6; ♀ 238.9 g ± 3 g).

Food intake also showed no significant difference from the controls (♂ 9.4 ± I.0 g/I00 g body weight/day; ♀ 8.I ± 0.6 g/I00 g body weight/day).

Hemoglobin concentration decreased significantly I g in M_2 and M_3 groups. (Controls: ♂ I3.5 ± 0.3 g %; ♀ I5.0 ± 0.I g %).

Red blood cell count. No significant difference from the controls (♂ 7.36 · I0⁶ ± 4.I · I0³/mm³; ♀ 6.69 · I0⁶ ± I.6·I0³).

Colour index in the groups M_I, M_2 and M_3 decreased significantly 0.I2 below the controls (♂ 0.58 ± 0.02; ♀ 0.7I ± 0.0I).

White blood cell count. All groups exhibited significant increases (3-4,000) in comparison with the controls (♂ 7,390 ± 229/mm³ ; ♀ 7,500 ± 542).

Erythrosedimentation rate. No difference from the controls (♂ I.5 ± 0.3 mm/Ist hour; ♀ 2.2 ± 0.I mm/Ist hour).

Hematocrit studied in three groups (F_I, F_2, F_3) decreased significantly (3) in comparison with the controls (42 ± 0.8).

Coagulation time resulted significantly prolonged (I') in three (F_I, F_2, F_3) out of the 6 groups studied (controls: ♂ 4'I3" ± 8"; ♀ 2'38" ± 4").

Blood urea nitrogen in group F_2 decreased significantly 4 mg % below the controls (♂ 4I.8 ± 2.4 mg %; ♀ 20.9 ± I.2).

Blood sugar was decreased about I2 mg in two groups (F_I, F_2) in comparison with the controls (♂ 46.2 ± 5.2 mg %; ♀ I4.7 ± 3.8 mg %).

SGOT. No variation in all 6 groups studied compared with controls (♂ I27 ± I5.I U.; ♀ 234 ± 38.2 U.).

SGPT. Decreased some 8 U. in groups M_2, M_3 and F_2 below the controls (♂ 28 ± 3.I U.; ♀ 38 ± 2.I U.)

Acid Phosphatase. No variation in comparison with the controls (♂ I0.9 ± I.4; ♀ 7.6 ± I.2)

Alkaline Phosphatase. Decreased significantly some 30 U. in groups M_2 and F_3 below the controls (♂ 52.3 ± 7.9 U.; ♀ 53.9 ± 7.7 U.)

Urine analysis for pH, glucose, albumin, blood, uro-bilinogen and ketone bodies : all 6 groups studied have given results comparable with the controls.

Body weight as well as weight of several organs (liver, kidney, adrenals, heart, spleen, testicles and ovaries) did not change significantly in treated groups.

Histological examinations of tissues listed above have shown no microscopic changes.(+)

ANTIGENICITY TESTS

Attempts have also been made, using three different procedures, to reveal possible antigenic properties of PHEG.

Schultz-Dale test on guinea pig isolated ileum: Tyrode solution, thermoregulated bath (37°C), tension I g, amplification x 9 (2,8).

Passive cutaneous anaphylaxis according to Ovary (7).
Ist i.v. injection with blood serum from guinea pigs previously treated with PHEG.
2nd i.v. injection after 4 hours, with I mg PHEG (in I ml of 0.5% Evans Blue).

Hemoagglutination with sheep tanned red cells according to Boyden (I).
Immunization patterns, number of animals and results are summarized in Fig. 2.

ACUTE HEMODYNAMIC STUDIES

First of all, the hemodynamic effect of low doses of i.v. PHEG has been studied in normal animals, since it was known that small amounts of SPG give rise to a hemodynamic picture similar to acute cor pulmonale.

_____

(+) We are greatly indebted to Prof. Pellegrino (Director, Istituto di Patologia Generale, University of Siena Medical School) for his co-operation in this part of our study.

POLY-N^5-(2-HYDROXYETHYL)-L-GLUTAMINE   335

ANTIGENICITY TESTS

	Guinea pigs No	Immunization patterns				Schultz–Dale	P.C.A	Hemoagglutination
		I	II	III	VIII			
		day				Positive tests No		
PHEG	24	20mgi.v.				0/24	0/24	0/12
	23	20mgs.c adj				0/23	0/23	0/12
	23	5mgi.v.	10mgi.v.	20mgi.v.		0/23	0/23	0/12
	36	1mgi.d. adj.			1mgs.c. adj.	——	0/36	——
BSA(V)	12	1mgi.d. adj.			1mgs.c. adj.	——	11/12	——
	11	20mgi.v.				8/11	10/11	——

Treatment period = 3 weeks
i.v.= intravenous
i.d.= intradermal

s.c.= subcutaneous
adj= complete Freund adjuvant

In a preliminary group of 5 cats prepared for continous recording of arterial pressure in the femoral artery and thermal dilution curves in the left atrium (3)(2 ml of saline at room temperature injected into the right atrium as indicator), we have seen that i.v. 3% PHEG solutions (3.7 ml/kg of body weight, injection speed of 3.75 ml/min) did not cause statistically significant changes in arterial blood pressure (systolic –Mx–, diastolic –Mn–, and differential –Δ–) nor in cardiac output ($\dot{Q}$), mean transit time ($\bar{t}$) and central blood volume (CBV).

Effects of PHEG infusion after bleeding have been studied. In I4 animals prepared as above, controlled bleeding from the femoral artery decreased significantly all the parameters considered above, except CBV. The discrepancy confirmed by variance analysis is certainly related to the expected, individually differing reactions to hemorrhage. In 4 animals, reinfusion of saline after bleeding failed to restore entirely Mn, $\dot{Q}$ and $\bar{t}$, which were affected, as usually, by bleeding. On the other hand, in 5 animals, reinfusion of PHEG after bleeding restored entirely all the hemodynamic variables considered here (Fig. 3).

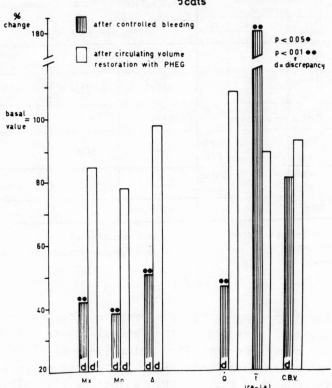

BLEEDING- 3% PHEG
Arterial blood pressure – Cardiac output
5 cats

Bleeding volume index has also been calculated (5,9).
This calculation is based on the following procedures and
definitions :

H_{Ia} : indicates bleeding volume which lowers mean arterial
blood pressure to 50 mm of Hg

H_{Ib} : is the additional bleeding volume which lowers mean
arterial blood pressure to 10 mm of Hg

H_I : the total bleeding volume $(H_{Ia} + H_{Ib})$

H_{It} : the theoretical bleeding volume calculated per kilo of
body weight of each animal species.

H_2 : the total bleeding volume in animals which have been deprived of H_{Ia} and which have been reinfused with an equal amount of blood or blood substitute.

H_2/H_{It} x I00 is the bleeding volume index (BVI). When blood or ideal blood substitutes are reinfused, BVI is equal to I00 or more.

4 out of I0 cats reinfused with saline after hemorrhage of H_{Ia} did not survive. Average BVI of the remaining 6 cats was 37. Figure 4 shows other Bleeding Volume Indices obtained with dextran and PHEG at two different concentrations.

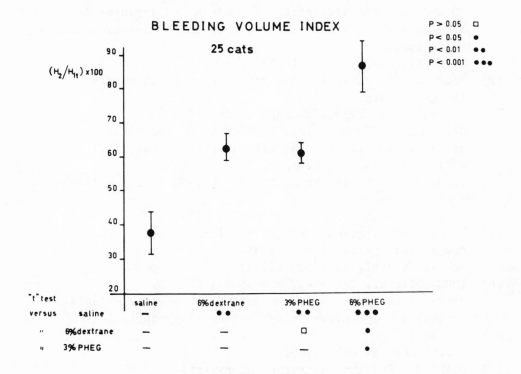

CONCLUSIONS

Poly-N⁵-(2-hydroxyethyl)-L-glutamate (PHEG) is a white, solid substance with an average molecular weight of 50,000, water-soluble, stable in autoclave-sterilization; its solutions develop no electrical charge at physiological pH and it has an oncotic pressure higher than B.S.A.

Preliminary acute and subacute toxicity tests are satis- factory. Several antigenicity tests also have been negative.

Finally,acute hemodynamic studies (based on calculation
of blood pressure, cardiac output and mean transit time, as
well as bleeding volume index) indicate that PHEG can help
circulation at least temporarily, if properly reinfused after
hemorrhage.

The present results seem to encourage further studies of
PHEG in view of its application as a plasma expander in
clinical therapy of shock.

REFERENCES

(1)   BOYDEN S.V. The adsorption of proteins on erythrocytes
       treated with tannic acid and subsequent hemo-agglutination
       by antiprotein sera.
       J. Exptl. Med. 93: 106 (1951)
(2)   DALE H.H. The anaphylactic reaction of plain muscle in
       the guunea pig.
       J. Pharmacol. Exptl. Therap. 4: 167 (1913)
(3)   GEROLA A., TSYBENKO V.A., BARTORELLI C. Registrazione
       di curve di diluizione termica in piccoli animali.
       Boll. Soc. Ital. Biol. Sper. 42: 1174 (1966)
(4)   KENNY A.D. Evaluation of Sodium Poly-α_{I}-L-glutamate as
       a plasma expander.
       Proc. Soc. Exp. Biol. Med. 100: 778 (1959)
(5)   LAWSON H. The measurement of bleeding volume in the dog
       for studies on blood substitutes.
       Am. J. Physiol. 140: 420 (1943)
(6)   LUPU-LOTAN N., YARON A., BERGER A., SELA M.
       Conformation changes in the nonionizable water-soluble
       synthetic polypeptide Poly-N^5-(3-hydroxypropyl)-L-
       glutamine.
       Biopolymers 3: 625 (1965)
(7)   OVARY Z. Passive cutaneous anaphylaxis.
       Immunological Methods, p. 259-283. Ed. Ackroyd J.F.
       Oxford: Blackwell.
(8)   SCHULTZ W.H. Physiological studies in anaphylaxis. I.
       The reaction of smooth muscle of the guinea pig sens-
       itized with horse serum.
       J. Pharmacol. Exptl. Therap. I: 549 (1910)
(9)   THOMPSON W.L., WAYT D.H., WALTON R.P.
       Bleeding volume indices of hydroxyethyl starch, dextran
       blood and glucose.
       Proc. Soc. Exp. Biol. Med. 115: 474 (1964)

AUTHOR INDEX

(Underscored numbers indicate complete papers in this volume.)

SUBJECT INDEX

347

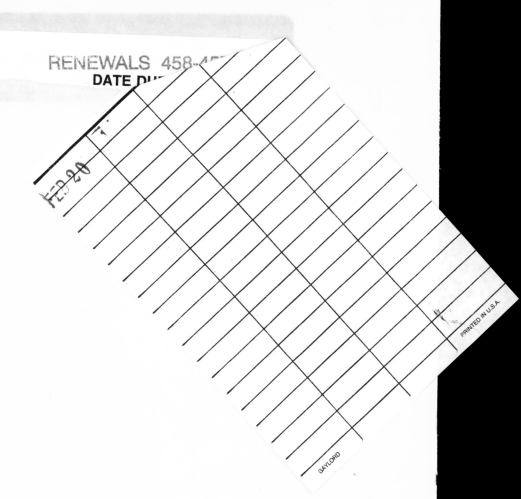